Masking America,
1918–1919

ALSO BY KERRY SEGRAVE
AND FROM MCFARLAND

*Taming the Automobile: Early Regulation
of Motor Vehicles in America, 1895–1903* (2024)

*Dying for Chocolate: Cordelia Botkin and the 1898
Poisoned Candy Murders* (Exposit, 2021)

Women and Bicycles in America, 1868–1900 (2020)

*The National Security League, 1914–1922:
Wall Street and the War Machine* (2020)

The Electric Car in America, 1890–1922: A Social History (2019)

*"Masquerading in Male Attire": Women Passing
as Men in America, 1844–1920* (2018)

*The Women Who Got America Talking:
Early Telephone Operators, 1878–1922* (2017)

*The Hatpin Menace: American Women Armed
and Fashionable, 1887–1920* (2016)

*Police Violence in America, 1869–1920:
256 Incidents Involving Death or Injury* (2016)

Chewing Gum in America, 1850–1920: The Rise of an Industry (2015)

Policewomen: A History, 2d ed. (2014)

*Beware the Masher: Sexual Harassment
in American Public Places, 1880–1930* (2014)

Wiretapping and Electronic Surveillance in America, 1862–1920 (2014)

*American Television Abroad: Hollywood's Attempt
to Dominate World Television* (1998; paperback 2013)

Payola in the Music Industry: A History, 1880–1991 (1994; paperback 2013)

*The Sexual Harassment of Women
in the Workplace, 1600 to 1993* (1994; paperback 2013)

*Women Serial and Mass Murderers: Profiles of 85
Killers Worldwide, 1580–1990* (1992; 2013)

Extras of Early Hollywood: A History of the Crowd, 1913–1945 (2013)

Parking Cars in America, 1910–1945: A History (2012)

*Vision Aids in America: A Social History of Eyewear
and Sight Correction Since 1900* (2011)

*Begging in America, 1850–1940: The Needy, the Frauds,
the Charities and the Law* (2011)

*America Brushes Up: The Use and Marketing of Toothpaste
and Toothbrushes in the Twentieth Century* (2010)

Lynchings of Women in the United States: The Recorded Cases, 1851–1946 (2010)

Movies at Home: How Hollywood Came to Television (1999; paperback 2009)

Tipping: An American Social History of Gratuities (1998; paperback 2009)

Masking America, 1918–1919

Efforts to Control the Great Influenza Pandemic

KERRY SEGRAVE

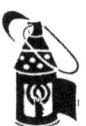

McFarland & Company, Inc., Publishers
Jefferson, North Carolina

ISBN (print) 978-1-4766-9449-8
ISBN (ebook) 978-1-4766-5189-7

LIBRARY OF CONGRESS AND BRITISH LIBRARY
CATALOGUING DATA ARE AVAILABLE

Library of Congress Control Number 2024031983

© 2024 Kerry Segrave. All rights reserved

*No part of this book may be reproduced or transmitted in any form
or by any means, electronic or mechanical, including photocopying
or recording, or by any information storage and retrieval system,
without permission in writing from the publisher.*

Front cover image: New York conductorettes
wearing masks, October 16, 1918 (National Archives)

Printed in the United States of America

*McFarland & Company, Inc., Publishers
Box 611, Jefferson, North Carolina 28640
www.mcfarlandpub.com*

Table of Contents

Preface 1
Introduction 3

1. Influenza and Masking: Origins   7
2. Vaccinations   20
3. New England   40
4. Middle Atlantic   51
5. South Atlantic   71
6. East South Central   96
7. West South Central   106
8. East North Central   113
9. West North Central   140
10. Mountain   167
11. Pacific   198

Chapter Notes   241
Bibliography   259
Index   277

Preface

This book looks at the steps that health and political officials in America took in 1918 and 1919 to eliminate or reduce the effect of the Spanish influenza pandemic on American residents. The emphasis is on the steps taken regarding masking the population. However, all the other steps the officials took are mentioned. The federal government did not impose any steps on Americans because each state or territory was responsible for health care in its jurisdiction. The federal authorities could control external borders and block the arrival of ships, for example. Still, internally, they could do no more than recommend what steps to take to the state and local jurisdictions. Therefore, the book deals with the situation on a state-by-state basis, with those states or territories grouped following the practice of the United States Census Bureau.

The first steps taken did not involve masking but were, for most, part of a second wave of restrictions applied after it became apparent that the first group of restrictions had no effect. Most masking rules were imposed on a county or city basis rather than on the entire state. Because influenza went through communities on a "wave" basis, increasing then decreasing then increasing, et cetera, authorities, by choosing with care the points in time they used to make comparisons, could falsely claim to have achieved success.

Some states had the power to impose restrictions on a statewide basis. In other states, that power was absent, and restrictions had to be imposed locally, either by county, city, or town. States with the power to impose restrictions statewide often did so at the beginning, but then backed away and left rescinding restrictions and any reimposition to the local officials. Reasons were never advanced for such action, but it likely was due to the opposition to those restrictions.

Even if effective measures existed to combat the flu in that period, the fractionated health system regarding jurisdictions made it unlikely to achieve success. When, for example, Kansas City, Missouri, had different restrictions in place compared to Kansas City, Kansas, it negated any benefits derived from the restrictions. And the outcome was the same negation when either Kansas City had different restrictions compared to other communities in their respective states.

This book was researched using online databases, with the Library of Congress's "Chronicling America" being the most useful. Also used were newspapers.com, newspaperarchive.com, and various other online newspaper databases.

Introduction

Chapter 1 looks briefly at the origins of the 1918 Spanish flu pandemic and the origins of masking the public, or as many liked to say at the time, opening the back door, placing chicken wire over it, and hoping that kept the mosquitoes outside.

Vaccines are the topic of Chapter 2. The pandemic began, in terms of intense media coverage, around the middle of September 1918. At the beginning of October, health and political authorities began to take concerted action. Amazingly, the first "flu vaccines" were injected into people's arms on October 1, 1918, in Wilmington, Delaware.

New England states are covered in Chapter 3. It was a region free of compulsory mask wearing, except for Boston, wherein the city's police had to wear them on duty under certain circumstances. The reference to no mandatory masking is to official health and political authorities. The military all over America imposed mandatory masking at their military installations, camps, cantonments, and draft offices nationwide. And there were many since World War I was still underway. As well, individual employers often forced their employees to wear face coverings. The federal government often did the same in one of the few areas inside the country that it had the power to do so—the United States Post Office.

The Middle Atlantic states are discussed in Chapter 4. Notably, the New York City health commissioner, Dr. Royal S. Copeland, imposed no masking rules on his city, nor did he impose the usual shutdowns, including those suggested by Rupert Blue, surgeon general of the United States Public Health Service. While Blue had no power to compel, he could and did recommend. The majority of states almost automatically followed and imposed his detailed recommendations.

Chapter 5 covers the South Atlantic states. In Washington, D.C., the authorities went so far as to provide the countless telephone receivers in government offices with flu masks of their own. D.C. Commissioner Louis Brownlow had views opposite Copeland's and was extreme in his approach to restrictions. In Kings Mountain, North Carolina, all stores, including food stores, closed for a week. They could take phone orders and deliver, but in America at that time, according to the 1920 census, only 35 percent of households had a telephone. The other option was to go to the grocery store, stand outside, and yell your order out. They would prepare it and leave it outside their front door if they heard you. That, perhaps, illustrated the folly of having small communities write their laws for something that was a national problem.

Chapter 6 features the East South Central states, including Roanoke, Alabama, and Vidalia, Mississippi. In both communities, people had to wear masks everywhere, away from their homes. In Paris, Kentucky, all barbers had to be masked. The occupation of barber was the hardest hit. There were many instances of barbers being compelled to wear masks, but only rarely were hairdressers mentioned.

Chapter 7 covers the West South Central states. In Shreveport, Louisiana, all postal employees who interacted with the public wore masks. Also, every operator with Bell Telephone was compelled to wear a mask, which was an example of civic officials encouraging such action in the hope that the example would spread throughout the community and thus allow them to avoid imposing such measures. Monroe, Louisiana, compressed its business hours, as did many communities. Density and crowding were everywhere viewed as threats. Yet these towns cut their hours by up to a half and forced people into a narrow choice of hours, thereby increasing the density and crowding in stores—the very density they purported to fear.

In the East North Central states, the subject of Chapter 8, Dr. James Inches, Detroit health commissioner, candidly admitted he had no belief in the shutdowns or masking, but he implemented some measures in his city because of pressure placed on him. His experiences illustrated the infighting among state and local health and political officials who tried to take credit while avoiding blame. In Lima, Ohio, officials imposed a 50-square-foot minimum floor space per customer in businesses. Indianapolis passed a harsh masking law, but intense lobbying and resistance caused the authorities to rescind it. Chicago passed no mask mandate laws, but officials exerted a lot of persuasion to try to achieve a masking regulation.

Chapter 9 covers the West North Central states. Dr. F.B. Strauss, the Bismarck, North Dakota, health commissioner, was notable among the petty tyrants and bureaucrats gone authoritarian. Aberdeen, South Dakota, mandated masking but had to backtrack after heavy pressure from citizens. Des Moines, Iowa, also mandated masking. But it took only days for the order to be changed, altered, implemented, and repealed. Once again, citizen pressure prevailed.

Mountain states are covered in Chapter 10, wherein Helena, Montana, was another place where resistance forced authorities to back down after ordering mask wearing. In Denver, Colorado, heavy resistance forced a masking reversal by the officials. In Utah, there was a battle between Salt Lake City and Ogden. When the former lifted restrictions, the latter viewed the move as premature. For a short time, Ogden deployed armed guards to police the roads into their city. Nobody was allowed in if they did not have a health certificate issued no more than 24 hours before the time of proposed entry to Ogden. Tucson, Arizona, passed a law limiting the distance schoolchildren kept from each other to at least three feet. Tucson also enforced a mask law, arresting 50 people in one day for violating the order, resulting from raids on hotel lobbies. Phoenix imposed a masking law that lasted only a week, the victim of citizen pressure.

Chapter 11 covers the Pacific states and territories. It was the most extreme region by far. Four of the five jurisdictions imposed masking laws—only Hawaii escaped. Seattle police were forced to wear masks all the time while on duty. On November 3, the Washington State Board of Health ordered statewide masking. It was the only state that attempted to impose masking statewide. It was ignored in many parts of the state and rescinded on November 11. Pendleton, Oregon, imposed the four-foot rule for all people in all business interactions. Only people such as barbers, dentists, and servers were allowed to get closer; when they did so, they had to wear masks. In California, many communities imposed mask mandates, none more draconian or bizarre than in San Francisco. That mandate required people to be masked wherever two or more people congregated. An exception was in your residence if the household size was one or two. If your household size was three or more (say, two parents and one child), all had to be masked everywhere, even at home. The ordinance didn't make an exemption for the time spent sleeping.

One of the most striking features of the 1918 pandemic, compared to that of 2020, was that nobody who lost income in 1918 got any of the money back. All the shutdowns imposed on people, some of which took place with only a day or two of notice, inflicted financial damages on all those affected. Every worker laid off or locked out did not receive any compensation. Every business that shuttered lost income, to a greater or lesser degree. The sole exception was the teachers, who, in some states, were fully paid for any periods they were locked out. When a cinema was shut down with only a few days, or even a few hours, of notice, not only did the cinema owner lose future business, but also the owner was often out of pocket for contracts with film distributors that went into the future. Those losses perhaps reinforced some of the protest movements that sprang up at various times in various places. Those protests cut short some of the harsher measures imposed by the authorities. However, the authorities never admitted they had been wrong or mistaken in any of the insane measures they inflicted on their population. That, of course, was remarkably similar to the 2020 episode.

One of the main reasons fueling mask wearing, whether the jurisdictions imposed it or an attempt was made to accomplish the same thing through hectoring, whining, and persuasion by the authorities, was that the first round of lockdowns had not worked, and reimposing them for a second time, after they had already been removed in so many places, was viewed by officials as likely to generate even more opposition and resistance. It was held out as a hope to businesses that there would be no curtailment of their hours, no minimum space requirements, or more drastic measures if only businesses would join in with the authorities and champion face coverings. And in many cases, businesses did join in to urge masking. In a more general sense, masking was getting good press from 1916 through 1918 because of the invention and use of the gas mask in World War I. There was constant press about how good the American gas masks were. Also, ordinary people, all the way through November 1918, were encouraged and urged to save peach (and other fruit) pits and walnut (and other nut) shells and drop them off at collection points. They were ground up and used for the charcoal base of gas masks. And then people of science, who were the ones who should have known better, and everybody else, came to believe and dispense the idea that the chicken wire spread across the open back door would keep all the mosquitoes outside.

1

Influenza and Masking: Origins

Where did the Spanish influenza pandemic that struck North America in late September 1918 originate? In the summer of that year, Europe had already noticed it, and articles began to appear in the American press. As was usually the case, those articles claimed there was no reason to worry. One such news story appeared in print on July 16 and proclaimed in its subhead that "New York doctors feel certain epidemic which started in Spain will not come here." According to the article, the medical experts of the day said that New York was in little danger of an epidemic of influenza, which started in Spain and spread to the German armies. The story admitted that, while no one knew much about the disease, most of the doctors believed "it is only the common grip" (another name, along with *grippe*, for the flu back then) and that its perseverance in Spain and Germany was due to the poorly nourished condition of the people. Commissioner Royal Copeland of the New York City Health Department said there was no cause for alarm and that he had heard of no new cases of influenza or grip. "I think the epidemic in Spain is a mild duplicate of the one we had in this country in 1889 and 1890, where everyone was ill from grip, then a new disease."[1]

Copeland added, "There is nothing for us to worry about. If the reports from Germany are true, saying soldiers are dying from the disease, it means that the resistance of the German people is low. Any disease, even so simple a thing as measles, may cause death if people are not strong." Dr. Daniel D. Hubbard of the health board said he thought the disease was nothing new. "I believe it old-fashioned grip and I do not believe that New York is in danger. There is little doubt the epidemic is flourishing in the German armies because the men are in poor physical condition." Dr. John J. Hill, assistant superintendent at Bellevue Hospital in New York, said he had heard of no new "Spanish influenza" cases in New York. "We have not had any cases. I think many of the cases of influenza reported are grip." A few physicians tried distinguishing between the two words, but most did not. "Both were infectious viral respiratory diseases."[2]

Early in August, another article reported on the disease, noting that the Spanish influenza pandemic appeared over a considerable part of Europe. Attention was given to it a few weeks after its outbreak in Spain. There was no doubt that it was a very severe form in Germany, Austria, and the territories occupied by the Central Powers during the last two years. Malnutrition and "war weariness" were said to be principal factors. The disease was also raging in England. A comparison was made to the 1890 flu pandemic (often called Russian flu at the time). Over the previous ten days in England, the sickness had severely interfered with society. Office staff was crippled by absenteeism. In Northumberland, so many miners were affected that coal production (vital for war work) was decreasing. Up to 70 percent of them were absent from work. The term *la grippe* was applied to the disease in the early 1700s. And in England, between 1709 and 1732, it received the name *influenza*.[3]

Dr. Royal S. Copeland, New York City health commissioner, said on August 16 that about 24 cases of influenza had been discovered on ships arriving in the Port of New York from Europe in the past four weeks: "We have not felt and do not feel any anxiety about what people call 'Spanish influenza,' and we considered it so unimportant that it did not seem necessary to make a public discussion of the situation. But we have taken all precautionary measures." Dr. L.I. Harris, director of the Bureau for the Guidance of the Public, issued some guidelines for the public: Don't use a roller towel in public places such as hotel toilets, restaurant toilets, and so on. Don't use common drinking cups, glasses, forks, or spoons. Avoid contact with people who cough or sneeze; "if you must be affectionate don't kiss them on the mouth." Don't spit in public places (a big problem in that era). Burn or boil the bed and personal linen of people suffering from the so-called common cold. See that your home and workplace have sufficient ventilation. Avoid the dust from dry sweeping.[4]

On September 10, about 100 sailors from the merchant marine who had been stationed aboard training vessels in Boston harbor were found to be suffering from influenza. They were removed from their ships for treatment and taken to tents on the grounds of the Brooks Hospital.[5]

Officials in Washington, D.C., announced on September 11 that the "strange, prostrating malady which recently ravaged the German army and later spread into France and England ... has been brought to some of the American Atlantic coast cities." People returning on American transport vessels had brought it over. Little means were available to combat the disease, except by "absolute quarantine," and that "obviously is impossible at this time because it would require interruption of intercourse between communities as drastic as was resorted to in the dread days of yellow fever in the South." Officials added that preventive measures were considered the best weapons to avoid the sickness. As the disease was new to American physicians, "the government may take the menace in hand by issuing county-wide warnings and general instructions of how to avoid the infections, if possible, and how best to combat it if it be contracted." And finally, "Spanish influenza, although short-lived and of practically no permanent serious results, is a most distressing ailment which prostrates the sufferers for a few days, during which he suffers the acme of discomfort."[6]

In Camp Lee, Petersburg, Virginia, it was reported on September 17 that 500 cases of Spanish influenza had developed there. It had been necessary to build temporary hospitals in the camp to accommodate the sick. The authorities believed rookies from seacoast cities brought the flu to the base. The base was a cantonment, and some 8,000 people were sleeping outside, under canvas, because there were not enough barracks.[7]

Three days later, the announcement was made about outbreaks of Spanish flu in five additional army training camps, making nine camps in which the illness had been discovered. The total cases to date were 9,313 (11 deaths). Camp Devens, Massachusetts, reported the most significant number of cases (6,583). Camp Devens also cited 43 new cases of pneumonia, "which medical officers believe resulted from the flu epidemic." In response to a request from the United States Public Health Service, health authorities in many states sent word that day as to the development and spread of the pandemic. Two vessels with influenza aboard were quarantined at Newport News, Virginia, "and in all parts of the country steps were taken by health officials to check the spread of the disease."[8]

Dispatches from cantonments in various parts of the country, as of September 22, told the same story of the spread of the virus—everywhere, the military was stricken in large numbers, with small numbers of deaths, but those were also increasing. But the report said, "The disease is not spreading nearly so rapidly in the civilian population." The New York City Department of Health had received reports of only 20 cases. The numbers in military facilities were in the hundreds at each location, even in the thousands. For example, the Great Lakes Naval Training Station near Chicago had about 3,600 men infected. United States Surgeon Rupert Blue warned, "Please maintain the best physical conditions possible and avoid crowded places where there is danger from sneezing, coughing, and spitting. People stricken with chills, fevers, headache, backache, and reddening of the eyes will please go to bed immediately and call a physician." Dr. Copeland worried about misdiagnosis (the tendency to find the same thing as everybody else because everybody else was finding it). "The diagnosticians must not expect to find a new symptom complex, and those who have in the past seen a large number of cases of influenza will readily recognize the cases which seem now to be correct.... The picture generally speaking is the familiar one which has been prevented year after year in the typical cases of influenza."[9]

A general summary article published on September 30 noted that early in May 1918, dispatches from Madrid told of a mysterious disorder raging through Spain in the form and character of the grippe. Not long after, a similar disease took hold in Switzerland and, at the same time, penetrated France, England, and Norway. Early in August, people carried the condition from Europe on ocean liners, and it began appearing in the United States. Over the past two weeks, the occurrence of the sickness in the civilian population and among the soldiers in the cantonments had increased so significantly in number that federal, state, and municipal health bureaus were then mobilizing all their forces to combat the Spanish flu—what they recognize to be an approaching pandemic. Herein, it was described as the same as the grippe, only more severe and more likely to lead to pneumonia than the less virulent form of flu, which went by the name of the grippe. And it was noted, "The designation of the new malady as 'Spanish influenza' is purely arbitrary.... It is fairly certain that Spanish influenza, if different from the familiar grippe, originated in the German camps." The article remarked that through all the wars of history, disease generated by unsanitary herding of men in the camps of belligerents had always produced pandemics, which before that time had been little or not at all known to many of the populations affected. America had been "practically exempt" from direct contact with the disease until the arrival in the Port of New York of the Norwegian liner

Bergensfjord on August 12, which had more than 200 cases of sickness resembling influenza during the voyage. On August 16, at the Port of New York, a ship arriving from one of the Scandinavian countries reported 11 more cases of Spanish flu. On August 18, a passenger liner at the Port of New York reported that 21 cases of Spanish influenza had developed among the passengers and crew on her voyage.[10]

The Library of Congress maintains an extensive online database with millions of pages of American newspapers dating back to the 1700s. The search term "influenza" on this database produced the following number of hits for 1914–1922, respectively. The numbers were 1,843, 2,043, 2,688, 1,643, 41,377, 40,174, 25,729, 6,300, and 9,078. The three most extensive years by far were 1918–1920. For 1918, the number of hits for August was 224, while the number for September was 2,002. Breaking the number of hits for September into three equal parts produced 28 hits for September 1 to 10 and 478 hits for September 11 to 20. The number of hits for September 21 to 30 was 1,496. September 17 was the first single day with over 50 hits (52), and it stayed there, with a few exceptions, for many months to come. Thus, for the media, Spanish influenza arrived in America in mid–September 1918.[11]

For public health officials, bureaucrats, and political authorities, the official arrival of the pandemic came on October 2, when United States Surgeon General Dr. Rupert Blue issued his pronouncement. After that, strange and ineffective preventive measures were undertaken. The country's main cities issued the most drastic orders to combat the flu, closing saloons, theaters, schools, churches, and places of amusement and prohibiting public gatherings of all kinds in every community where the flu had developed. Following Blue's advice, in whole or in part, cities such as Washington, Philadelphia, Pittsburgh, Boston, and Omaha, to name a few, quickly shut down to some extent. Blue explained that no national authority existed for such a closing but that state and local boards had the power to act. While some state boards, he said, had complete control to cover their entire states with such an order, in other states, only county and municipal officials could legally act.[12]

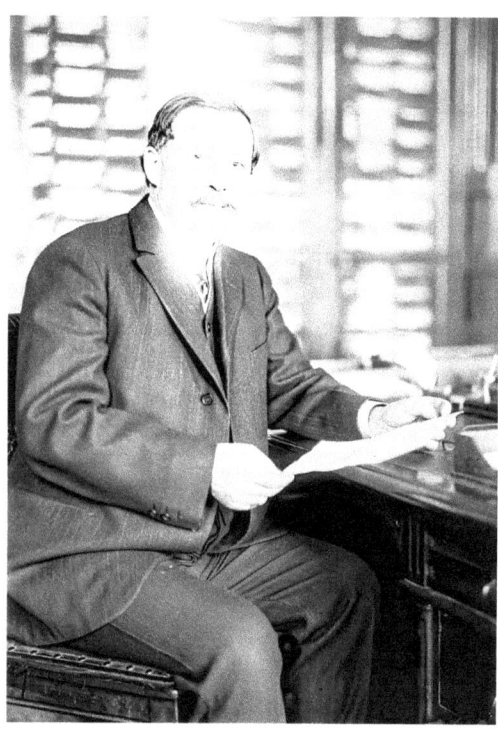

Rupert Blue in 1914. The New York City Health Commissioner, Copeland, was one of the health professionals who resisted, to some extent, the prevailing wisdom.

Rupert Blue gave a lengthy interview published on October 18, 1918. It was in question-and-answer format about the disease, how it started, its causes, symptoms, how it spread, and so forth. In that piece, Blue said almost nothing about masks. Even attendants (nonmedical) looking after a sick person in the home were not advised to wear masks—only that an apron or gown should be worn over the ordinary clothing. Blue did say that nurses and doctors in attendance on patients should wear a mask. When the surgeon general was asked how to guard against the flu, he suggested a proper proportion of work, play and rest in a person's life, keeping the body well clothed and eating sufficient, wholesome, and properly selected food. There was a close relationship between the spread of a disease like influenza and overcrowded homes—people should, if possible, make every effort to reduce home overcrowding. The value of fresh air through open windows could not be overemphasized. When crowding was unavoidable, as in streetcars, care should be taken to keep the face turned to avoid inhaling directly the air breathed out by another person.[13]

Rupert Blue was right that the federal government had no role except in an advisory capacity. A weak attempt was made to address the problem and end the situation. Even that was almost a full year into the pandemic. In mid–September 1919,

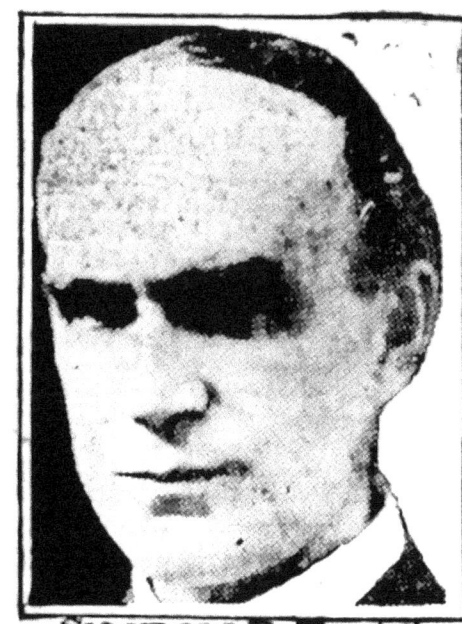
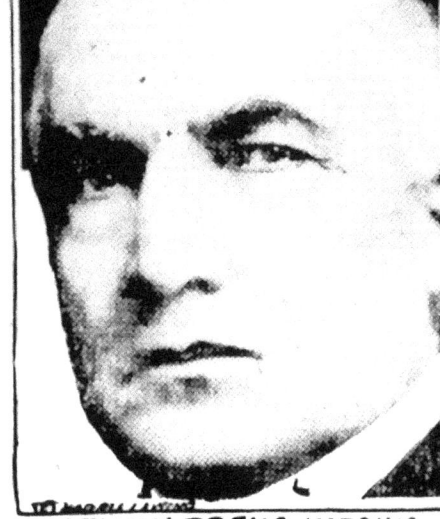

Simeon Fess and Warren Harding, Ohio, sponsored a bill to spend some money on influenza research to help in the event of another epidemic. It also would have established federal controls instead of each of the 50 states deciding its own course. The bill went nowhere.

the United States Congress attempted to give Blue some power. Two Ohio politicians sponsored a bill introduced to both houses of Congress. Representative Simeon Fess and U.S. Senator Warren Harding (who would go on to win the U.S. Presidency in 1920) introduced a bill that would have appropriated $5 million to fight influenza and put Blue's United States Public Health Service in charge of the anti-flu fight. One of the critical issues that the Fess-Harding bill hoped to tackle was to isolate the virus causing the disease, thus making an actual vaccine possible. Several months later, Fess said he saw "little interest for it" in Congress. The bill died in committee, going nowhere.[14]

Throughout the entire 1918–1920 Spanish influenza pandemic, the medical profession failed to isolate the virus, nor did they have a test to diagnose it. A well-known syndicated columnist of the time, Dr. William Brady, had plenty of critics of his medical column. In one of his columns in March 1919, he addressed how a mild case of influenza was diagnosed. He wrote, "There is no absolutely infallible test by which a physician can determine that this mild respiratory infection is, and this other mild respiratory infection is not, influenza. It is wholly a matter of judgment."[15]

Dr. S.L. Burton was the state medical director of the Modern Woodmen of America in New Mexico, a fraternal benefit (insurance) company. He reported, in February 1920, that the bacillus causing Spanish influenza "has not been isolated." He also said, "I do not believe vaccination protected a single person from contracting the disease." However, vaccinated people may have a milder form of the disease than the unvaccinated. Burton did not mention crowds or masks in his paper on the facts of influenza.[16]

The mask was used in many situations during the 2020 coronavirus pandemic, and it was used extensively during the 1918 Spanish flu pandemic. World War I was ongoing when the flu became an emergency and was likely a significant factor in the spread and contagion of the affliction. And we can thank that same war for being the catalyst for introducing more pedestrian mask use in public health emergencies back in 1918 and a century later.

When the war was underway and poisonous gases were introduced as weapons, it was only natural that coverings to protect people were brought into play—a variation of sorts of the somewhat uncommon industrial mask. Masks were used in industrial situations for years before World War I. For example, workers toiling near grinding machines faced minute particles of dust and metals and sometimes received masks to protect themselves. Surgeons in operating theaters had been using masks for two or three decades by the start of the war. However, their function was not primarily to be used against infectious diseases.

Gas masks received much media publicity, one reason being their novelty appeal. As the war dragged on, the civilian population and military personnel used more and more gas masks in modified form. Children often had to wear these gadgets as they went to and from school. However, they were usually many miles away from any military activity. When the Spanish flu arrived near the tail end of the war, the use of gas masks among the military was well known to the general public and documented by the media. Because of the publicity, those gas masks in modified form had already spread a little among the civilian population. Suppose a gas mask could save soldiers from harm. Why couldn't those masks, if changed, protect people from a different respiratory problem?

The time was right to introduce the mask, in its final modified form, to the general population to battle the flu. And so, the mask wars began in earnest in America. A century later, America repeated the same mask wars. Perhaps nothing more clearly illustrated the old idea that "those who don't know history are doomed to repeat it" than those mask wars.

A photo appeared in the press at the beginning of June 1916 that depicted a group of Scotsmen who were soldiers fighting the war in the north of France and were wearing "gas masks." These appeared to have the same sophistication and utility as pillowcases with eye holes did for kids out collecting candy at Halloween.[17]

A 1916 photo from February 27 depicted several French schoolchildren from Rheims wearing masks to protect against German poison gases. In the picture, only one child is very clear. His face covering seemed to be nothing more than a scarf or a towel wrapped around his lower face.[18]

A few months later, a brief account remarked that in the war zone in Europe, the children wore gas masks to school to protect themselves against the deadly vapor should any of it float to their neighborhood from the battlefields. But, as in the case of caps, overcoats, and other apparel, children often left their masks off.[19]

A reporter explained to readers that many believed the gas mask was an invention of the current war, but they were wrong. When the Germans introduced poisonous gases in attacks, the Allies initially could not cope with the weapon. After

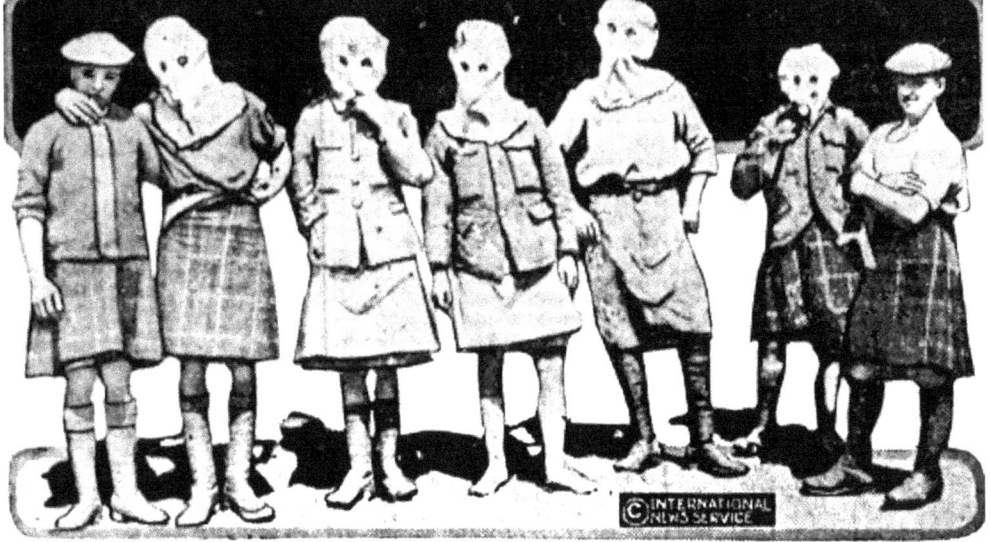

A group of Scottish soldiers in 1916 wearing early versions of gas masks.

a few such attacks, the Allies turned to industry and found a means of negating the use of poisonous gas by using a gas mask. Many industries had used such masks for many years. A photo appeared with the article, showing two women wearing their masks who were handling dangerous chemicals at the Bush Terminal in New York. Those masks were designed to protect workers from deadly fumes and sparks. These, at least, looked like they were effective.[20]

A nearly full-page article appeared in January 1918 titled "The Girl in the Gas Mask." It featured photos of female workers wearing such masks. What gave the feature a certain novelty was that for the first time, women could do such dangerous work in such high numbers. Industry filled many positions with women because men were working as soldiers. The reporter who wrote this article jokingly remarked that "The Girl in the Gas Mask" wore a mask before she entered "the industrial world to take up these dangerous occupations, but for a different purpose—to preserve and intensify their beauty." But now they were wearing them for a different reason: to preserve life. Even then, before the Spanish flu pandemic had begun, the journalist

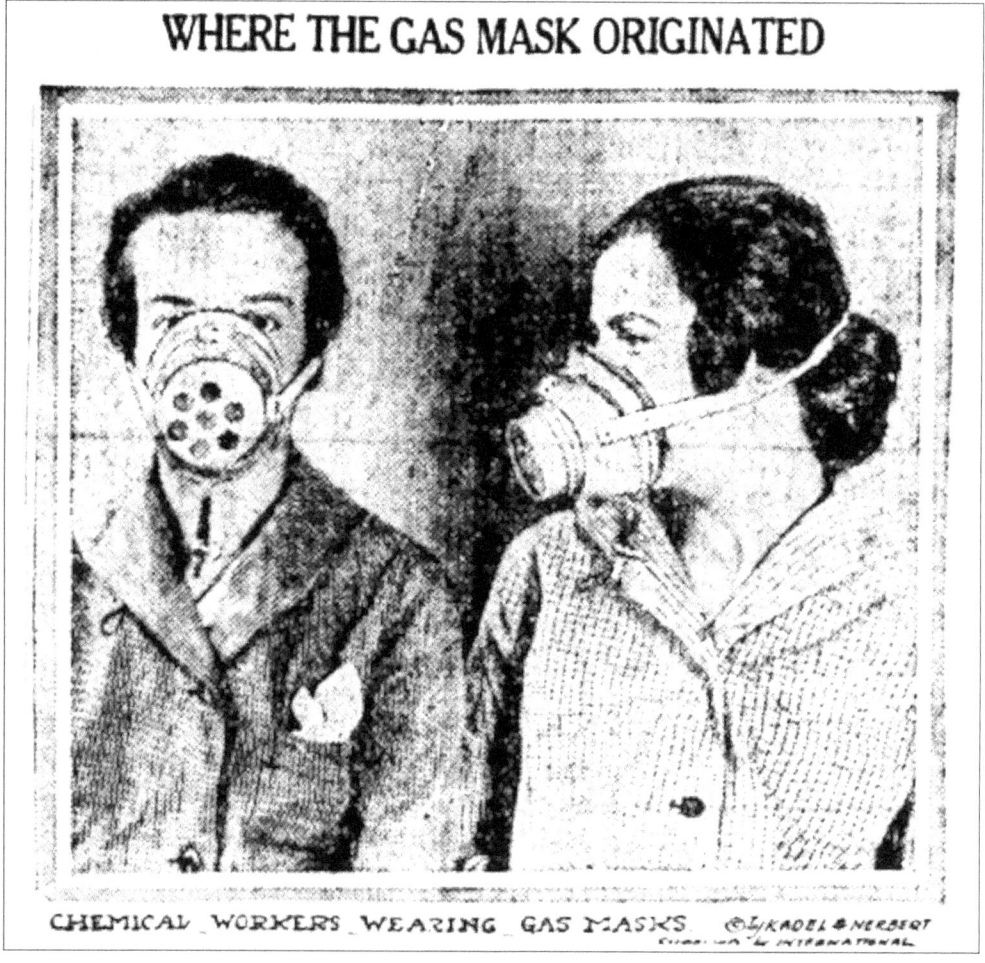

Women war workers wearing protective masks due to their work in a chemical plant.

PLAY BASEBALL IN GAS MASKS

Not in the least inconvenienced, these American boys in training for the "big game over there" are playing ball in their gas masks. Throughout the training camps in this country gas mask drills and tests are held almost daily and when the American boy gets overseas he can manipulate a gas mask to perfection and can adjust it just like the "old-timers." The usual time in adjusting a gas mask is six seconds, although after a little training it can be put into position in the twinkling of an eye.

This photograph shows a number of American soldiers playing a baseball game. So easy was it to wear a gas mask—and, by extension, a flu mask—that these men donned them easily and played a full game of baseball wearing them. Or so they would have you believe.

looked to extend the mask's scope. He noted that gasoline fumes often overwhelmed automobile owners and others working in closed or improperly ventilated garages, causing asphyxiation before they knew the danger and "that the danger of a 'gasoline death' easily can be avoided by wearing a gas mask."[21]

A different, almost full-page article gave a lengthy report on poison in warfare. One section dealt with gas masks and painted the product as effective, lifesaving, and so on, as other articles had done. Gas masks received good press. The article mentioned that French schoolchildren wore masks. It included several pictures, with the oddest one being three horses outfitted with "anti-gas nose bags," which looked about as effective as the crazy contraptions seen on the Scotsmen.[22]

An unidentified "gas expert" pontificated that gas would win the war and that "we are rapidly approaching the time when it will be necessary to wear masks constantly." People were constantly inventing new gases, and the "greatest danger from gas arises from removing the masks too early." Such talk, of course, helped lay the groundwork for wearing masks during the flu pandemic.[23]

Swiss newspapers reported that their troops on the Alsatian frontier had begun to suffer from German poison gas floating back from the western front toward the Rhine. The civilian population along the Rhine was warned to provide themselves with gas masks. Schoolchildren in Mulheim and Freiburg were also said to wear gas masks daily.[24]

In June 1918, it was reported that train passengers passing through Nanking province in China received masks to protect themselves from a variety of plague said to be "raging" in the district.[25]

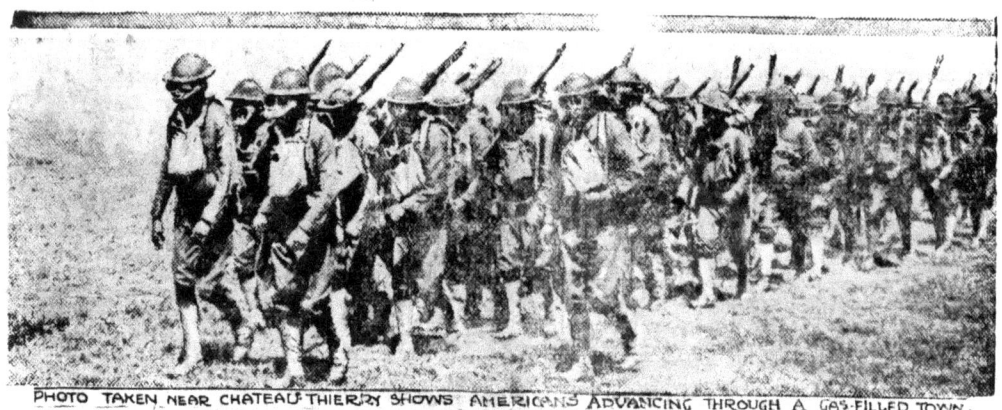

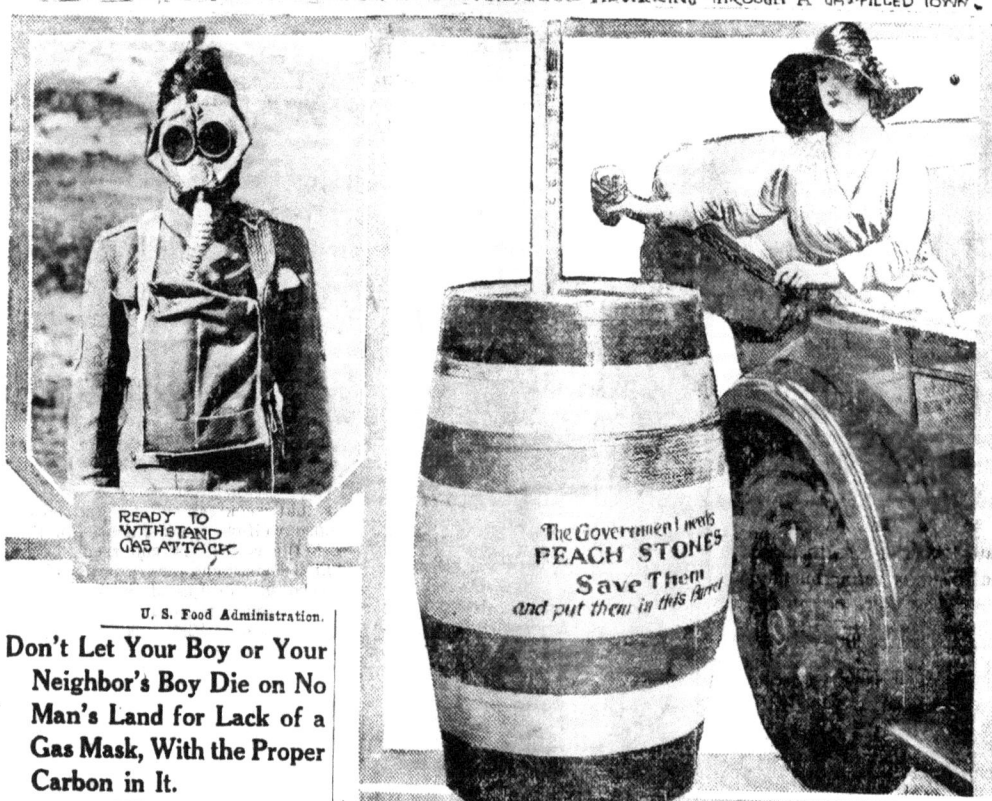

Contributing to the public's increased awareness of gas masks were the never-ending campaigns and drives to save and donate fruit pits and nut shells. These items were ground up and used to produce carbon for the mask filters. Those drives took place all over America and lasted into November 1918. The photograph is from Owensboro, Kentucky.

On June 14, 1918, still before the pandemic, it was announced at Camp Meade, Maryland, that more intensive training concerning gas attacks was underway. Officers and men were to wear masks for long periods every day. In the office, for example, letter dictation would occur with both the man dictating the letter and the receiver of the dictation wearing masks. And men would "learn how to sleep with masks on and even how to eat with the least possible exposure to the open air." It was training and social control that could more easily be imposed on the citizenry later during the Spanish flu since it had been publicized and practiced to an extent on some of the population.[26]

With the start of the pandemic unofficially (by the media) and officially (by state and local authorities) starting during the last half of September 1918, the influence of gas masks was still evident. From the nation's capital came a report on September 26 that the Washington, D.C., chapter of the Red Cross had announced the "newest" means of combating the spread of the disease "in the form of a germ mask. The device is a modified form of the gas mask." Four layers of thin, clean gauze, arranged to cover the mouth and nose of the wearer, acted as a filter against germs. It was reported that the Potomac division of the Red Cross had ordered 45,000 of the masks for use by the soldiers in training near Washington and patients at the Walter Reed Hospital there. "Prominent women of Washington" were making those masks at the local surgical dressing station of the Red Cross. If the "contrivance" proved effective, it was expected to be adopted more widely.[27]

Another account declared that the Washington Red Cross workers were making "miniature gas masks" at a rate of one every five minutes. Among the most prominent of the volunteer workers toiling away was reportedly Mrs. McAdoo, wife of William McAdoo, then United States Secretary of the Treasury.[28]

As the use of flu masks spread, the comparison and analogy to gas masks quickly faded away but still appeared now and then. A couple of weeks later, a report noted that in its effort to safeguard against the spread of the flu among the thousands of war workers in the various departments, bureaus, boards, and commissions in the capital region, all telephone instruments were then "wearing gas masks." The "sanitary corps" inspected all the war work establishments, placing "medicated gauze" on all the telephones' mouthpieces.[29]

It was reported that thousands of citizens in Lexington, Kentucky, were wearing anti-influenza "gas masks" as of October 2, 1918. A few weeks after that, a mini-editorial from a Maryland paper declared, "Now let's all put on our gas masks or flu muzzles, quit talking, and fight harder."[30]

In May 1917, a group of five volunteers started the production of gas masks in America. From then until the signing of the World War I truce in November 1918, America produced five million masks, three million extra canisters, 500,000 horse gas masks, and many mustard gas suits, globes, ointments, and antidotes. The 1918 model gas mask, said Colonel Bradley Dewey, commanding officer of the gas defense, showed a design improvement, overcoming the discomforts of earlier models and adding "tenfold efficiency."[31]

The Kolynos company was a massive manufacturer of consumer products at the time of the pandemic. Primarily, it made oral care products, such as toothpaste.

Making a Kolynos Gas Mask To Fight Spanish Influenza When Exposed to Infection

Take two small pieces of absorbent cotton. Gently form each into an oval shape, of a size to pass easily into the entrance of the nostrils. Wet them with Kolynos Liquid and put one in each nostril. They will be held in place by the curving wings of the nose and the pocket at its point.

By this means *germ-laden air is filtered and at every inhalation the air passages are disinfected with the vapor of Kolynos Liquid.*

The beneficent effect will be immediately felt in the throat, the bronchial tubes and the lungs.

Combine with this the regular brushing of the teeth, *three times daily,* with Kolynos Dental Cream, that the mouth and throat may also have a high degree of resistance to infection.

DON'T DELAY! If not already a Kolynos user, take these precautionary measures today!

You will find Kolynos Dental Cream and Kolynos Liquid for sale in drug and department Stores generally.

The Kolynos Company
New Haven, Conn.
U. S. A.

Founded in 1908, it merged into Colgate-Palmolive in 1995. Its consumer items were well known to the citizenry, and the company went on to sponsor many national radio programs in the 1930s and 1940s. It placed a large ad in a Washington, D.C., newspaper on November 5 headlined, "Making a Kolynos Gas Mask to Fight Spanish Influenza." It supplied instructions and reminded the reader that Kolynos Liquid was necessary to make the device. The article also noted that brushing the teeth three times a day with Kolynos toothpaste might also confer a high degree of resistance to infection.[32]

Opposite: An ad for the Kolynos company. It was a major producer in its day of consumer products, especially mouth care. The ad instructed the reader on how to make a "gas mask" for protection from the Spanish flu. It also hyped other Kolynos products.

2

Vaccinations

With the influenza pandemic getting total and daily coverage by the media around mid–September 1918, it was unlikely that the question of being vaccinated to avoid catching the ailment would surface very quickly. Yet it did. On September 26 of that year, an article from Boston declared that much interest was manifested in experiments being made with a new flu vaccine produced there at Tufts College laboratories in Massachusetts. Nurses at Boston City Hospital and students at Tufts Medical School had reportedly already been inoculated. According to the report, "officials said that a day or two would show whether the product would effectively prevent further epidemic spread."[1]

The Delaware Hospital in Wilmington held an influenza clinic from 5 p.m. to 6 p.m. on October 1 to administer flu vaccines to anyone who wanted to receive them. The report said that the vaccine "is believed by many to immunize the patient against an attack of grip or influenza." Administered in four doses to the patient every eight to ten days, "it has also been used with some success in treating and curing the disease, although the results are by no means certain. In treating the disease it is used at shorter intervals of three or four days." The treatment theory was the same as that underlying vaccines to prevent typhoid fever, which was very successful and required of all men entering the U.S. Army. At the vaccine clinic in Wilmington, the vaccine was not free but sold at the hospital for $2.50 a shot. However, there was no charge for administering the vaccine, which was said to be in limited supply.[2]

One day later, another article observed that New York City scientists working under the supervision of Dr. William H. Parke had discovered an "effective serum for the prevention of Spanish influenza." Preparations were underway for it to be manufactured in quantity. It was to be distributed to physicians as quickly as possible. New York City Health Commissioner Royal S. Copeland's report stated that the vaccine developed in the New York City labs was an entirely independent product from the recently announced federal public health service vaccine. Copeland sent a telegram to U.S. Surgeon General Rupert Blue, asking for details of his discovery and stressing that the New York City treatment was "purely a preventive" and not for curative use.[3]

Copeland explained that tests of his vaccine had given a "promise of success." As a result, the vaccine was being prepared for physicians to use. It would be ready for distribution in "small quantities" in a few days. The serum "discovered" by Dr. Parke, "the health expert," was made from "influenza germs" obtained from people in the early stages of the disorder, combined with "bacilli procured at autopsies upon bodies of victims of the disease." Copeland stressed that it was not a cure.[4]

"Vaccines" were developed at a fast and furious rate in October 1918. On October 8, J.S. McBride, the Seattle health commissioner in Washington state, announced that local health and naval officials at Bremerton had developed a successful Spanish influenza serum.[5]

A couple of days later, the public health service in the nation's capital was investigating all aspects of seeking an effective vaccine. But an announcement by the agency stated that as of that date, in early October, it could not recommend any vaccine that it felt would be successful.[6]

Finally, a vaccine emerged that would last through the entire pandemic. Dr. William James Mayo of the famous Mayo Brothers Clinic announced on October 12 that a serum had been developed at the Mayo Brothers laboratory. He said, "Out of a thousand cases of influenza treated, it has prevented a single case of pneumonia developing." He added that the serum had not been perfected and that experiments were continuing.[7]

A couple of days later, Dr. Edward C. Rosenow of the Mayo Brothers Clinic in Rochester, Minnesota, responded to an inquiry from the Cincinnati Health Board for information. He wired Dr. William Peters, the local health officer, that he was working on an influenza serum. He said preliminary results were favorable, but "nothing definite as yet has been found." He promised to send supplies of the vaccine to Peters if it proved successful. During the flu pandemic, the terms *vaccine* and *serum* meant the same thing.[8]

At the same time, Salem, Oregon, announced that it would use the Rosenow-originated vaccine in a campaign against the Spanish flu. Rosenow told the Chicago Influenza Emergency Commission of his experiments with the vaccine, which he had used to treat 20,000 people. The Chicago Commission at once named a committee of physicians to take charge of the manufacture and use of all vaccines in Chicago, including the Rosenow/Mayo one. Rosenow was to provide a supply sufficient for 100,000 doses from his labs in Rochester. While the vaccine was designed to provide immunity from the disease, Rosenow was "unwilling to make specific claims as to its value. He believes it aided greatly in suppressing the spread of influenza at Rochester."[9]

Rosenow was the chief bacteriologist at the Mayo Clinic. By October 17, it was reported that he had 100,000 doses of the vaccine ready to arrive in Chicago on Saturday, October 19, and that they would immediately be distributed in thickly populated areas of the city. Additional vaccine was to be manufactured in the laboratories of the Chicago Health Department under the direction of a committee of "prominent" pathologists and bacteriologists appointed a day earlier by the "pneumonia-influenza commission." The committee was also responsible for the vaccine's distribution and administration. Another committee, composed of "bankers and wealthy business men," was appointed to raise funds to make the distribution without cost to the public. It was reported that the Mayo vaccine was intended to make people immune and had recently been given to 20,000 people in Rochester, Minnesota, "resulting in a great reduction in the spread of the epidemic." Reportedly, not one death resulted after the vaccine was given, "although many of those inoculated had previously been sufferers." Because of the absence of knowledge of the germ, which had taken such a toll on lives, Rosenow included in his vaccine "all the forms of pneumonia germs, streptococci, and other unidentified organisms to create a mobilization of antibodies." According to the doctor, the patient became immune for a limited time after the first injection. To bring about "complete immunization," three injections were necessary at intervals of one week.[10]

As of October 17, some vaccines in Chicago had been sent to Grand Forks, North Dakota, and were slated to be used there by its physicians. This account claimed that the material had "proved to be exceedingly efficacious," without giving specifics.[11]

Meanwhile, officials in New York reported on their vaccine, citing "favorable results" from the first trials in cantonments (temporary quarters for troops). Those results, explained Copeland, gave him every reason to believe the treatment had succeeded. The preparation, made by Dr. William Parke, contained only one bacillus—the germ of the "old-fashioned grippe." *Grip* and *grippe* were common words used in that period for influenza. Parke, director of the New York City Bureau of Laboratories, stated in his report, "The fact that the influenza vaccine produces immunity to the disease is the strongest possible indication that Pfeiffer's bacillus (the germ of the grippe) is the cause of the disease. If we can prevent the initial disease (influenza) we need not worry about complications (pneumonia)." The New York City Health Department announced that the vaccine would be available in the city immediately.[12]

Amazingly, a vaccine was available in some drugstores; that is, if the ad from McSwain Brothers Prescription Druggists in Paris, Tennessee, was to be believed. Their ad in a local newspaper, the *Parisian*, on October 18, proclaimed it was on offer. No details were given as to whose vaccine it was or whether it was free. Another newspaper, the *El Paso Herald*, on October 19, contained a small advertisement for an influenza vaccine, apparently originating from Dr. Edward Auer's Laboratory.[13]

Although several vaccines were being developed in the first half of October 1918, none had any traction. All had faded away by the end of October, except for the Mayo Clinic vaccine, which dominated the field until it was shown to be useless. An article in the *Evening World* of New York City began with a letter to the paper's editor: "The prophylactic vaccine action against pneumonia and influenza looks very promising, and any physician requesting material will be supplied." It was signed "W.J. Mayo." The *World* newspaper suggested that several New York City hospitals experiment within the next few days with the vaccine created at the Mayo lab, "which has saved between 15,000 and 20,000 persons afflicted with influenza." At the request of the Chicago Health Department, Dr. Rosenow had gone to Chicago to aid in preparation for the extensive use of the treatment there, which was said to be already well underway. Charles B. Grimshaw, superintendent of New York's Roosevelt Hospital, said, "Anything that Dr. Mayo recommends is worthy of investigation, and if it proved to be the medium of relieving the present epidemic, it would be little short of a godsend." Grimshaw explained that his hospital had been trying a different vaccine treatment among the nurses "with a view to preventing infection." Of the 60 vaccinated nurses, five developed influenza. Of the 90 unvaccinated nurses, 25 contracted the disease. Grimshaw concluded, "Perhaps Dr. Mayo's vaccine will touch a better preventive average than this."[14]

On October 21 in Chicago, the city health department began to administer the Mayo vaccine. A shipment of 100,000 doses had been received from the Mayo Brothers Clinic in Rochester, Minnesota, and other shipments were to follow. The Chicago Health Department also began manufacturing the vaccine, soon allowing the city to distribute 100,000 doses daily. It continued to be presented as a preventive for illness, not a cure. The treatment in Chicago consisted of three doses administered by subcutaneous injection. To obtain the material, the health departments of the various cities and towns of Illinois had to apply to Dr. St. Clair Drake, head of the state health department in Springfield.[15]

Fargo, North Dakota, received a vaccine shipment from Rochester on October 23 at the city's Agriculture College. It was noted that the treatment would be received in sufficient quantity to permit its use in Fargo and at the college. The report stated, "The serum has been used successfully both as a preventative and as an inoculation by the United States government." The statement was untrue, as the government had not used any vaccines.[16]

Other vaccines outside of Mayo continued to make a brief flurry on occasion. New York City's preventive flu vaccine, courtesy of Dr. Copeland, was reportedly made available to the public starting on October 22 at the health centers and clinics of the city's health department, with the addresses of all those centers and clinics being helpfully published in the article. Two or three injections were necessary at intervals of two days to receive a complete treatment.[17]

Dr. Charles F. Dalton, secretary of the Vermont Board of Health, announced on October 23 that a vaccine to prevent influenza was being distributed to physicians in Vermont and thus administered to their patients. Dr. Timothy Leary of Tufts College made the vaccine from a formula. Still, through scientific research and many experiments, the local scientists at the Vermont laboratory had "perfected a serum to such an extent that its efficiency was much greater than when used with the Leary formula alone." One injection was given each day for three successive days. Dalton wanted it understood that he and his Vermont Board of Health did not view the vaccine as a "guaranteed preventive" as the treatment was still experimental. But he added, "It has already been used in Massachusetts and other states with excellent results."[18]

Some corporations and firms engaged in war work in New York City had begun to combat the flu, or so they hoped, by inoculating their officials and workers with vaccines. The United States Steel Corporation led the way. The first man from that organization to be vaccinated on October 24 was Elbert H. Gary, chair of the firm. Before the office closed for the day, the entire office force of 125 people had been inoculated. A reporter noted, "It was optional with the employees whether they should accept the serum, but there wasn't a man among the lot who didn't follow the leaders." Five doctors from various hospitals administered the shots. A second injection was given a few days later, and then a third. The next day, other big employers in the area were reportedly ready to follow U.S. Steel's example, but they were not named. Gary had previously wired U.S. President Woodrow Wilson regarding the vaccine, saying his firm would go to any expense to keep up the workers' efficiency in carrying on the war effort. At Camp Dix (later Fort Dix) in New Jersey, 10,000 soldiers received shots, which partly demonstrated the vaccine's success as a preventive. Out of that number, not a single case of pneumonia had developed from the flu.[19]

The Quincy County exemption board in Illinois ordered enough flu vaccine for 200 men of class one of the draft who were to be inducted into the army. The Illinois Department of Health distributed the vaccine free to local military boards, but the supply was reportedly limited. The Quincy exemption board made the vaccine compulsory for the men going to a cantonment and free for others in class one who requested it.[20]

A conference of public health officials met in Pittsburgh on October 22 to discuss the "advisability of inoculating every resident of that city with a newly 'discovered' serum as a preventive agent" against the Spanish flu. Those officials were members of the Alleghany County Medical Society and the Pittsburgh chapter of the Red Cross. After the conference, Health Director Davis stated that no decision had been reached.[21]

An article from Fairmont, West Virginia, on October 23 about physicians giving flu shots in the community carried the subhead "Local practitioners say they are certain it works." According to the account, "quite a number" of residents had been inoculated. Many of the city's "leading physicians" were advertising its use not only as a means of protecting the individual but as a means of preventing the further spread of sickness. Local doctors had on hand, reportedly, "quite a quantity" of the serum. Some physicians who were using it declared three shots were necessary for an entire course of treatment. In contrast, others insisted that four shots were required. Readers were assured that no sickness followed the shots and that patients went about their daily lives as usual. Then the unnamed reporter wandered into some significant untruths when he said, "The serum has the endorsement of the US government and is prepared and sold by all the leading drug houses in the country. A number of the larger cities in the United States are strongly recommending its use." So enamored with the vaccine were the physicians of Clarksburg, West Virginia, that 3,000 industrial workers, employees of the Weirton Steel Company, had been inoculated. The Hazel Atlas Glass Company and the Owens Bottle Machine Company employees had "consented" to be vaccinated with the serum, and the required number of doses had been ordered from Philadelphia.[22]

The State of Massachusetts, through its health commissioner, had appointed a committee composed of the "leading research physicians and authorities of the world" to investigate available vaccines. As a result of the investigation, the committee determined "that the state encourages the distribution of influenza vaccine intended for prophylactic use, but in such a manner as will secure scientific evidence of the possible value of the agent. The use of such vaccines is to be regarded as experimental. That the state shall neither furnish nor endorse any vaccine at present in use for the treatment of influenza." The committee was composed of such men as Dr. Rosenow, "recognized as the greatest research expert in the United States," Frederick P. Gay, George W. McCoy, George C. Whipple, William Davis and F.C. Frum.[23]

It was reported that Dr. Strauss, city health officer, would receive a supply of vaccine sufficient to inoculate every person in Bismarck, North Dakota, as soon as the Mayo Brothers Clinic in Rochester, Minnesota, could prepare and ship it. Strauss had wired for a supply of the vaccine a few days earlier. He received a return message from Rosenow stating that the store at his lab was inadequate to meet the heavy demand. Still, he would forward the order to Strauss as soon as possible. Strauss emphasized that a dose would be available to the public at no charge but that there would be a fee "to cover the actual work of inoculation."[24]

The Manufacturers' Association of East Chicago and Indiana Harbor decided to use the influenza vaccine on all employees at the various industries in the area at a meeting on October 23. The meeting was attended by members of the association, local physicians, and Dr. Paul M. Holmes of the United States Public Health Department. As a result, a "large quantity" of the vaccine was ordered. With a limited supply, inoculating those employees began the following day. In all cases where major industrial concerns vaccinated their employees, company executives made a unilateral decision, with the employees having no say. Often, though, accounts that presented such stories solemnly declared that the workers had given their "consent."[25]

The Oregon Board of Health announced at the same time that state and city health officials were preparing a prophylactic vaccine that would be ready for free distribution by doctors soon. In Seattle, Washington, 60,000 people had reportedly received shots, with the claim that "none had contracted the disease in a serious form." At the Skinner and Eddy shipyards in Seattle, 6,000 employees were inoculated. It was said that the shipyard hospital reported fewer cases of sickness than in any previous month. It was also noted that only two of the 1,200 men inoculated at the Bremerton, Washington, navy yard had contracted influenza. The vaccine being developed in Oregon was to be supplied to physicians only. The charge for a shot was expected to be just the cost of a regular visit to the doctor.[26]

The next area to lay claim to a vaccine was Oklahoma, with a journalist observing that the "pneumonia vaccine is now being manufactured in Tulsa at the Wright Laboratories by several prominent physicians and chemists of this city." Doctor A. Rautros, chemist, and Dr. J.D. Gilbert, of the City of Tulsa health department, returned home from Kansas City, where Mayor Hubbard had sent them a couple of days earlier to obtain a formula for "the wonderful vaccine that is producing such great results" in fighting Spanish influenza in eastern cities. Because of the "enormous demand" for the treatment in Kansas City, the pair from Tulsa could not obtain any, but after a conference with Dr. Abraham Sophian, "the eminent serum specialist" and a friend of Mayor Hubbard, they obtained the formula and explicit directions for manufacture. Work back home in Tulsa started at once. The vaccine was prepared from germs from people infected with the Spanish flu. The germs were grown in a culture medium. Then they were washed with a salt solution and killed with heat. Next, the solution was made into liquid form, and the vaccine was injected into the arm. According to this report, "Three different doses administered hypodermically at intervals of from three days to one week are effective in warding off the disease." Earlier, Rosenow had contacted Tulsa officials after a request for doses to Mayo. Rosenow told Tulsa that the supply at Rochester was inadequate to meet the demand.[27]

MAYOR RECEIVES SECOND "SHOT" OF NEW ANTI-INFLUENZA SERUM

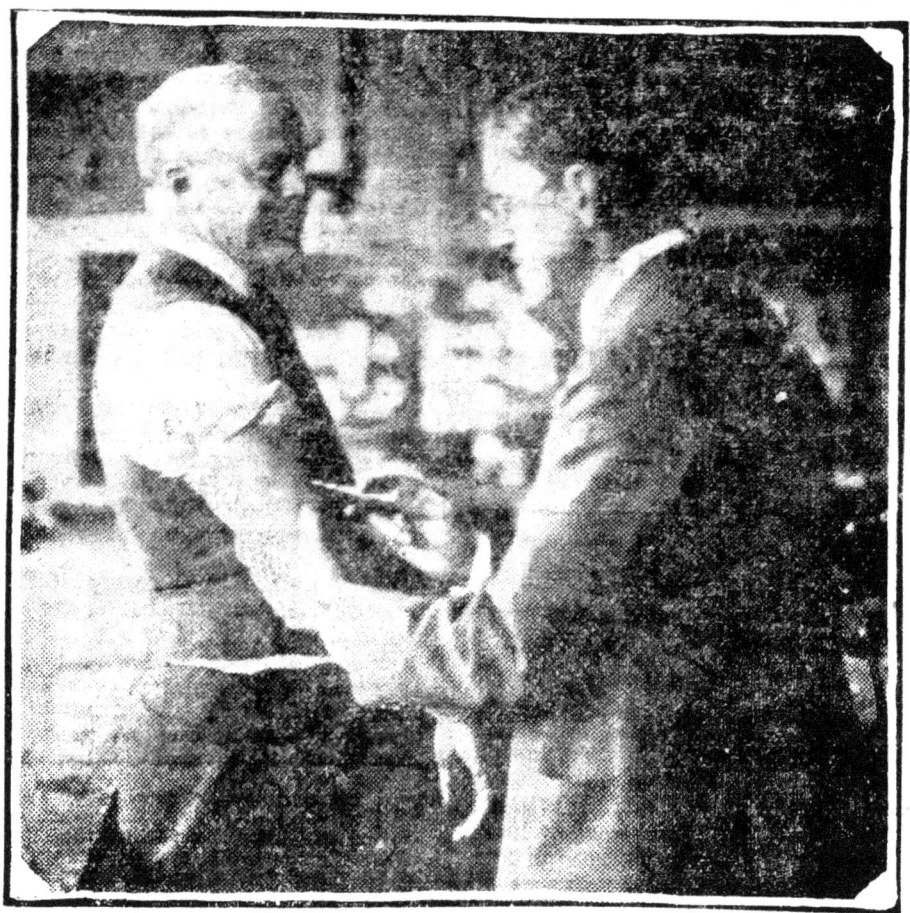

DR. TIMOTHY LEARY INOCULATING MAYOR PETERS WITH ANTI-INFLUENZA SERUM.

Boston Mayor Andrew Peters receives a flu shot from Dr. Timothy Leary and thus sets a "good example" for the public and signals virtue.

In the first days of October, when the disease first threatened Philadelphia, Dr. Timothy W. Bowes, Medical Director of the Philadelphia Electric Company, and his assistants "virtually kept the entire force of that corporation free from the epidemic grip or influenza." The company's workforce of 3,500 employees had "submitted" to injections, and of those, not one contracted the flu. Other corporations asked the Philadelphia Electric Company for aid, which was given, and Dr. Bowes and his assistants inoculated another 10,000 people who had no connection with his company at no charge. Those demands exhausted the company's medical department of Sherman Serum, and a messenger went to Detroit to get more. This article pointed out the differences between a vaccine and a serum. A vaccine was an injection that protected patients by giving them a milder and modified form of the disease. An example was the smallpox vaccine. A serum acted differently. In the blood serum (the liquid remaining after coagulation), there was a substance called opsonin that had the property of rendering the various disease-causing germs that got into the blood more easily destroyed by the phagocytes, or white corpuscles, which could be called the police of the blood. Diphtheritic serum was made by inoculating a young horse slightly with the virus, which sickened him. His blood killed the deadly germs and thus became more powerful. Then he was given a larger dose of diphtheria. And it also killed the germs, and the blood became even more robust, and so on, for several months. His blood serum became enormously filled with opsonin. Then his blood was taken, and some was injected into a child seriously ill with diphtheria.[28]

The federal government furnished the vaccine for munitions workers. It was to be administered to the Root and VanDervoort Ordinance Company employees and the Root and VanDervoort Engineering Company of Moline, Illinois. Within a day or two, the U.S. government and the Illinois health authorities requested that workers engaged in war work under government contracts take advantage of the preventive treatment for influenza. The flu had already struck those two plants "rather severely," and several employee deaths had occurred. Therefore, the company urged "that all workers submit to the vaccine treatment."[29]

An article from Arizona that favored the use of vaccines began by declaring the statement sometimes made by "misinformed laymen and by some physicians that there is much danger and no virtue in the use" of influenza shots, which prompted a reply from Dr. Orville H. Brown, Arizona superintendent of health, and Dr. Warner Watkins, of the pathology lab that was supplying the bulk of the vaccine then being used in Arizona. Their statement began by noting that the vaccine's use was experimental in that it had never before been used for that purpose on a large scale. The last influenza pandemic (1889–1890) was before the day of that class of vaccines. However, Brown and Watkins noted there were theoretical grounds on which to hope vaccines would be of value. One of the reasons they had for believing that was the U.S. Army's experience with pneumonia in the cantonments during the past year. Those soldiers were vaccinated against pneumonia as fast as Washington could produce the material. The army's medical department "has convinced themselves that ordinary lobar pneumonia can be largely prevented by this means. Vaccination against influenza is based on the same scientific basis as vaccination against ordinary pneumonia."[30]

Early in the epidemic, the Massachusetts Board of Health appointed two commissions to investigate the value of the influenza vaccine. They concluded that although the evidence was meager, it suggested that "the incidence of the disease among the vaccinated is smaller than among the unvaccinated." It also concluded that "the statistical evidence, so far as it goes, indicates a probability that the use of this influenza vaccine has some prophylactic value" and "there is no evidence that unfavorable results have followed the use of the vaccines." Finally, "the state encourages the distribution of influenza vaccine intended for prophylactic use." The Mayo Brothers vaccine was said to be "almost identical" to the one being made and used in Arizona. It was also observed that Dr. Rosenow, who prepared and distributed the vaccine for the Mayo Brothers Clinic, had reached conclusions "coinciding exactly" with those of Brown and Watkins. And the conclusion was that the preventive treatment should "by all means be used. It can do no harm and will either prevent influenza or diminish the severity of the attack. Taking the vaccine should not lead anyone to neglect the other precautions which have been recommended."[31]

There was nothing unusual about Rosenow urging more and greater use of vaccines, since he had created one and was the leading Mayo Brothers salesperson in flogging the product. It was a blatant conflict of interest. The "epidemic" became one about the middle of September 1918, concerning the media coverage. It became an "official" epidemic on about October 1, 1918, concerning actions of one kind or another instituted by state and local governments such as lockdowns, or euphemistically termed nonpharmaceutical interventions and closures. There was then no flu vaccine available. Yet the article reported in Arizona on October 26 cited conclusions from Massachusetts that could not have been reached in such a short period.

U.S. Surgeon General Rupert Blue reached a more thoughtful conclusion. Speaking in Washington on October 26, he noted that the use of vaccines in combating or treating Spanish influenza had yet to go beyond the experimental stage, as far as the U.S. Public Health Service had learned. Blue said, "It must be remembered that several different vaccines are now being tried. The reports so far received, however, do not permit any conclusion whatsoever regarding the efficacy of these vaccines or their relative merits. The Public Health Service is watching the experiments carefully but is not urging any form of vaccine treatment."[32]

A Louisiana newspaper gave over one-third of a page to an ad from the Morgan City (LA) Board of Health, signed by C.C. deGravelles (chair). The ad featured prominent medical people in the area singing the praises of vaccines. Dr. Duval was both a Touro Hospital pathologist and a Tulane University pathology professor. He declared he treated 678 people employed by the D.H. Holmes Company in New Orleans, and not a single case of Spanish flu developed where three doses were given. The employees of Dyer Brothers and Parker-Blake Company had been treated, and not a single case of influenza developed where three doses were administered. Dr. Allen Eustis, associate professor of medicine at Tulane, had been using the serum for the last three weeks "and believes that everyone should take it." Doctor G.B. Adams, a pathologist at Charity Hospital and assistant professor of pathology at Tulane, had given the treatment to more than 4,000 people and claimed that not 1 percent of them had developed influenza if three doses were given. Dr. Copeland, head of the New York Sanitary Board, "urges everyone to take the serum treatment." In Morgan City, there was no charge for administering the influenza vaccine. Those who could pay were charged for the cost of the serum, but it was free for those who could not afford the vaccine.[33]

The editor of a Connecticut newspaper sounded one negative note. He said there was no warrant for the idea that there was any serum that influenced the course of Spanish influenza favorably. He cited the remarks of Surgeon General Blue and then added, "The wholesale use of influenza serum among the employees of industrial plants is an experiment not warranted by previous results obtained in serum therapy and not justified by the experience recently obtained from such experimentation." He was OK with those involved being fully informed of the history of the serums. As the editor concluded, the use of a serum in the presence of the disease is one thing; "the use of the serum upon healthy men and women as a preventive is quite another thing. There is no worthy evidence as to the duration of immunity if any occurs.... The injection of a serum into the blood stream constitutes a violent shock to the system, which is sometimes attended by grave results, immediate or delayed."[34]

Another critical article appeared on November 1, 1918. It summarized the two committees set up early in October in Massachusetts by E.R. Kelly. The first group contained Rosenow and the others, who considered the evidence available on the prophylactic and therapeutic use of flu vaccines. The committee concluded, according to this report, that the evidence at hand "affords no trustworthy basis for regarding prophylactic vaccination against influenza as of value in preventing the spread of the disease, or of reducing its severity." The reporter suggested that further experimental evidence should be collected to augment the existing "meager" evidence. The second group reported that the weight of the evidence "indicates that the use of the influenza vaccine which we have investigated is without therapeutic benefit," although there was some evidence of "a probability that the use of this influenza vaccine has some prophylactic value." In summary, this report felt that Idaho should "neither furnish nor endorse any vaccine at present in use for the treatment of influenza."[35]

In an ad in a Seattle, Washington, paper on November 5 for the Bon Marché department store, a small section at the bottom pointed out that an influenza inoculation nurse was on site to administer flu shots during store hours. The program was in cooperation with the Seattle Health Department. Also noted in the ad was that the store's hours were limited to 10 a.m. until 3 p.m., a nonpharmaceutical intervention brought about by the epidemic—a lockdown of sorts. That meant that a store that was usually open 12 or more hours a day, with its customer base spread over those hours, had compressed its hours to just five per day, thus almost guaranteeing that customer density would be much more significant over those abbreviated hours and that the increased density would not limit the spread of the flu?[36]

Finally, in Bismarck, North Dakota, the city health officer, Dr. F.B. Strauss, announced that on November 7, his city had received its order of vaccines from the Mayo Brothers Clinic in Rochester. The doses had been placed in the hands of area physicians preparing to inoculate Bismarck citizens immediately. According to Strauss, this material "is said to have been very efficacious in preventing Spanish influenza or in eliminating the danger from influenza once the malady had been contracted." As city health officer, Strauss recommended the inoculation "of every Bismarck citizen as a means of preventing a recurrence of the recent plague."[37]

Reportedly, as of November 12, thousands of U.S. soldiers and war workers received injections of the pneumonia vaccine recently developed by the U.S. Army Medical School in Washington, D.C. One case of pneumonia occurred among the 10,000 soldiers injected at Camp Upton. The report stated that while the vaccine was created for the army, "the civilian population has quickly adopted it." It added, "After meeting with persistent opposition for smallpox and typhoid fever for years, the medical profession everywhere is now almost embarrassed by the popular demand for vaccination against pneumonia." The great success of this item resulted in the Army Medical School being prevailed upon to give another evidence of its ability by inventing a vaccine against influenza. It was useless for the institution to protest that influenza was an entirely different matter. Very little was known concerning the influenza germ because "it is too small to be seen through the most powerful microscope and cannot be tested upon animals either."[38]

Thus, the Army Medical School—under pressure—had come up with a new influenza vaccine, then only a few weeks old. While its success rate was unknown, "whatever it does, it cannot hurt the patient." The army had started work on its pneumonia vaccine over a year earlier, long before the pandemic began. According to the army's research, certain diseases could not be transmitted to the lower animals. Spanish influenza was said to be one, along with typhoid fever. A scientist could kill a mouse or a guinea pig by injecting it with either of those disorders but could not cause it to contract the disease. Then the army simplified the number of shots required for the typhoid treatment to be effective. A course of treatment of three or four doses over several months was considered excessive. So they reduced the typhoid treatment to one dose.[39]

As of November 14, Phoenix, Arizona, had been "closed" for six weeks. Talks were then being held about reopening the city. Dr. O.H. Brown, Arizona health officer, again suggested that general vaccination be permitted in Phoenix. However, Dr. Beauchamp, the City of Phoenix health officer, opposed the plan, stating that he would resign before he would countenance the general use of the influenza vaccine upon the public. Beauchamp insisted that the vaccine was in the experimental stage and that many of the most prominent physicians in the country, including Surgeon General Rupert Blue, did not favor the flu vaccine. Disputes such as this between state health officials and local health authorities (most major cities had a health officer) were common. It sometimes led to inaction as the two jurisdictions could not agree on some items.[40]

Schools in Crystal Falls, Michigan, reopened in mid–November after being closed for two weeks due to the flu. The reopening was partly due to the children receiving shots; it was reported that inoculating the pupils with anti-influenza serum had been "progressing nicely." The parents' response regarding sending their kids to the authorities for injection was reported as "very good." Many of the children were due for their third injection in the coming week.[41]

A story in a Phoenix newspaper on November 17 threw cold water on the vaccines then available. It was a reprint from a medical journal and debunked a newspaper article titled "Vaccine Blots out Flu." The story declared, on October 20, that about half the people of an unidentified town of 10,000 had been vaccinated, at least in part. There were seven cases of the disease in the community, all among unvaccinated people. In a nearby town with 400 unvaccinated inhabitants, there were 200 cases and 15 deaths. Also referenced was a physician who declared, "I have given over 1,000 inoculations with 100 percent protection and treated several hundred cases with no deaths." Not mentioned was the fact that the physician was a manufacturer of vaccines. In summary, the critical article observed that none of that so-called favorable evidence had ever been submitted to any scientific scrutiny, nor were any details provided. As presented in the critical article, the medical journal concluded, "Vaccination against epidemic influenza is in a wholly experimental stage. Nothing can be learned as to its real value from indiscriminate vaccination of the public.... Pending developments, nothing should be done by the medical profession that may arouse unwarranted hope among the public and be followed by disappointment and distrust of medical science and the medical profession."[42]

At that time, Phoenix had been in lockdown for six weeks. New regulations were imposed by a commission from the Maricopa County Medical Society of Drs. Ancil Martin, Kimball Bannister, and W.W. Watkins. The group met with Dr. H.K. Beauchamp of the City of Phoenix, Dr. A.B. Nichols of the county and Dr. Orville H. Brown of the State of Arizona, and then issued new recommendations. One of those recommendations wanted to see one free vaccination station established under medical supervision and control where a "careful record" of those inoculated could be kept, and other stations could be installed if required. The value of the flu vaccine, in general, was discussed, with the state health officer firmly favoring its use but opposed by Beauchamp, who declared he had no faith in the vaccine and added that he would not recommend it. Other physicians present at the meeting insisted that the use of the vaccine had tended to minimize the danger of the flu. The only decision reached concerning vaccination was that it should not be compulsory and that it should be administered, if at all, at no cost.[43]

In El Paso, Texas, doctors received consignments of Rosenow's vaccine late in November. The story admitted that while several places had tried the vaccine, it was still considered an experiment. Some locals had received it, but only those who had heard of it and asked for it. Considerable efficacy was claimed for the vaccine. The story in the Texas paper was that of the 15,000 people given shots in Rochester, Minnesota, not one had suffered from influenza or pneumonia. In one school, 350 kids were vaccinated, and not one had developed the disorder; 14 nurses at St. Mary's Hospital in Rochester had influenza before they received their shots, and no one developed the flu after injections. Another Rochester hospital reported that no pneumonia or influenza occurred among the 1,400 people vaccinated there. The problem with that data was that Rosenow had provided it all. He had developed the vaccine and was actively selling it on behalf of the Mayo Brothers Clinic, all in Rochester. That is, there was an enormous conflict of interest. Plus, Rosenow never provided any details for his numbers.[44]

The military hospital at Payne Field, near West Point, Mississippi, received some pneumonia vaccine and a consignment of influenza vaccine. Regarding that development, a military newspaper grumbled, "Along with all the other recruit horrors, which includes pneumonia vaccine, typhoid vaccine, paratyphoid vaccine, and smallpox vaccine, somebody in the wilds of the army medical research for something or other, has found another vaccine."[45]

A chiropractor named J.W. Hall of Exira, Iowa, took out a full-page ad in his local paper on November 28 criticizing what was being done in the name of the flu epidemic. Much of what he had to say remained relevant 100 years into the future. Of particular note were his observations and comments on vaccines and the mask.[46]

In Alma, Michigan, the city health department declared its determination to stop the flu epidemic in the city and said that it had "taken steps to vaccinate everyone or request that they wear a flu mask when attending public events." Along with that came the announcement that the ban, in effect for some weeks in Alma, had been lifted so that church services, movies, dances, and other public gatherings would again be held. It was said that movies had been the hardest hit. According to the report, some of the army camps had used vaccines "with a marked success." In Flint, Michigan, where it was used, "it gained wide favor." Shots were free to all who wanted them at Alma city hall from 11 a.m. to 1 p.m. and 7 p.m. to 8 p.m. After receiving the third and final shot—a complete treatment—the patient received a card from the health department that would permit them to attend any public gathering without wearing a flu mask. In other words, a health pass—sound familiar? Those who refused to take the shots had to wear a mask in public gatherings until the abatement of the present epidemic.[47]

Dr. Macfarlane was the local health officer in Cedar City, Iowa. He announced that he had on hand 250 doses of "the pure strain Spanish influenza vaccine" that Rosenow had discovered and that it was "highly recommended by the leading physicians throughout the country." Supposedly, it had proven to be "exceedingly effectual in Salt Lake City, as well as in all the large cities of the United States." An entire course of treatment consisted of three doses, 48 hours apart. Those doses were free in Cedar City, except for a one-dollar fee for administering the three shots.[48]

An advertisement placed by New Mexico Normal University (Las Vegas, NM) on November 29 informed the reader that potential students had to meet specific requirements to attend classes beginning for a new term in a few days: "only students who have been inoculated with anti-influenza serum or who have had influenza admitted. Arrangements have been made for the inoculation of students after they have returned to Las Vegas."[49]

George Shorten was the city health inspector for the Ogden, Utah, city board of health. His agency published an ad on December 3 in which Shorten and his board of health made an "unqualified recommendation" to have the flu shots as a preventive measure. The City of Ogden was offering the vaccine free to the public with city physician Dr. W.P. Brown giving the injections at the clinic located in the First National Bank Building.[50]

At the same time, Keokuk, Iowa, announced that the vaccine would be free to all who wanted it in a clinic set up just as soon as the city's order arrived from the Mayo Brothers labs in Rochester. At least three injections were required, with intervals of a few days between the shots. According to the story, the vaccine had "nothing much to do with influenza. It is a preventive measure against pneumonia. People do not die from influenza very much, but pneumonia which often follows influenza is very fatal, about one-third of the cases dying within a week or so."[51]

Vaccine claims were so exaggerated and false, much of the time, that the United States Public Health Service felt compelled to make a statement on the issue, which it did on December 7. It said that because of "the exaggerated and in some respects misleading statements that have appeared in the public press" concerning the value of bacterial vaccines in the prevention and treatment of influenza and pneumonia that

> **NEW MEXICO NORMAL UNIVERSITY**
> LAS VEGAS
>
> **High School and College Classes**
> BEGIN MONDAY, DECEMBER 2ND
>
> Only students who have been inoculated with anti-influenza serum or who have had the influenza admitted. Arrangements have been made for the inoculation of students after they have returned to Las Vegas.

New Mexico Normal University in Las Vegas, New Mexico, would only admit students who had received their flu shots when classes restarted. However, it did allow students who had contracted the disease and recovered. That is, it recognized natural immunity.

so often followed, it declared that "the evidence that has been presented thus far does not warrant the reposing of confidence in any influenza vaccine for either prophylactic or therapeutic purposes." The statement continued, "Several vaccine preparations made by the influenza bacillus, some from streptococci, some from various types of pneumococci and other organisms have been recommended and used in various localities and evidence has been advanced which has been held to show that the number of persons attacked has been less and the deaths fewer among the vaccinated than among those who had not been treated." Yet when the evidence was analyzed, "either there was no indication of protection or therapeutic value or there was no more than a suggestion that possibly some protection had been inferred."[52]

When Dr. Rosenow addressed the annual meeting of the American Public Health Association on December 10 in Chicago, he declared that 90 percent of the deaths from influenza and pneumonia were preventable with proper vaccine use. He insisted that the deaths from influenza and pneumonia among those who had been inoculated "were one-tenth those among the unvaccinated." The article that covered the event made no mention that Rosenow was the creator and chief salesperson of the best known of those vaccines.[53]

In his speech, Rosenow cited figures from Rochester, Minnesota. He said that after patients received the third shot, those vaccinated people contracted nine cases of flu per thousand people, as opposed to 220 per thousand among the unvaccinated. Over 21,000 people were given three shots, while 61,000 got no treatment. Deaths among the former group from influenza and pneumonia were one-third of the latter group. His use of the vaccine led to the decision that surgical patients in the Rochester hospital must be vaccinated prior to surgery. Based on such data, Dr. A. Asburgh of Idaho Springs, Colorado, had been using the vaccine in his community as "a preventive and as a cure in the early stages of influenza and pneumonia, with gratifying results." Three doses were required, seven days apart. In Chicago, the city ordered the vaccine in "vast quantities," and the city's population was "vaccinated by the thousands daily." Also noted was that "everyone leaving his home in Havre, Montana, must have a 'shot in the arm.'" And that "all employees of the Great Western sugar company in northern Colorado have been given the inoculation at their option, and not the expense of the company."[54]

Bismarck Health Officer F.B. Strauss warned his city's residents, "Another wave of flu hysteria, entirely without foundation, is sweeping over the capital city." He argued that "this hysteria does no good. In fact, it works harm." He thought there was no reason, unless things got worse, to close theaters. "He thought schools should remain open for normal and healthy kids; those who were manifestly sick should be kept home." But he urged "that everyone become inoculated with the anti-flu serum."[55]

And still, the new vaccines continued to arrive. The laboratories of the School of Medicine at the University of Missouri in Columbia produced and manufactured a new flu vaccine said to differ from any other, offering it for free distribution to registered physicians.[56]

In mid–December, Webster City, Iowa, received a "large supple" of pneumonia and influenza vaccine from the Mayo Brothers. Physicians in Webster City "strongly recommend" injections at no cost, with the vaccine to be given to all who requested it. They stated that having the shots rendered one immune to both illnesses. Three injections were required at one-week intervals. A supply ample for all of Hamilton County had been received, and the Hamilton County Medical Association recommended inoculation. The vaccine was the Rosenow one. There were not two separate vaccines. The vaccine was more frequently presented as good for the flu and pneumonia as time passed. Sometimes the treatment was offered just for pneumonia.

That confusion, mixed with the confusion of vaccine versus serum, made the situation unfathomable. Underlying that, and probably creating the confusion, was that none of these vaccines or serums were good. None prevented or cured anything.[57]

School Superintendent Henry C. Johnson of Ogden, Utah, wrote to Surgeon General Blue to ask about the value of the vaccine as a prophylactic measure for children of school age. The reply he received said, "Influenza vaccine still in experimental stage. Prophylactic value doubtful. Do not recommend use for school children."[58]

In mid–December, Kansas Board of Health officials announced the plan to create a flu vaccine at the state laboratories at the University of Kansas at Lawrence. Professor N.P. Sherwood, professor of bacteriology, had been sent to Rochester, Minnesota, to gather information on the "cooking" of flu germs in manufacturing serum. One reason for going to local production was what happened in the wake of the annual public health conference in Chicago. "A result of the Chicago conference serum, which has proven highly effective in one community, has failed to produce results in another community." Rosenow gave a glowing report at the meeting about the unbelievably good efficacy of the vaccine he had created for the Mayo Brothers, for whom he sold the concoction. Those radiant results referred to experiments he had conducted in Rochester. It worked to sell more vaccines, but strangely, other towns that bought and used his vaccine based on his results found that it did not work for them at all. They got no results. Bizarrely, rather than calling Rosenow out, new purchasers, such as Kansas, blamed it on geography. It was to be the purpose of the laboratory specialists at the University of Kansas "to prepare a vaccine especially adopted for use in this state.... Several preparations may be required to meet demands in various sections of Kansas.... The state will work on the generally accepted theory that none of the vaccines are generally effective and that a special serum may be required for a successful campaign against influenza in Kansas." Kansas was anxious to have a vaccine to avert a third wave of the Spanish flu, as the second wave had passed.[59]

More bad news hit the vaccine pushers just a week before Christmas in 1918, when an announcement appeared in many newspapers. A journalist reported, "Announcement is made this morning of a ruling issued by the local board of health, backed by the health department of the United States government that the serum, which had been so widely advertised as a preventive for Spanish influenza and administered by many physicians throughout the country is utterly devoid of any

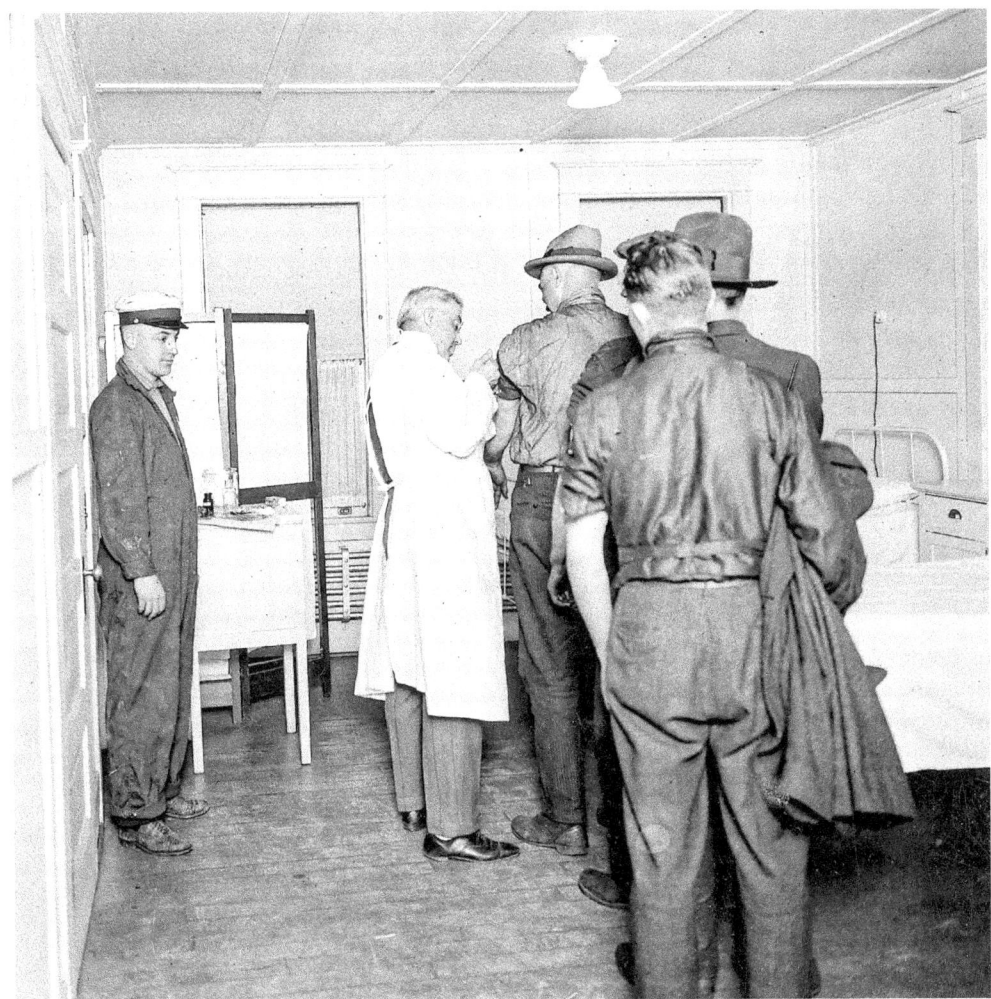

A number of hapless souls stand in line waiting to have their flu shots in Seattle.

virtue in providing the results claimed for it. It is looked upon as a most deplorable condition that thousands of people have been induced to take the serum and have paid a high price for it and have later been reported as victims of the disease and in many cases have been taken into the emergency hospitals." In Warren, Ohio, physicians were refusing to administer the vaccine to their patients. Members of the Warren Fire Department, who were inoculated with the serum, "were later victims of influenza and are testifying to its utter failure as a preventive."[60]

Only some people received the message or believed it. On the same day, Mayor Cooper of Canon City, Colorado, announced his city had purchased $100 worth of flu vaccine from the Mayo Brothers and had obtained a sufficient quantity from other sources to inoculate 2,000 people—thought to be ample for his community. Cooper thought the city would inoculate all those who wanted it for free. Dr. E.C. Webb, city health officer, remarked that about 2,500 people in the Canon City area had been vaccinated in the last three months and that perhaps 2,000 more would apply for the treatment if it were free.[61]

The battle for effective vaccines had been lost, but some would not admit defeat. Dr. W.A. von Zellen wrote a letter to the editor published on the op-ed page of a Michigan paper. It declared, "Notice is given to the people of Baraga County that they are too unprogressive in taking inoculation of the influenza serum ... everyone must wake up to the realization that he or she might be the next victim." He added, "Recognition should not be taken of criticisms against this vaccine, whether from the physicians or the laity, because this is the only recourse we have. When such eminent doctors as the Mayos and others of the best standing recommend this serum as prophylaxis, the people should abide by their assertions and decisions in preference to those of superficial, flighty egotists or ignorant aberrations." To conclude his scare piece, the doctor argued that the "US government uses this serum and makes it mandatory—why should not the rest of us do the same." The doctor conjured images of first the mother dying in the family, then the father, leaving a pile of orphans.[62]

On January 2, 1919, an editor with an Albuquerque paper discussed the vaccination issue. Referencing J. C. Perry, acting surgeon general of the U.S. Public Health Service, the editor declared, "The public health service had conducted several careful tests with influenza vaccine in various institutions, vaccinating half of the inmates and leaving the other half unvaccinated as a control. In every instance when influenza spread in the institution, its incidence among the vaccinated was practically the same as among the unvaccinated." The editor argued that the public health service had not discouraged using the influenza vaccine but was only stating that it could not recommend it as a preventive. The journalist then argued that life insurance companies were offering to pay for the vaccinations of their policyholders. The Occidental Life Company of Albuquerque had just received instructions to urge the vaccination of policyholders who were renewing their policies, with the firm bearing any expense. To prove his case, the editor argued that life insurance companies were not shouldering that expense "for the fun of it." Then he cited Dr. Fennell of the U.S. Army, who said vaccination had done wonders for the army and that the flu vaccine "bids fair to rival typhoid fever vaccination, about which there has been no doubt for some time." Fennell declared, "Laboratory methods that have stood the test of time were used to test the value of the vaccine, and the results have been particularly gratifying." The editor concluded, "No doctor who doesn't now urge vaccination is worthy of the public's confidence."[63]

Dr. Karl F. Meyer of the Hooper Institute of Medical Research at the University of California stated that the serums used in influenza were useless. He said, "Serums have not yet been introduced which produce immunity from Spanish influenza. The serums now employed are of no use whatsoever. Even the vaccine formerly employed successfully against pneumonia is not giving satisfactory results in influenza."[64]

Dr. G.W. McCoy, director of the hygienic laboratory of the public health service in Washington, D.C., remarked that "there is no serum that I know of which is of the slightest value in preventing influenza, nor is there a serum that is of any use whatever in the treatment of the disease." He made that statement after carefully examining vaccine and serum use in all parts of the United States, particularly in Pelham Bay, New York, "and the army camps where the mortality was great."[65]

Stories about vaccines were very prevalent in 1918 and into January 1919, but then the articles dropped off. Too many people had spoken out about the uselessness of the product. A few places still ignored the evidence and urged its use. Free vaccination to prevent the flu was soon ready for all people in Montana who wanted it, according to an announcement from the state board of health at the end of August 1919. The announcement followed the return of Dr. E.D. Hitchcock, a state bacteriologist doing research work at the Mayo Clinic. Montana was to manufacture the vaccine from cultures taken from patients in Montana. Hitchcock said that while the influenza organism was of the same species in all the states, its virulence differed according to the locality. Therefore, vaccines produced in Montana would be suited to the conditions in the region.[66]

When a couple of cases of Spanish influenza surfaced in Topeka, Kansas, in September 1919, worries arose about the coming year's possible caseload, and thoughts turned to what measures to take. The plan that had been thoroughly considered the previous spring for the state to manufacture an anti-influenza serum was dropped. Dr. Tom D. Tuttle of the Kansas Health Department said, "Such a serum has not been perfected to such an extent as would warrant the state manufacture of it."[67]

Three weeks later, it was reported that Dr. A.R. Lewis, Oklahoma health commissioner, had ordered 2,000 doses of the "Rosenow influenza vaccine" to be distributed among people in the state who could not afford to pay for the treatment. Dr. W.E. Sanderson of Altus, OK, said he had inoculated 4,000 people after they became ill with the flu. Of those 4,000 vaccinated people, only five died. None of those to whom he administered the vaccine before they became ill got sick. So far in 1919, he declared he had 20 cases of the flu and vaccinated all of them, and all were "improving."[68]

The state board of health in Louisville, Kentucky, began, on October 30, 1919, the daily culture of some trillion anti-influenza germs. Their capacity was five gallons of serum a day. Dr. Edward Rosenow was in charge, assisted by Dr. B.F. Sturdivant. Mayo Brothers loaned Rosenow's services to Kentucky because, in the previus year, the state had made a more extensive test of the Rosenow-Mayo serum than any other state. During the Kentucky outbreak in the last year, Kentucky procured from the Mayo lab sufficient vaccine to inoculate 500,000 people and distributed it to area physicians. That anti-influenza vaccine had a lowly origin, commencing with ordinary beef broth cooked in a regular bathtub, heated by steam coils. The broth then went to a centrifugal separating machine, where it was freed from impurities and sediment. Then it was placed in three-quart bottles and sterilized under pressure. The influenza germ was then introduced. Sputum from a person afflicted with the disease was placed on a glass slide. The bacteriologist inserted the slide into a microscope and selected "bugs adapted for propagation." A section on the slide, approximately one-fourth of an inch square, was placed in a vial containing five ounces of the broth and allowed to stand for 24 hours. At the end of that period, the broth became cloudy with numerous bacilli. The three-quart bottles were opened, and one ounce of the culture was poured in. Bottles were sealed and allowed to stand for 24 hours. During that time, the bacilli had multiplied sufficiently to permit the production of the finished vaccine. Next, the broth was placed in a jar connected by a rubber hose to a centrifugal machine that revolved about 35,000 times a minute. It was fed by gravity into the bottom of a tube whose rotary motion separated the vaccine, forcing the clarified broth out at the top and into another receptacle. The pasty serum clung to the side of the cylinder. The paste was then "killed" by introducing chemicals and was ready for use. When it was placed into bottles, the vaccine was forwarded to physicians. Twenty-one drops were sufficient for a single dose. Sturdivant commented that the vaccine "is not so much influenza preventive as a pneumonia preventive…. It may not be the best thing, but it is the best we know."[69]

Into 1920, there were even fewer mentions of the vaccine, although there were still a few adherents. Its time had come and gone. "In January of that year, the state board of health in Illinois voted not to recommend the use of influenza or any other mixed vaccine to prevent pneumonia or influenza."[70]

In New York City that month, Dr. Royal S. Copeland, city health commissioner, gave a brief outline of new cases in his city and grumbled, "The new outbreak of Spanish influenza has reached the proportions of an epidemic in New York City." It hadn't, but he was one of the many fear mongers of the day who would not let go. Various health authorities held a conference on what was to be done. The Department of Health, after "extensive experiments with vaccines against influenza since the epidemic of 1918, has decided that vaccine possesses no virtue as a preventive of the disease, and as a result will not recommend its use in combating the present epidemic. The department, however, will furnish the vaccine to physicians or persons who desire to use it." Dr. Copeland described one experiment that led the department to abandon the influenza vaccine. In an establishment employing 3,000 people, 1,500 workers were vaccinated against the flu, and 1,500 were not. The comparison later showed an approximate 5 percent absence from work in each group, with the record of the vaccinated being one-tenth of 1 percent worse than that of the unvaccinated.[71]

An editor with a Kentucky newspaper remarked early in 1920 that the flu had again hit in epidemic form in his area. Concerning influenza shots, he referred to a statement from T. Atchison Frazer, a health officer in Marion, Kentucky. "Yet not perfect though proven of sufficient value that every person should take it. It is harmless and ... no harm can come from its use."[72]

Panic continued to rule in Paris, Tennessee, where the city board of health put a lockdown of various businesses into effect in March 1920. The city and county health boards advised everyone to take the influenza vaccine. "It will not in every case prevent the influenza but will make a milder form and often prevent pneumonia."[73]

As late as October 1920, the Oklahoma City Health Department warned about influenza. It informed its readers that an abundant supply of vaccine for influenza treatment was available and would be provided free to all who desired the treatment.[74]

3

New England

Connecticut

With the flu pandemic underway and the media feeding a mass hysteria, one of the first announcements of the widespread and mandated use of masks came from Bridgeport, Connecticut. On or around September 13, 1918, the authorities ordered all doctors, interns, ambulance drivers, and nurses of the city hospitals in Bridgeport to wear masks when attending to victims of the Spanish flu. A public announcement of the order was made on September 27, when a further bulletin came from New Haven and Hartford stating that they were implementing similar orders. Dr. J.F. Keegan of the Emergency Hospital in Bridgeport said the masks were saturated with formaldehyde and "proof against the influenza germ." He added, "The masks are in no way similar to the gas masks worn by the soldiers at the front, but are small light affairs of gauze, which cover the nose and mouth and are adjusted by straps which go over the ears."[1]

A few weeks later, people were mainly "urged" to wear face coverings, if they were mentioned at all, at least in some jurisdictions. Mandatory wearing had been limited to hospitals and a few other areas, such as barbershops. That would slowly change throughout the epidemic until there was almost always a mandated order to cover the face. Rarely would it be left to simple "urgings." Even outside of hospitals, medical personnel had to be urged. While attending influenza cases, the Connecticut Department of Health encouraged physicians and nurses to wear masks. It was explained that those should be adjusted to the face before entering a sick room and not removed or otherwise touched by the hands until the attendant left the room. Then, the hands should be thoroughly washed in an antiseptic solution, and the mask should be sterilized. Medical personnel wearing their coverings for an extended period were advised to change their masks at two-hour intervals unless the masks were wet. In which case, they should be changed at shorter intervals. When changed, the covering that was removed needed to be sterilized. Sterilization of masks could be accomplished, it was said, by boiling them for five minutes. A used mask should be tightly wrapped in paper until it could be boiled.[2]

The Bridgeport health officer, Dr. Walter H. Brown, spoke at a "number of the theatres" in his city on the evening of October 11, warning people of the dangers of the disease and instructing them on how to avoid it. The Bridgeport Health Department ordered that the patriotic gatherings planned to be held at several places in the city should not be held.[3]

A few days later, Dr. Brown was usurped in Bridgeport by Dr. Sears, assistant surgeon of the United States Public Health Service, who had been given charge of checking the epidemic in Connecticut. Sears assured Brown that as soon as a sufficient quantity of vaccine could be obtained, it would be sent to Bridgeport for use by physicians. In talking with Brown, Sears said he agreed with how the campaign against the disease was being conducted in the community. According to a reporter, Sears also said that "the blanket orders given in some towns for the closing of theatres and public places has not done much good, and he did not see the necessity of closing the places in Bridgeport at this time."[4]

The Connecticut Department of Health organized a flying squadron composed of several of the best platform speakers from the City of Bridgeport to assist in fighting influenza. Brown addressed the group at a meeting on October 16. Members of the flying squadron were slated to speak at theaters, churches, and all public places to have people obey the rules to help stamp out the disease. The words of wisdom the speakers were expected to deliver concerning prevention included avoiding the cougher, sneezer, or spitter. People were advised not to use common towels or drinking cups, to wash their hands before eating, and to keep their fingers out of their mouths. People were told not to be spreaders and to smother every cough or sneeze. Face masks were not mentioned.[5]

A strong disagreement arose among the doctors of Fairfield, Connecticut, over the closing of the schools in the town on account of the flu. At a joint meeting, the school board and health board decided not to close the schools. Dr. George E. Thielcke, Fairfield health officer, considered it unnecessary at the current time. In Bridgeport, the night schools were ordered to be reopened, and classes resumed after four weeks of closure.[6]

In New Haven, on September 30, it was reported that health authorities had a conference as a measure against the spread of influenza. It was expected that recommendations would be made that every person attending a gathering or theatrical performance and those who, in the course of their duties, were brought into "close speaking contact" with others wear a muslin face mask. Following that, all Yale military and naval unit members were provided with such masks.[7]

Early in October, orders were issued to close soda water fountains. Then, a day or so later, all liquor saloons were ordered to close until further notice. Barbers were requested to wear masks while at work on customers, and all those caring for the sick were required to wear the "regulation muslin mask."[8]

On October 11, the Connecticut Department of Health announced directions for making gauze face masks, "which should be worn by all persons attending cases of influenza or pneumonia." Most newspapers in most of the nation would publish these instructions, or variations, at some point, usually during the last three months of 1918. In this case, and most others, the instructions for mask care were given and were the same. "These masks should be changed at two or three-hour intervals and oftener if wet. They should then be immediately boiled for five minutes, burned, or wrapped securely in a paper bag or newspaper until they can be boiled."[9]

A newspaper editor with a New Britain, Connecticut, newspaper wrote an editorial on the influenza epidemic on September 19, 1919, on what he termed the disease's first anniversary. He argued that a gauze mask "is a strong ally of humanity against the spread of the disease." The mask stopped the germ from entering the mask wearer's system. Also, it prevented the germ from exiting the system of someone with the disease. He noted that it had been said that a mask worn by someone who had the disease and discarded it full of the germs could be worn with perfect safety by anyone, as far as the flu was concerned, after it had been exposed for ten minutes to the open air. If that was the case, why did all the "experts" insist a mask be worn only for a few hours and then boiled for five to 30 minutes, depending on the "expert?" If the flu epidemic should return to the editor's area, he concluded that if "the people should be forced upon the first appearance of the disease to wear the masks there would be no epidemic here."[10]

Vermont

The Vermont Board of Health, on the afternoon of October 4, decided to close all public gathering places. It was the state's most drastic action ever taken as a preventive measure. Schools, churches, and amusement areas were all closed. Vermont was following the advice laid out by Dr. Rupert Blue, the surgeon general of the United States Public Health Service. Many states followed Blue's advice to the letter, more or less, and most of them imposed their closures within about seven days of Blue's issuing the guidance. The order in Vermont was effective immediately and signed by Charles F. Dalton, Secretary of the Vermont Board of Health.[11]

A couple of weeks later, the Vermont Board of Health issued an order forbidding the holding of political or nonpolitical conventions. A few days later, the state board declared that the statewide shutdown would continue until at least November 3, following a meeting the board held in Montpelier. On November 3, if the influenza situation throughout the entire state improved, the shutdown as a blanket order would be lifted. Still, it would remain in effect in such communities as conditions warranted.

One month later, on November 6, after a meeting of businesspeople with the state board of health officials, the board declared the statewide ban to be off. Churches would open the following Sunday, while schools would resume on Monday. Dr. R.M. Pelton, the local health officer in Richford, Vermont, was notified that the shutdown order had been removed for the state, except in isolated areas. Therefore, Richford churches could open on the coming Sunday, with schools opening on Monday. A significant reason for the early vacating of the closure orders was lobbying by businesspeople.[12]

For some communities, the fear induced by the authorities could not be so quickly dissipated just by removing the shutdown order. In Richford, there were a large number of children absent from schools when they reopened. The kids were not sick, but parents who were still fearful kept them home. Getting the kids back in school was essential because they had to make up for the time lost during the shutdown. The health officer, Dr. Pelton, was pressed into duty. In an interview with the local newspaper, he said that the disease had run its course and little danger remained. Therefore, Dr. Pelton said, parents should "send the children to school."[13]

Shutdowns plagued some communities in Vermont for months to come. East Fairfield schools in the village were still closed as of December 13. Fairfax lifted the closure order but later reimposed it. It was removed for the second time on February 14, 1919.[14]

There was very little mention of masks in Vermont. An article in Rutland on October 7 stated, "Attendants on cases, nurses or relatives, may do something to avoid contracting it by wearing a few thicknesses of ordinary strip gauze over the mouth and nose when attending cases."[15]

A week later, the same newspaper published an article from the United States Public Health Service about how to deal with influenza. It was an article published in dozens of newspapers during the last couple of weeks in October. It barely mentioned masks. At one point, it stated that "nurses and attendants will do well to guard against breathing in dangerous disease germs by wearing a simple fold of gauze or mask while near the patient." No other use of a mask was mentioned or advocated. Another piece of advice declared, "When crowding is unavoidable, as in street cars, care should be taken to keep the face turned so as not to inhale directly the air breathed out by another person." But there was no mention of using a mask in that situation.[16]

The United States Public Health Service returned in September 1919 with an article that warned municipalities about the dangers associated with any return of the disease over the coming winter season. It said diplomatically, "The use of face masks has not been attended with the success predicted for them."[17]

Rhode Island

As of October 5, Rhode Island had stopped all public assemblies. All theaters and cinemas were closed, as were the schools, both public and private. Dances, public and private, were also entirely suspended. Churches were also closed, but only after they agreed to a "request" from the Rhode Island Board of Health, as opposed to obeying an order imposed on the other entities subject to a closure order. The board of health held a special meeting on October 17. After a prolonged discussion, they decided to remove the ban on public gatherings. Thus, churches could open on Sunday, the 20th, and schools on the following day.[18]

Like Vermont, Rhode Island paid little attention to flu masks. The United States Public Health Service article advising on the disease, cited in Vermont, was published in Rhode Island and probably every other state in the union. The article highlighted another fact that remained true throughout the Spanish flu pandemic. There was no test for the disease; a doctor diagnosed it by eyeballing a potential sufferer.[19]

Maine

In Maine, both daily papers published the order of the Bangor Board of Health closing all churches, schools, theaters, clubs, and other places of public assemblage "in terms explicit, emphatic and without any qualifications whatever." There was a worry, on October 5, that some people in the state were still unaware of the order. At the same time, Maine had made influenza a reportable and quarantinable disease. That meant that physicians had to immediately report cases under their supervision to the local health authorities, who would immediately quarantine the home where the condition was present. In most of America at the time of the Spanish flu outbreak, influenza was not a reportable disease, which hampered any response to the infection, with cases not being promptly reported or not reported at all. Advice at this early stage was for people to avoid sneezers. No mention was made of masks. In Maine, the state board of health did not have the power to order statewide closures, so it was left to the various local health boards to impose closure orders. On November 4, cinemas and churches were allowed to reopen.[20]

In Lewiston, Maine, closures took place earlier. At a meeting on September 27, physicians, members of the board of health, the superintendent of schools, and Mayor Lemaire decided to close all dance halls. Local theaters and streetcars would also be aired and fumigated each day. Additional cars would be put into service during rush hours to limit congestion. Nurses were required to wear masks at the local hospitals. In Portland, all public gathering places were ordered to shut down a day or two after Lewiston imposed its closures.[21]

Dr. William C. Woodward was the health commissioner for the City of Boston. In that capacity, he gave some general advice to the people of Maine. He remarked that anyone attending a sick person should wear a gauze mask and change it every few hours, with the used one being boiled before it was reused. He went a little further in advocating that anyone who had to go in the presence of the sick, not just attendants, should cover their face with a mask or some similar protection, with a handkerchief being "better than nothing."[22]

In Belfast, Maine, as of October 11, masks for use in influenza cases had been made at the Red Cross rooms. Where needed, they were available at the City Drug Store for free distribution. Their use was urged to prevent infection.[23]

The Bangor newspaper covered the final session of the American Public Health Association, which had taken place in Chicago and ended on December 12. It portrayed an equally divided opinion on specific topics, with health officers from large cities differing from those from rural communities. The health commissioner, Dr. J.W. Inches of Detroit, led the argument against closing public meetings, schools, theaters, and stores. However, he admitted his state compelled him to adopt some restrictive measures. He ridiculed the use of masks as not a feasible measure in the larger cities. On the other side, four physicians who held that closing public meetings in rural districts was efficacious were listed by name. The paper did not report on the committee struck by the convention to reach some definite conclusions. Nor did it say when those actual recommendations were released several days after the convention ended.[24]

Late in December, there was a minor scare in Portland when a slight increase in cases led some to believe that more restrictions might have to be imposed. Dr. Tetreau, the city's health officer, favored using masks. A reporter remarked on an article that appeared in a national weekly publication regarding the use of those masks, with "the trend of the article being that the mask had many disadvantages."[25]

In the fall of 1919, a Bangor newspaper printed a piece from the United States Public Health Service that made some predictions for the coming flu season. And, as noted before, this piece tactfully stated that masks had not attained the success predicted for them.[26]

New Hampshire

In mid–October, Portsmouth, New Hampshire, decided to continue the Spanish influenza quarantine for at least another week, with the churches, schools, theaters, and all public meetings suspended. The public health service office made the decision at Portsmouth city hall by order of Dr. Stone. As in most of the rest of New England, face masks played very little or no role at all in how the authorities dealt with the influenza crisis.[27]

Massachusetts

As early as September 20, the Ayer, Massachusetts, community was already under closure orders. In addition to placarding homes in which cases of influenza existed as a means of warning the public, the Ayer Board of Health declared a quarantine against Camp Devens, applying to all men not engaged in the necessary or administrative business of the camp. They also closed moving picture theaters and places of public entertainment. The quarantine against the military installation at Camp Devens illustrated the difficulties many communities had with such facilities when they were adjacent to a community. Such camps and cantonments existed all over the nation, sometimes as a part of an existing military installation, sometimes on their own. Cases of influenza tended to hit these areas first before spreading out to the local communities. At this early stage, the town of Ayer listed six suggestions for dealing with the outbreak: (1) Sleep and eat regularly. Get plenty of fresh air and sunshine. Keep the bowels open. (2) Spray the nose and throat at least daily with a simple solution such as boric acid or salt and water. Wash the hands frequently; the more often, the better. (3) Keep out of crowds. (4) Call a physician in case of chills, bodily pains, or "ordinary cold" symptoms. (5) Isolate a person ill with influenza in the home as much as possible. Minimize contact with such a case except for the one caring for the ill person. (6) Follow any instructions that your public health nurse may give you.[28]

The City of Des Moines, Iowa, sent an urgent request to Dr. William C. Woodward, City of Boston health commissioner, early in October, asking for his advice on how he was dealing with the disease in Boston. Before taking up his Boston post, Woodward had held a similar position in Washington, D.C., for 15 or 20 years. Des Moines selected Boston in part because it was experiencing a large number of cases of the Spanish flu. In his reply, Woodward declared that he believed schools should be closed. He felt that saved children from possible infection in schools and on their way to and from school. It also released school doctors and nurses for work under the direction of the city. He also felt that theaters, including cinemas, should be closed. In addition to possibly defective ventilation, they were ordinarily devoid of the germicidal effect of direct sunlight. Churches, Woodward argued, should be requested to reduce services to the "absolute minimum." They differed from theaters because they ordinarily afforded a larger floor area and air space per person, had more exposure to sunlight, and were occupied for shorter periods. Also, they played a role in "steadying those inclined to panic and those bereaved. Closing would probably alienate large and uninstructed elements in the population and lead to highly undesirable opposition now and in future." He argued that factories that maintained proper sanitary standards should not be closed, although no reasons were given. However, soda water fountains and saloons should be closed "because of crowding and of interchanging of infective mucous on glasses and similar articles." He allowed that the sale of liquor should continue, but only in bottles, not in glasses in restaurants, as part of a meal. Woodward viewed vaccines as experimental, unwise, and "liable to lead to a fiasco and will discredit vaccines generally." He favored placarding quarantined homes as tending to eliminate unnecessary visits to sickrooms "and for general educational value." Concerning masks, Woodward stated, "Urge conscientious use of masks. They certainly tend to protect attendants from infective mucous from patients and are a constant reminder of the need for care."[29]

By the end of September, measures to prevent the spread of influenza were in force everywhere throughout Massachusetts. Virtually every city had barred public gatherings of all kinds. The New England branch of the Red Cross distributed large numbers of gauze masks for physicians' protection.[30]

A curiosity appeared in a Fall River newspaper in September 1919 that claimed Charlie Chaplin had stopped the flu. At least, that was what motion picture producers told a reporter. The reasoning was that influenza had been raging for many weeks. In the west, people wore flu masks while film houses and regular theaters were closed. Department stores suffered. The filmmakers agreed to produce no new material for a time to save the situation financially. Then Chaplin's second film of the year was released. The theater managers said, "We could not keep the houses closed. The people would not stand it. So we reopened them—and nothing happened. There was no more flu than there had been. A ghost had been laid."[31]

On October 2, 1918, the Holyoke Massachusetts Red Cross Society completed 200 influenza masks for the Holyoke Board of Health, the number considered sufficient for the time. It was reported that those masks had been of great value in letting doctors and nurses work around flu patients without infection. The local Red Cross chapter also had an order on file to produce 2,000 masks for the state headquarters. Any members of the general public who wished for a mask were told to contact the local Red Cross office.[32]

An editorial in a Boston newspaper on September 18, 1918, urged the reader to use common sense in dealing with the epidemic and that the simple rules of cleanliness and personal hygiene were a person's best protection. Masks were not in use then, even among doctors and nurses. But this editor already had the idea, for he declared, "We should keep out of crowds, indoors or out, whenever possible; and when impossible, it is well to have a clean handkerchief to hold over the mouth and nostrils as a mask."[33]

On September 28, Dr. William Woodward, Boston health commissioner, asked a reporter to stress to his readers the "necessity" of using gauze masks in the vicinity of patients. He said, "We are having a pattern made of a gauze mask—a plain, simple mask which any woman can make—and when it is completed we are going to ask the newspapers to print the directions for making." But they had to wait until that was ready. In the meantime, Woodward said, "Make any kind of a mask, any kind of a covering for the nose and mouth and use it immediately and at all times. Even a handkerchief held in place over the face is better than nothing, only take care to remove the mask immediately upon its becoming damp or moist from the breath or perspiration."[34]

That same month, an emergency hospital was established at Corey Hill, near Brookline. It was in the open air for the worst of the influenza cases. According to the report, the attendants' safety was mainly due to using gauze masks. From the beginning, every person who approached a patient was required to wear several folds of gauze over the mouth and nose. The report said, "A regular inspector of masks sees that everyone wears a mask and changes it every two hours. The inspector also is

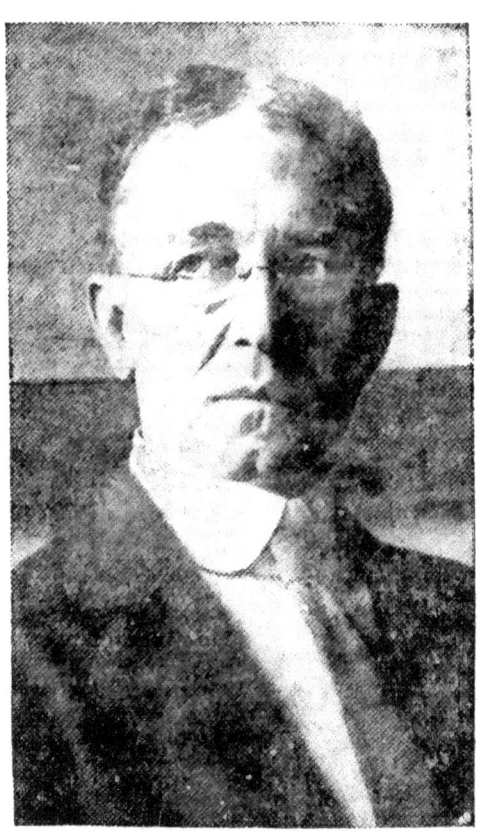

DR. WILLIAM C. WOODWARD, Boston's new health officer appointed by Mayor Peters.
(Photo copyright by Int. Film Service, Inc.)

Dr. William C. Woodward, for 24 years the health officer of Washington, will come to Boston the first week in August to become health officer of this city, having recently been appointed to that position by Mayor Peters at a salary of $7500. Dr. Woodward is recognized as one of the most capable and efficient health officers in the country.

This July 1918 photograph shows Dr. Woodward on the occasion of his appointment to the post of Boston Health Commissioner, to take effect the following month. One of his first major acts took place in September, when he signed the lockdown order for Boston. It was similar to many in use across the nation. This one pretended to be only for only ten days or so. But all such orders could be, and usually were, extended. Giving it a short period was done so as not to rile the public unduly.

responsible for keeping a supply of masks always on hand and for burning the old ones." A photo of another open-air camp at Lawrence, Massachusetts, showed an armed guard wearing a mask overseeing the place. Imagine internment camps for sick people. The fresh air idea was behind many other "precautions," such as streetcars being forced to open or remove all windows, even during rainstorms or snowfalls.[35]

Health officials kept hammering away at the value of masks. A couple of days later. One doctor said, "If those caring for patients will only wear the masks which the Red Cross is giving away and will intelligently follow the instructions, a great many lives will be saved." He added, "But the instructions must be followed to the letter. The mask must be sterilized as soon as the nurse leaves the sick room, and it must not be thrown carelessly aside because when it is next used it may be put on the wrong side out, thus making its use more dangerous than its absence. These masks are being made by the Red Cross in unlimited numbers, and every person who can use one may obtain it by applying to any Red Cross station."[36]

Aside from health professionals, one of the best-known early uses of flu masks came from Boston, Massachusetts, on the evening of October 4, 1918. At roll call in Boston police stations that evening, every Boston police officer was given a gauze

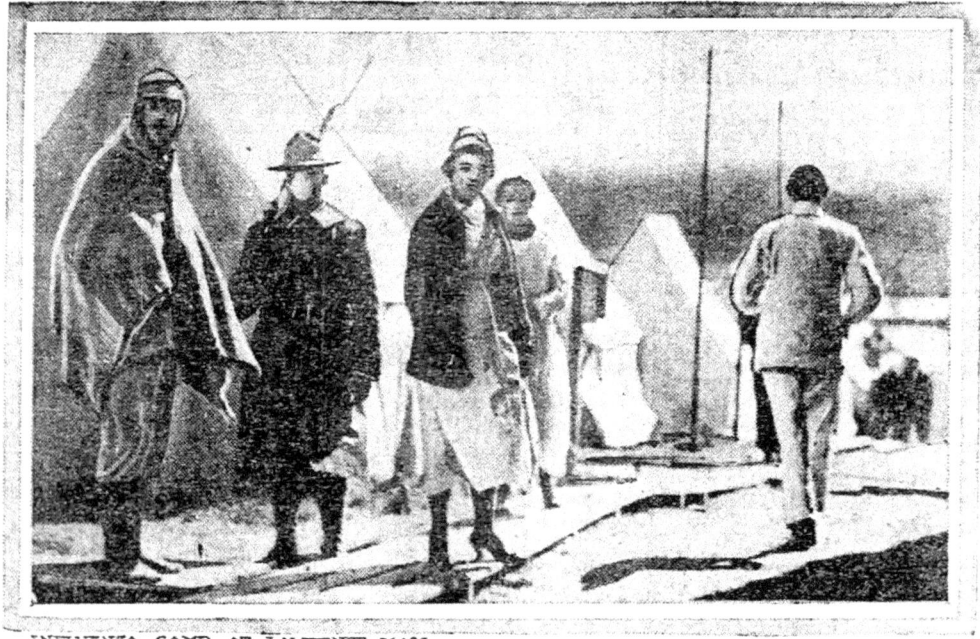

Open Air Camp for Influenza Cure

INFLUENZA CAMP AT LAWRENCE, MASS

AS fresh air is considered the only means of effectually preventing influenza and is also a large factor in the cure of the disease, it has been found necessary to establish fresh air camps for victims in many localities. This photo shows a scene at the open air influenza camp at Lawrence, Mass. The open air treatment for the influenza patients was decided upon as the best way of curbing the epidemic. Note the armed guard wearing an influenza mask.

This photograph shows the open-air flu treatment center. Note the armed and masked guard. The use of masks by the military was almost universal in America. One reason was that the military was obedient. Another reason was to set an example for the civilian population.

mask that he was expected to wear if he should be called into a residence where there were patients with influenza or if he should be needed for ambulance work. The officers were cautioned to burn the masks after using them and to obtain others from their desk sergeants. Many newspapers in America carried the story and photo of a masked Boston police officer. Most of those brief accounts led the reader to believe the police officer had to wear his mask all the time when on duty, not just under the minimal circumstances outlined by the force.[37]

At the end of December, Dr. Woodward came out with advice for coughers and sneezers. He explained that coughing, sneezing, laughing, and talking expelled flu germs. Those germs were thrown out at the level of the mouth for a distance of several feet and then floated in the air for a time. He reiterated, "Anyone having the disease, or who may possibly have it, should always hold before his mouth when coughing or sneezing a cloth or piece of paper or something to prevent these droplets from escaping into the surrounding air. These cloths should be burnt or boiled at once to kill the germs." When the epidemic waned in New England, Woodward still did not advocate using flu masks for the general public.[38]

And that was true for New England as a whole. There was no

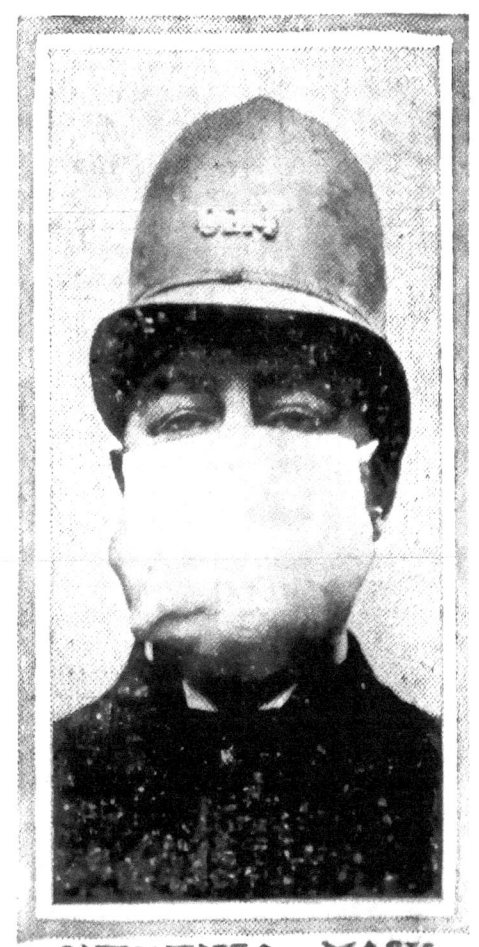

Boston Police Wear Influenza Mask While on Duty.

INFLUENZA MASK.

Seventeen hundred germ masks have been issued to the police of Boston, according to a report from that city. Because of the tremendous strides in the influenza epidemic there, this precaution has been taken by the authorities. The mask is a fold of antiseptic gauze which is placed over the mouth and nose when exposed to infection. The photo shows a Boston patrolman wearing a mask.

This photograph of a masked Boston police officer appeared in many newspapers across America. In most captions on that photograph, the reader was left with the impression that all officers wore masks all the time while on duty. In reality, they only wore them when they knew they had to enter an influenza home or had ambulance duty. The vast majority of their duty time was maskless.

enforced mask wearing anywhere in the region. Except for health professionals, no one was compelled to wear a mask in the civilian population, except for the Boston police, in limited situations. Military people in the camps and cantonments around the country were usually required to wear masks; they were also subjected to forced influenza vaccines, which were, then, junk science. Since the influenza virus was not isolated during the pandemic, it was not clear what was injected into the arms of many soldiers and civilians.

4

Middle Atlantic

New Jersey

Closure orders were imposed quickly in New Jersey. In a Hopewell newspaper on October 9, featured ads placed by a theater and several churches stated that they were all closed due to the influenza quarantine.[1]

Just as quickly as closure orders were imposed in New Jersey, they were removed. On October 25, the New Jersey Board of Health lifted all the restrictions. Every agency in New Brunswick affected by the closing order lost no time in reopening. The motion picture houses, closed for two weeks, were crowded with film buffs on the night of October 25, and the saloons did a booming business, along with the soda fountains. A reporter described the situation, "Many people expressed joy at the opening of the theatres, churches, saloons and other places affected. The saloon men especially welcomed the lifting order. On the part of many who have been in close touch with the situation there was a feeling that it might have been wiser to continue the prohibition a few days longer, the physicians and clergymen especially holding the view that no sacrifices of pleasure or convenience were too great to make in the interests of public health safety. Yet all over the city last night there was a general feeling of relief." All the schools were to reopen on the following Monday.[2]

In Clifton, New Jersey, the local board of health ordered all dentists and barbers in the city to wear gauze masks. The Red Cross would furnish the masks. Members of those professions were to wear masks while performing their duties.[3]

Like New England, New Jersey did not bother with masks to any extent. An Asbury Park newspaper published a piece on general advice about the flu situation from the United States Public Health Service in mid–October. It was the standard piece that appeared everywhere, which made no mention of masks at all except that medical personnel should use them when attending to the sick, along with other attendants.[4]

New York State

New York City announced the establishment of a rigid quarantine on September 11, 1918, at the Port of New York. Dr. Royal S. Copeland, New York City health commissioner, explained that they had launched an anti-spitting crusade to try to prevent the spread of Spanish influenza in the city. According to Copeland, a steamship from France had landed there with 25 people suffering from the disease. He also pointed out that "there is no known cure" for the illness.[5]

The quarantine proved ineffectual, and by October 11, shutdowns were put in place all over New York State on a place-by-place basis. The usual suspects in Buffalo—schools, churches, and theaters—were closed on that date. A day later, Mayor George S. Buck of Buffalo increased the list of places shuttered to include five- and ten-cent stores, soda fountains, pool rooms, bowling alleys, and every gathering of more than ten people. Buffalo acting health commissioner, Dr. Franklin C. Gram, and the "epidemic control committee" appealed to all citizens to wear masks over their noses and mouths. Gram especially wanted to see every doctor, undertaker, police officer, firefighter, letter carrier, and so on continuously exposed to the public wearing a gauze mask. Chief Garvin of the police department and Chief Murphy of the fire department explained that they had no such orders. Still, the demand to wear masks would be executed as soon as orders were received from the health department.

A Buffalo newspaper featured a photo on page one showing the public how to wear a mask correctly. Garvin wanted the police, firefighters, and others to wear masks "to educate the public on the value of" using masks. According to this story, "Experts declare that if everyone in Buffalo wore such a mask for a week or ten days the epidemic here would be over." In discussing preventive means at a meeting of the epidemic control committee, it was suggested that every person in the city wear a mask. The committee recommended wearing a mask but did not phrase it as an order because the committee decided to first appeal for public support. "If everyone in the country would go masked at all times the epidemic would be conquered in the United States in a week or ten days," declared Dr. Charles

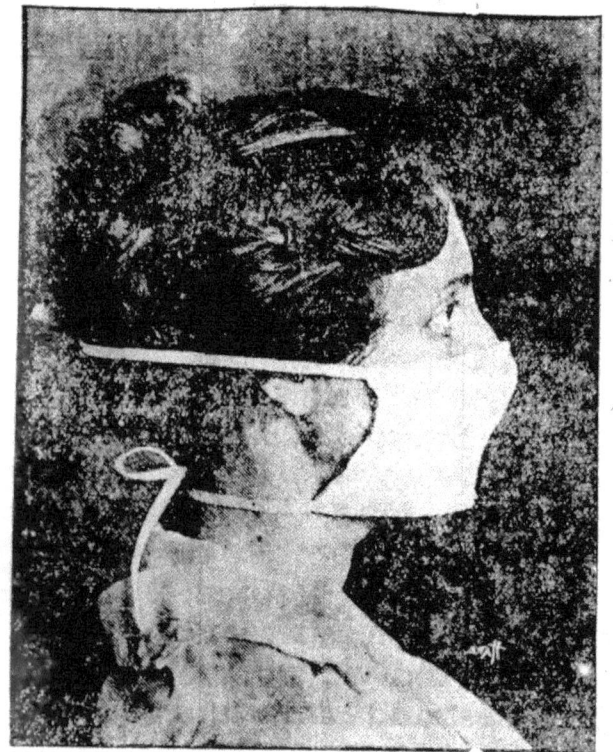

To get the public used to the idea of masking, many newspapers, such as this one in Buffalo, published detailed instructions on how to make one. Many also published photographs of masked individuals for the public's enlightenment.

G. Stockton, a committee member. Finlay H. Greene, general chair of the committee and leader of the influenza public education campaign in Buffalo, announced that masks were then being distributed to all drugstores in the city for exhibition. "From these sample masks, the pattern can be obtained. Anybody can make a mask easily. Physicians urge that all citizens cooperate in stamping out the epidemic by wearing masks. This applies to well and sick."[6]

Closure orders were imposed and removed in communities all over New York State. In Tonawanda, the shutdown was lifted on October 31, with the saloons taking advantage of the change that night. Churches were to hold services the following Sunday, and schools were to reopen on Monday. Cinemas resumed business on November 1. The health authorities fumigated all locations. Akron, New York, lifted the closure orders on November 4 and reopened schools after a five-week closure. However, Niagara Falls Health Officer Scott decided the ban should remain in effect for at least another week. And on November 1 in Batavia, the health officer removed the closure order that had been in effect for three weeks.[7]

Niagara Falls, New York, lifted their closure orders a few days later. Then, on November 18, the city's health officer, Walter Scott, reimposed the quarantine by banning all "unnecessary" public gatherings, dances, and store sales.[8]

When Elmira, New York, imposed closure orders on October 14, it shut down schools, theaters, saloons (where lunches were not served), clubs, and fraternal organizations and discontinued public meetings. It was noted that in "many cities," gauze masks are being worn as prevention against the contraction of influenza. The method was discussed at the meeting, which imposed the closure orders. A reporter said, "It is not improbable that wearing of masks may be ordered in Elmira."[9]

Two days later, it was reported that barbers at the Sanitary Barber Shop on East Water Street in Elmira had adopted the flu mask and were wearing them to protect the patrons of the shop from the epidemic.[10]

As Buffalo contemplated its lockdown, a meeting was held on the afternoon of October 7 to consider the matter. Besides the acting health commissioner, Dr. Franklin C. Gram, the others attending the meeting were Buffalo Mayor Buck; Ernest C. Hartwell, superintendent of schools; Henry C. Miles, president of the Buffalo Chamber of Commerce; medical inspectors from the city's health department; several "prominent" Buffalo physicians; representatives of Buffalo's main manufacturing concerns; the commanding officers of military installation Fort Porter; and a representative of the cinemas. The same newspaper page had two photos with images of masked people, as it tried to keep the issue before the public. One shot was of workers with the New York Red Cross making masks. The second was an image of many masked Chicago street cleaners being inspected by equally masked superiors before heading out for their shift.[11]

As a result of the meeting, no closure was ordered, at least for the time being, with the committee opting for a campaign of public education revolving around hygiene with the citizens adopting a "voluntary quarantine" of the city, with an enforced quarantine to come if the situation got worse. No mention was made of face coverings except that patients suffering from influenza should wear a mask.[12]

As things worsened in Buffalo, little was left to lock down that would not stir up a general rebellion. Therefore, the Buffalo Health Department emphasized the

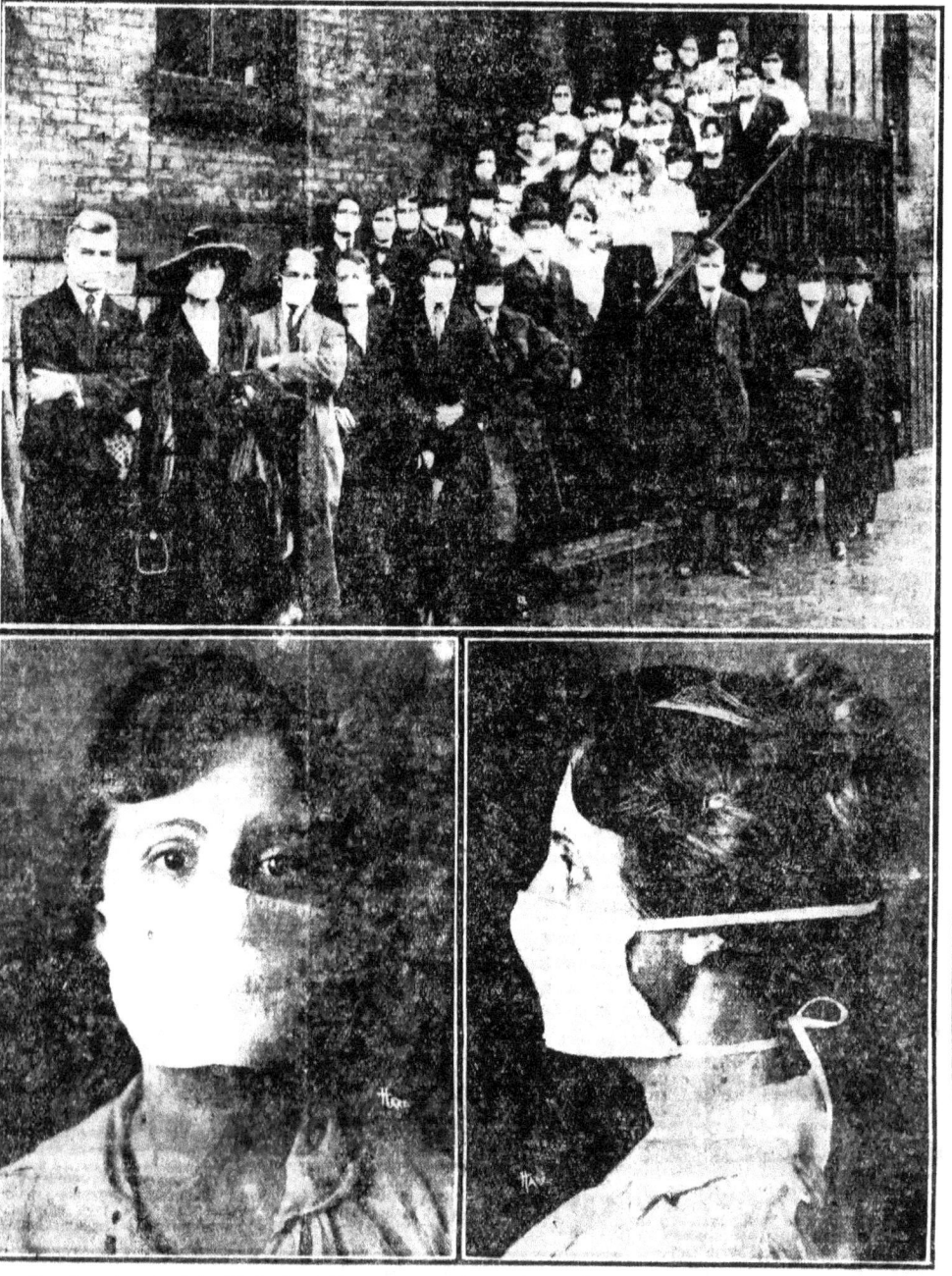

The department of health is furnishing gauze masks to city employes, and suggesting their use by everyone check the spread of influenza. The lower pictures show the proper method of wearing mask. The upper picre is of department health employes.

Buffalo went all out on a public relations campaign to get the public to wear masks. This photograph shows a person modeling one, while *above* her is a group photograph of Buffalo Department of Health employees wearing masks to convince the public to follow suit.

recommendation that well and sick people alike wear simple gauze masks. The health department and its advisory physicians stated that the general wearing of masks would quickly stamp out the disease and permit the resumption of business. "All depends on public cooperation," declared a journalist. The health department first listed precautions that were easy for all to observe: "Wear a gauze or cloth mask over nose and mouth. IF YOU DO, THE GERM CANNOT GET IN."[13]

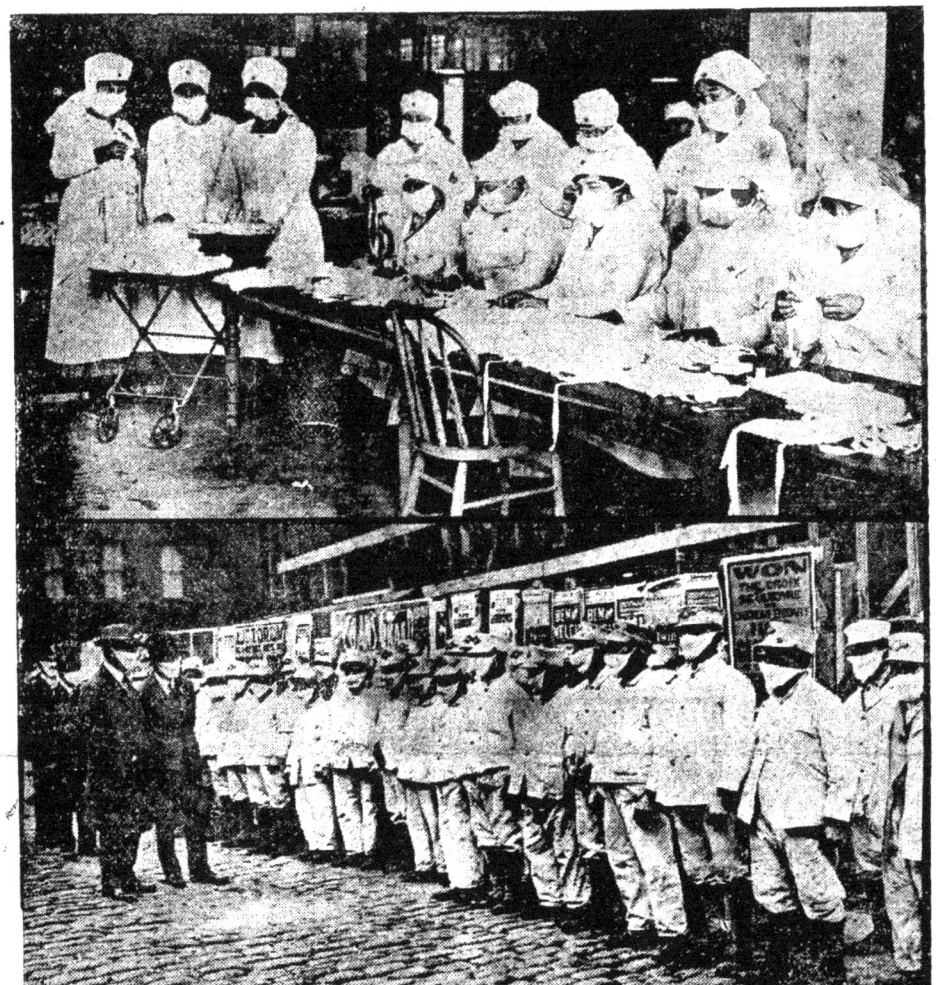

INFLUENZA EPIDEMIC SPREADS THROUGHOUT COUNTRY.

The epidemic of influenza, which, for a time, promised to confine itself within limited bounds, now is reported prevalent in forty-six states. Despite stringent precautions, the epidemic has taken a strong hold and has brought the entire nation to an alarming position. The larger communities have taken special precaution to prevent a spread of the disease. In Chicago, the street cleaners have been furnished with gauze masks to protect them and keep them from carrying whatever germs they might have in their systems. Red Cross headquarters in New York is a busy place. The upper photo shows the women at work, while the lower photo shows the Chicago street cleaners being inspected before going out to do their work.

This photograph from Buffalo depicts women volunteers at a Red Cross center making masks, while *below* is a line of Chicago street sweepers being inspected by their masked superiors before heading out to work.

On October 12, the epidemic control committee discussed a mandatory order for wearing masks. Although every physician at the meeting agreed that mask wearing would stop the epidemic, the call for all people to wear face coverings was a request rather than a command. A reporter said, "The committee desires public cooperation.... But masking is a new thing. It is effective but peculiar." And he added, "Should Buffalo as a whole don masks it will blaze the way for the entire country to fight the epidemic this way." Masks were on display at all drug stores. Dr. Dewitt C. Sherman of the committee suggested that women wear a double-heavy veil over the nose and mouth if preferred. The local Red Cross quickly made enough masks to equip the Buffalo Health Department. Those masks were then treated with zinc sulfate as a germicide. It was not uncommon in 1918 and 1919 for masks to be saturated with some germicide or what was believed to be a germicide. On the day following the Industrial Physicians and Surgeons Association of Buffalo meeting, it was expected that thousands of employees of Buffalo industrial plants would be wearing gauze masks, both factory hands and office staff. At the meeting, all in attendance wore face masks as they entered the room. Dr. William G. Bissell dwelled at length on the efficiency of the mask. However, he agreed that wearing one in the open air was unnecessary. He was the main speaker at the event. Suppose that the city officials were too fearful of imposing a masking mandate on their population. In that case, they could and would try to do it through the back door by coercing companies into being the villains who imposed the masking orders. Companies were led to believe that they would not have their plants shut down only if their workers wore masks and the situation did not worsen.[14]

By October 14, the use of masks in Buffalo had significantly increased. Masks had been distributed to upward of 50,000 workers, and thousands more were subjected to "oily spray treatments" for the nose and mouth. Such treatments were not common in America, but some places employed them. Also, the Buffalo Police Department donned masks as Chief Henry J. Girvin issued an order that uniformed men go about their duties with their masks in place. Health Commissioner Gram explained that the mask was a simple contrivance. He said, "It has already been explained how to make masks by taking a piece of gauze, cheese cloth, or a part of an old shirt or sleeve, as long as it is thoroughly laundered, tying a few strings to it and putting it over the mouth and nose." Added Gram, "It is not necessary to take cheese cloth or any particular kind of cloth, nor is it necessary to tie strings to it. One of the best masks is an ordinary clean handkerchief tied over the face in the manner described. Handkerchiefs have many advantages in other ways. They are laundered and usually large enough to be tied over the face without the attachment of strings. They can be rendered sterile by running a hot iron over them unless they are sufficiently dirty to boil and wash. In addition to other qualities, there is usually also a good supply of handkerchiefs in the possession of every individual." The Larkin Company in Buffalo had 8,000 masks for its employees. The day before, at the Curtiss plant, many people had worn masks, and more wore them each day. Pierce-Arrow and Buffalo Forge used oil spray for throats and noses. The other large plants that expressed a desire to cooperate with the city health department in forcing their employees to wear masks were the Seneca Iron and Steel Company, the Buffalo Drydock Company, the American Chemical and Aniline Company, and others.[15]

In an article published on October 15, a subhead proclaimed, "mask-wearing proves great aid in curbing the spread of disease," without producing any evidence. With emphasis placed on face masks, it became much easier for the health authorities and civic leaders to blame the public for any failures in the decrease in the number of flu cases. With the closures of schools, churches, and other places, it was impossible to blame them for failures. Closure orders were almost universally obeyed. Of the 112 church organizations in the city, there had not been a single complaint against the closure order, and all had complied. A few smaller saloons had sometimes disobeyed closure orders, but they were few. Health Commissioner Gram stated that whether the check in advance of the disease would conquer it "depends on public cooperation.... If all citizens should wear masks it will. It is up to the public to support the department and the doctors of the city. Mask-wearing in the factories, stores, and in public places will accomplish this support." Reportedly, masks were even more numerous that day in Buffalo than in previous days. Police officers wore them, and so did soldiers from Fort Porter; barbers in many big shops wore them. The National Biscuit Company ordered its employees to wear them. Women at Liberty Bond booths wore masks, and a big hotel ordered its employees to wear face coverings. Gram asserted that if all establishments serving food ordered their employees to be masked, "benefits will result." To emphasize how all this was the fault of the public—and not health and civic officials for initiating ineffective laws and coercive attempts—this article contained a small, boxed section that stated bluntly, under the heading "wear a mask," that "persons failing to mask who contract influenza can lay blame on their carelessness or stupidity. It is an effective means of prevention. New cases soon would cease if all wore masks."[16]

A day later, Commissioner Gram ordered all barbershops to instruct their barbers to wear masks. They were given two days to comply with the order, or their shops would be shuttered. Hotels, restaurants, and public eating places were to direct their employees to mask. Gram insisted that servers especially had to wear face coverings.[17]

A couple of days later, the question of protecting telephone receivers was discussed. It was decided that masks were the best protection, that covering the receiver with a handkerchief was a valuable aid, and that a tissue covering was helpful if removed after each use. The epidemic control committee requested that the physicians of Buffalo set a good example by wearing masks in their offices and when visiting patients outside, which implied that the physicians were not all wearing masks even then.[18]

Days later, Dr. Gram was still urging the use of masks and said, "There is ample authority for their use." But he was unable or unwilling to follow the path of authority and announce a public mandate for all in the city to be forced to mask up. And so, his advice fell on many deaf ears, including some physicians in his town. Gram did manage to coerce some companies into imposing masks on their employees, but that was much easier, as all capitalist companies were run on a rigid authoritarian structure.[19]

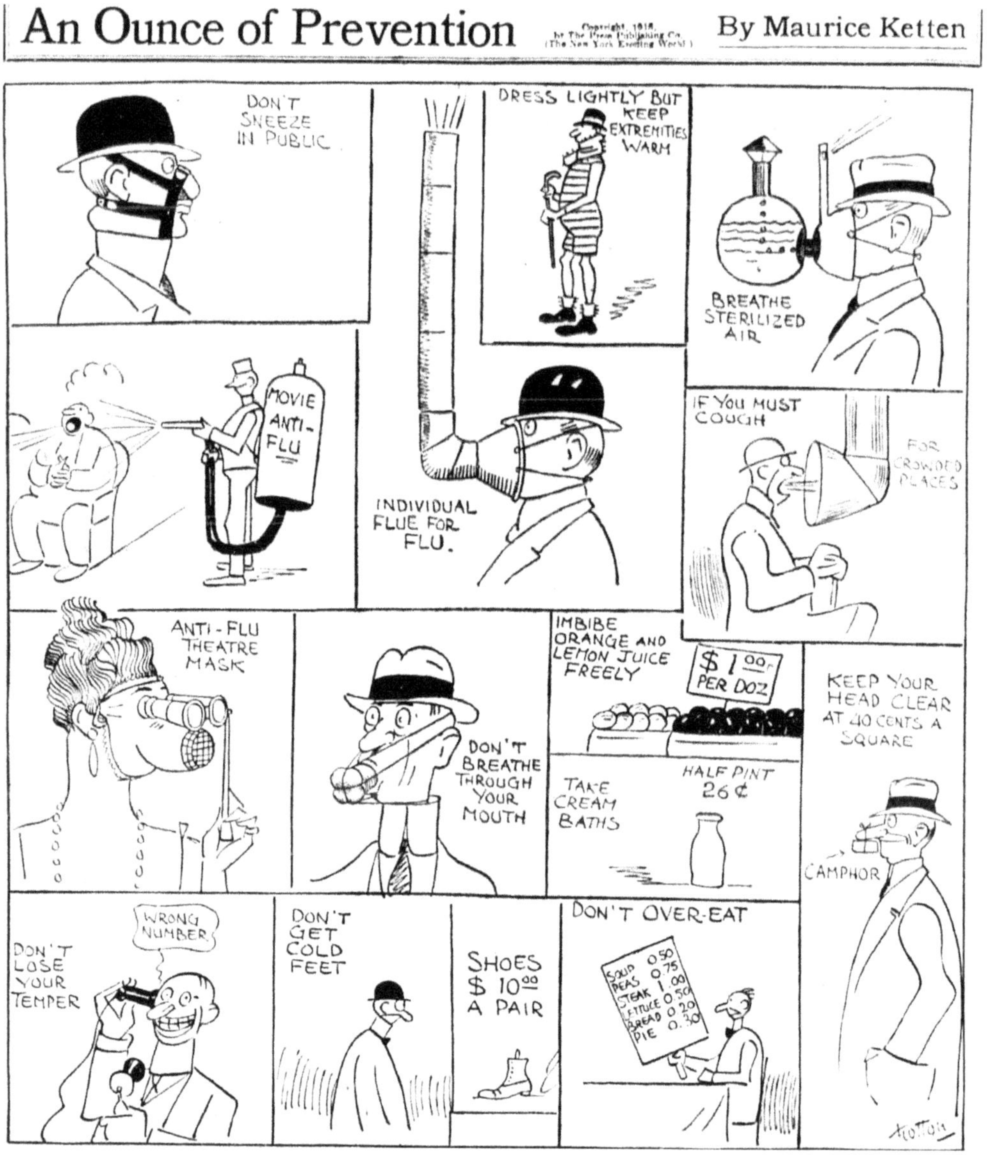

An Ounce of Prevention 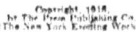 By Maurice Ketten

An editorial cartoon by Maurice Ketten in New York City mocked the efforts being forced on the public by the authorities.

Brooklyn's largest hospital, the Kings County Hospital, refused to use the flu mask. Staff members were permitted to mingle with the influenza patients with no face covering. The same was valid for visitors. Dr. J. Fitzgerald was superintendent of the facility and said that he did not see any reason, as of October 4, to change his opinion that using masks was unnecessary. In his view, based on years of experience, masks were not only not helpful but even dangerous. When the reporter asked around, he did not find Fitzgerald's opinion shared at the other Brooklyn hospitals.[20]

When the *Brooklyn Eagle* newspaper editorialized on the epidemic on October

On With the Mask!

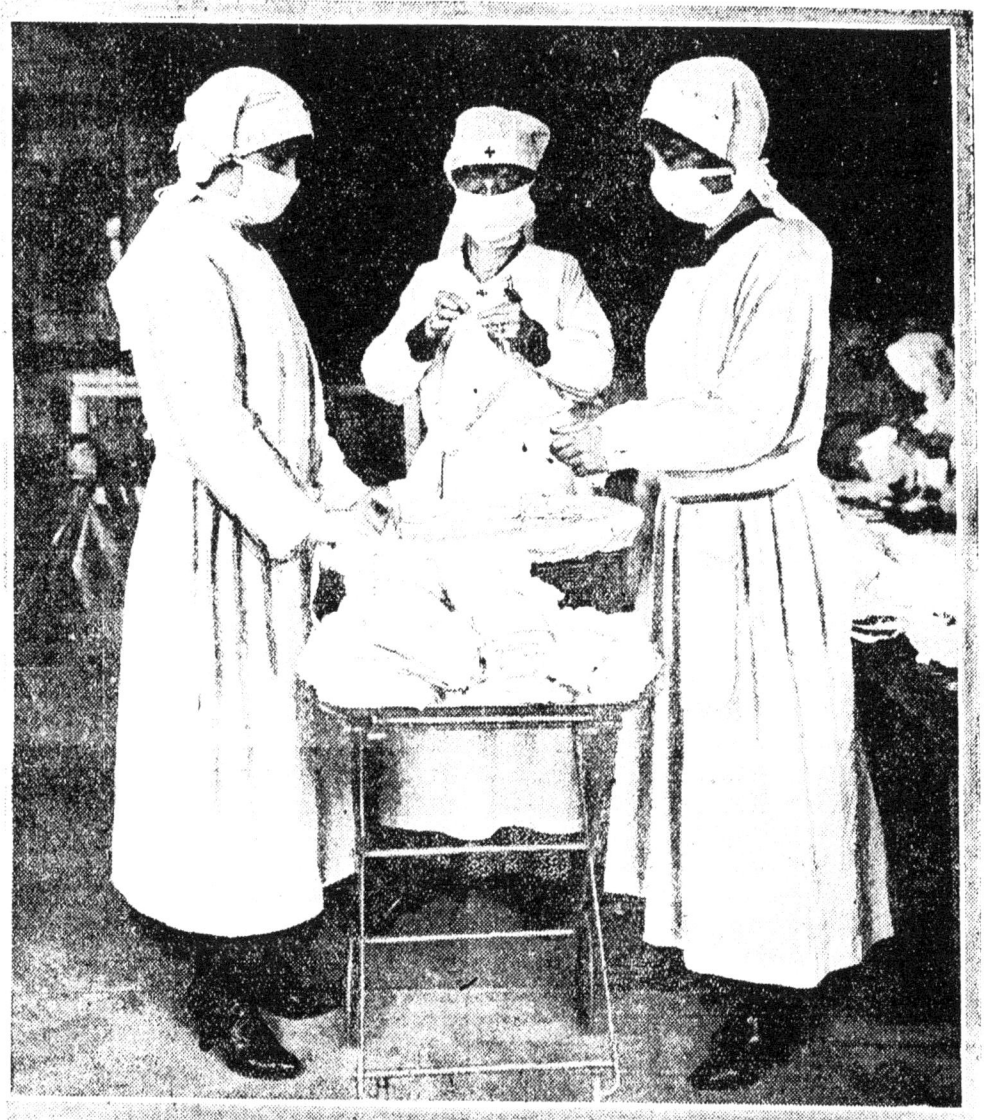

At the Red Cross model workroom, 20 East 38th Street, women workers are engaged—and busily, for they turned out 35,000 in four days—in making anti-influenza masks for use in the hospitals and training camps
—Photo by Paul Thompson

Three workers at the Red Cross in New York making masks. All these workers called in by urgent appeals in virtually all American communities to make the face coverings were women and volunteers. None of them were paid for their work.

13, it noted that "in Jersey City, the barbers are required to wear face masks. That precaution is perhaps extreme for travel in the street cars and subways, but the spread of the epidemic could be checked much more quickly if it were to be enforced." The editor also went on to observe that Royal Copeland, as health commissioner of New

York City, was "taking less drastic measures to control the epidemic than are other afflicted cities."[21]

When the *New York Times* editorialized on the influenza quarantine at the start of October, the editor mentioned a wedding at which some of the wedding party had been wearing masks. The editor said, "the precaution taken was the wearing of gauze masks.... But the entire community, and all who have the disease, in many cases unknown to themselves, perhaps, cannot wear masks." The quarantine was a vital tool for this editor, as opposed to the impractical face covering.[22]

As health commissioner of New York City, Dr. Royal S. Copeland refused to shut down any facilities. Schools and churches remained open. Theaters also remained open, although he shut some smaller ones because their ventilation was inadequate. Rules were put in place for hygienic procedures. Copeland also changed the schedule for employees of businesses and large offices, whereby employees were required to leave at slightly different hours of the day to stagger worker outflow and thus, at least a little, reduce congestion and crowding on the public transit system.[23]

The most drastic measures Copeland took came on October 13, when he said the danger of infection from and to barbers was great. So he asked the barbers to wear masks. He also said that dance halls presented a danger because many military personnel frequented those places, so he asked that the owners voluntarily close the establishments until further notice.[24]

When the Abraham and Straus department store in Brooklyn ran an ad on October 15, which covered over half a page, it featured a small item in the ad that declared, "Health Board Head Advises all Women to WEAR VEILS." In the smaller text, the ad stated that Health Commissioner Copeland said, "I heartily favor every woman wearing a heavy chiffon veil all the time she is on the street. It may become necessary to order everyone in New York to adopt this measure. These veils are rather thick and would serve as an almost absolute preventive. Let's forget style and stop this epidemic." Abraham sold those veils. The problem with the ad was that it was a complete lie.

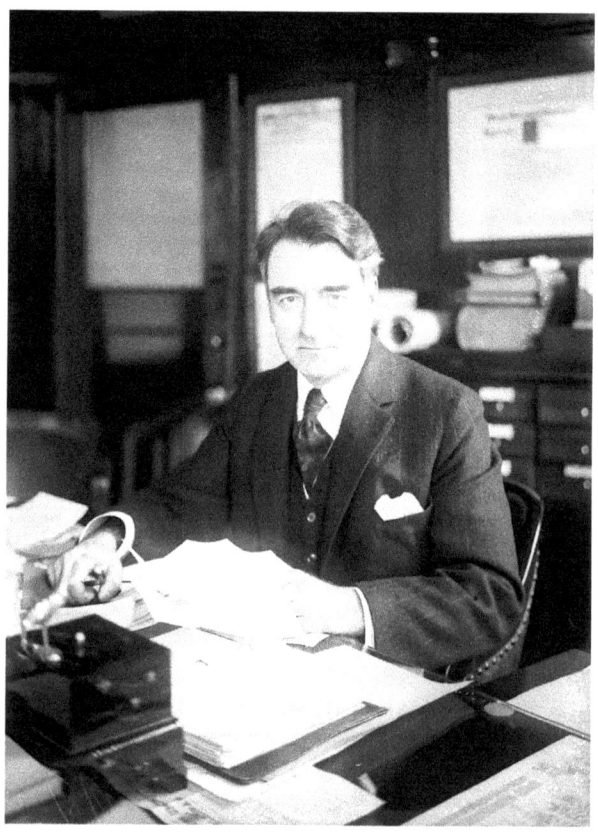

Dr. Royal S. Copeland, New York City Health Commissioner, photo circa 1915–1920.

Copeland never said a word about chiffon veils or about wearing them. That led to dozens and dozens of newspapers picking up the story and running it as a news item. One was the *Des Moines Register* (IA), which featured the item set off in a box on page 1. The headline for the piece was "New York Health Boss says Chiffon Veil is Safe Mask against Flu."[25]

Pennsylvania

The first application of drastic rules and regulations came on October 4 in Pennsylvania, with the effects of the measures widely felt in all cities. All churches and Sunday schools had to be kept closed. All saloons were closed until further notice. Theaters and motion picture places had to close their doors. Only close relatives of the deceased could attend funerals. Dance halls were shuttered, and all public meetings had to be postponed. It was all due to the drastic action the state health department and various city health bureaus took to prevent the spread of Spanish influenza. The Pennsylvania Department of Health issued the closing orders for the entire state on the evening of September 30 but left the question of closing churches, Sunday schools, and public schools to the discretion of local health officials. Dr. J.M. Raunick, Harrisburg health officer, announced that, for the present, the public schools in Harrisburg would be kept open as he felt it was better to have the children in the school system where they could be medically supervised. All kids who were coughing or sneezing would be sent home immediately. The churches in Harrisburg were closed. Hotel cafés that served lunch could stay open if no alcohol was served. Dr. B.F. Royer, Pennsylvania state commissioner of health, made the first order to close all amusement houses and saloons in the state.[26]

A day later, in Harrisburg, all schools were ordered shut, court sessions were discontinued for two weeks, soda fountains were ordered closed, and no ice cream was to be sold, except with meals served at restaurants, hotels, or in take-home cartons. According to this report, there was little dissatisfaction expressed anywhere over the orders. However, it was admitted that the closing of establishments hit many businesses hard. Dr. Raunick explained that the sale of ice cream and a piece of pie in restaurants and hotels was barred as a single order, but ice cream could be sold with meals. Raunick stated, "Those who have been affected and in some instances greatly inconvenienced by the direct order are everywhere willingly and cheerfully obeying the requirements."[27]

That Raunick had been less than truthful about full cooperation from everybody became apparent two days later when he announced that some saloon keepers had refused to obey the order to close, locking the front doors but doing business by using a rear entrance to the bars. Prosecutions would be brought, he said, with the maximum penalty being a fine of $100, 30 days in jail, or both. Dr. B.F. Royer issued a supplementary order on October 7 to the local health bureaus concerning the sale of alcoholic beverages as follows: "Consult with leading medical men and make provision for sale through drug stores on registered physicians' prescriptions of alcoholic stimulants and make provision for wholesale and bottling houses to supply retail needs for this purpose alone." Royer added, "One sneeze in a street car may infect a whole city. Kissing is another prolific method of infection, and this practice should be stopped except in cases where it is indispensable to happiness. Kissing between members of the gentle sex can certainly be abolished without hardship." A report from Coleville, Pennsylvania, remarked that Peter Eustuf and Steve Justima were fined $50 each for selling liquor against state orders, and 11 men caught in their places were fined five dollars each. Pennsylvania had also imposed anti-congregating rules, but there was no legal definition of the term.[28]

The Harrisburg city council put forward a suggestion to fumigate streetcars at the end of the line after each trip. Raunick told reporters he did not deem that necessary since the streetcar company was complying with his order to fumigate each car nightly.[29]

Stores in Harrisburg were open later on Saturday nights than on other nights. Late openings on Saturday nights were a common practice all over America. It acknowledged that people worked long hours but often finished work on Saturdays sometime in the afternoon and thus had some free time to shop. On October 10, Raunick and city health officials requested all stores to close on Saturday evenings at the same time as during the rest of the week. They worried about the potential danger of the crowds that filled the downtown stores on Saturday nights. This measure was put to the stores in the "nature of a request," although more robust measures were threatened. Raunick declared that residents of Harrisburg should abstain from crowding the stores during the epidemic. He said, "A lot of the effort of our closing orders is lost if people insist upon crowding the stores, especially when they have no intention of doing any shopping. Keep out of the stores unless you want to buy something and then don't linger after your errand's finished."[30]

It only took one day for one of the city's department stores, Bowman's, to take out an ad touting that it would close on Saturdays at 6 p.m. rather than anywhere from nine to midnight, as was then the custom. Bowman's tried to spin it as something it was doing for the benefit of its employees, and it even took advantage of the situation to hype special prices.[31]

One more day after that, it was reported that Harrisburg would be closed "tight as a box" after six thirty that Saturday night. Raunick had requested that all business places shut up shop by 6:30 p.m. and remain closed until Monday morning. Even barbershops and cigar stores were included in the early closing "request." The only exceptions were eating places and drugstores, which could remain open.[32]

When Raunick was faced with the suggestion that he order the quarantine of all houses where influenza existed, he declined. However, the doctor pointed out that it would be impractical with more than 7,000 cases in Harrisburg, as enforcement would be impossible. So, he urged that "everybody must be his own Quarantine officer." He added, "But I strongly urge that every person suffering from a cold remain home within his home or on the premises. Every employer should send home every employee suffering from a cold or symptoms of influenza."[33]

On October 16, after observing no decrease in the number of new cases and new deaths from the flu, Dr. Raunick again "requested" all stores to close on Saturday no later than 6:30 p.m., with the same exemptions for restaurants and drugstores. He also stated that he would issue an order to the Harrisburg Railways Company (streetcars) requiring at least half the windows in each of its cars in service to be kept open. That was an order and not a request. About the streetcars, the doctor explained, "The request of the [health] bureau has not been generally complied with and there has been some trouble reported to me." He thought removing the panes of glass in the cars might even be necessary if no other way was found to keep the passengers from closing them.[34]

A dozen youngsters reportedly followed a traveling salesperson as he got off a train. He was wearing a mask. "It's a gas mask," one kid in the crowd kidded the salesperson. He wore a white gauze mask that covered his nose and the lower part of his face. "What is it?" they yelled. "Influenza, you boobs. Don't you know every body is wearing 'em now."[35]

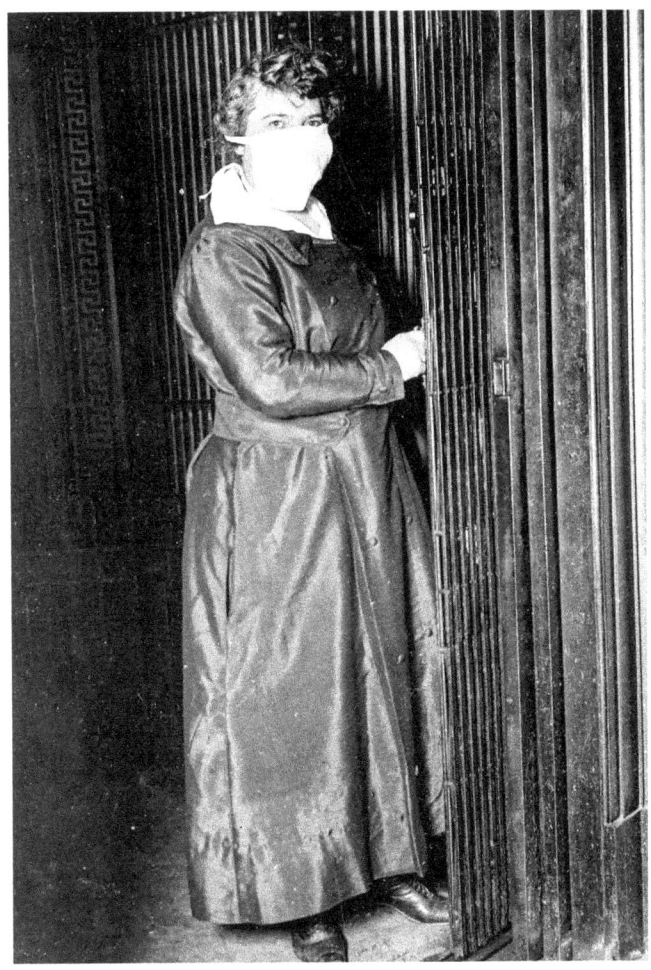

New York City elevator operator, October 16, 1918.

Because of the exorbitant prices being charged by some druggists in Harrisburg when they were filling physicians' prescriptions for whiskey, Dr. Raunick announced a new arrangement to supply whiskey for "worthy families." People needing whiskey were to go to a "reputable physician," get a prescription for the quantity needed (a maximum of eight ounces), then call with the prescription at one of the named and listed places. The article listed four: the Harrisburg Hospital, the Emergency Hospital, the Red Cross headquarters, and the City of Harrisburg Health Bureau. All those places would be supplied for free as several wholesale liquor dealers had "donated a sufficient supply."[36]

On October 18, Raunick announced that the stores would be requested to close by 6:30 p.m. for the third straight Saturday. The same exemptions remained, but the doctor remarked that those places could sell only drugs and food—no other commodities could be sold. The Red Cross urged nurses on duty in influenza cases to wear masks. A brief mention was made herein of the people rendered destitute by the epidemic, but only to the extent that Associated Aid Charities of Harrisburg had stepped up its appeal for donations to help "the worthy poor."[37]

October 20 and 21 saw a lessening of the epidemic with a drop in the death rate and a decrease in the number of new cases. Raunick said it was still too early to do anything and that all forms of control would remain in place. He regarded the situation as "stationary." A photo of the city's Emergency Hospital showed the nurses in the children's ward wearing masks and the windows wide open. The hospital had been created out of a school.[38]

Late in October, Dr. B. Franklin Royer, the acting Pennsylvania state commissioner of health, announced that as of October 30, the bans against amusement places, saloons, and public meetings were lifted in Harrisburg. Nothing had then been decided for the rest of the state. A telegram sent that morning to Pennsylvania Governor Martin Brumbaugh by Pennsylvania state Senator Edwin H. Vare urged the governor to use his influence to permit the saloons and theaters in Philadelphia to open.[39]

Health and police officials again called attention to the order prohibiting any Halloween celebrations in 1918. The police were ordered to disperse any crowds that gathered during the next few days.[40]

Following a conference with representatives from business, ministers, and members of the medical profession, the Harrisburg Health Department reported to a special session of the City Council that it was inadvisable to lift the flu restraining orders in Harrisburg before early November. However, if conditions continued to improve, Raunick said he might be open to an earlier lifting of the bans. Meanwhile, an announcement on November 1 stated that the Pennsylvania state ban on amusement places, saloons, and public meetings was to be lifted in the City of Pittsburgh on Saturday, November 9.[41]

Action by President Judge Landis of the Lancaster (PA) County Courts in issuing an injunction against the restrictive measures imposed by the Pennsylvania State Department of Health against Lancaster City for disregard of the anti-liquor sale provision of the flu ban was denounced by the acting health commissioner, B.F. Royer as "an unwarranted assumption of judicial authority." Royer said he desired to warn other municipalities against taking the Lancaster decision as precedent because he said he would use "every means at the control of the commonwealth to enforce the orders." However, since the slated lifting of the ban for Lancaster was a day or two away, Royer explained he would not fight the case in court.[42]

In Philadelphia, influenza was first reported by the Fourth Naval District on September 12, 1918. The state board of health closed churches, schools, saloons, and amusement places in Philadelphia, as they had throughout the state. During the ban in Philadelphia, the various business enterprises affected lost an estimated $1.5 billion. Cinemas lost $250,000, legitimate theaters lost $200,000, saloons lost $350,000, and transit companies lost an estimated $250,000. Department stores and other retailers also lost business (although they had not been closed) because, as a journalist noted, "most persons hesitated to take a chance of going to places where there was the slightest indication of crowds."[43]

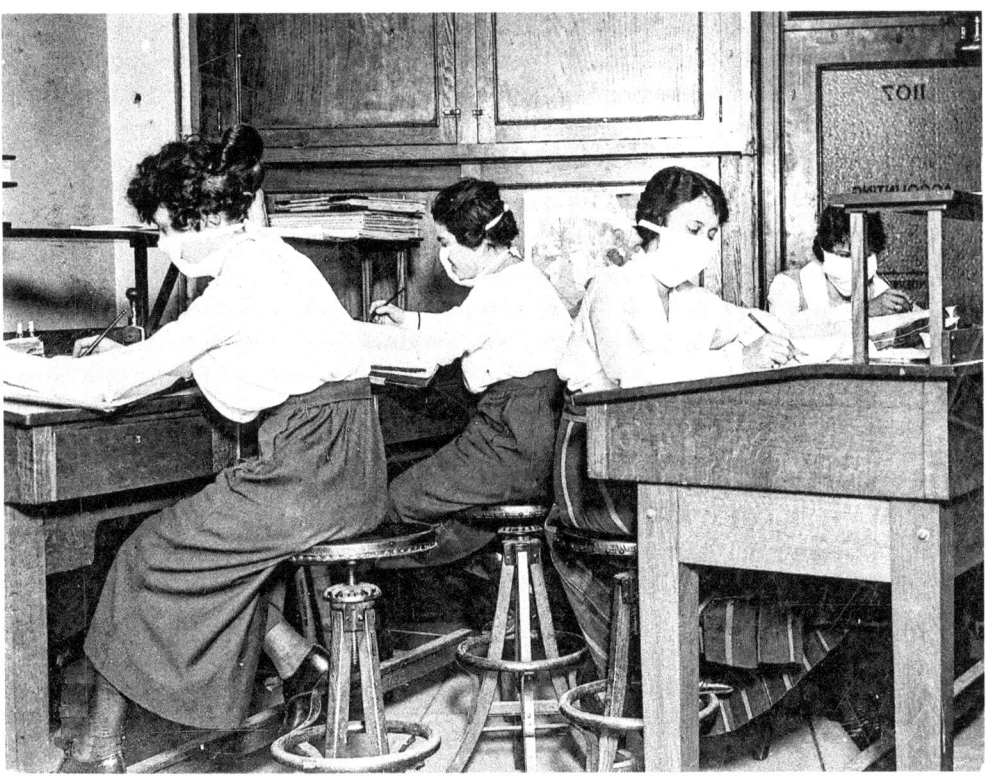

New York City clerks at work, October 16, 1918.

Royer placed the City of Lancaster, Pennsylvania, under quarantine on the night of November 1 for failing to observe the closing ban on sales of liquor. At almost the same time, Mayor E.V. Babcock of Pittsburgh issued a proclamation raising the ban in defiance of the state. Royer's order, sanctioned by the state attorney general, forbade trains or trolley cars to allow passengers to enter or leave the city. "The action is the most drastic ever taken by a state official," said a reporter. In his proclamation, Dr. Royer declared that all common carriers must stop allowing passengers in or out of Lancaster. "This action is taken for the purpose of protecting the people living outside of the city of Lancaster from any possible further dissemination of influenza due to premature relaxing of restrictions; for the purpose of protecting other municipalities from similar lawlessness under the protection of duly constituted authorities which might result from the precedent which the city of Lancaster would establish; and for the purpose of preserving the dignity and efficiency of the laws which have been adopted by the Commonwealth for the protection of the lives and health of its people." Concerning Pittsburgh Mayor Babcock, Royer said he would defer action until after he had conferred with the state attorney general and the United States Public Health Service, which he claimed backed him on the Lancaster move. Regarding Babcock's proclamation, he said, "It sounds like an invitation on the part of the Mayor of a great city to invite lawlessness and disorder.... It is very unfortunate ... the Mayor of a great city should not stand solidly back of the state and show a greater willingness to enforce orders."[44]

At noon on Tuesday, November 5, the restrictions that had been in effect in Harrisburg were lifted. Immediately, all theaters, cinemas, soda fountains, poolrooms, and other public places reopened. Bans were also lifted on saloons, but as that day was Election Day, saloon reopenings were delayed for one day. Practically all business places that had been closed had been fumigated. The churches also reopened. However, prosecutions were planned in Pittsburgh against owners of cinemas and saloons that had opened on November 4, in advance of the November 9 lifting of the ban there. Thus ended four weeks and some of the restrictions in Harrisburg.[45]

When Mayor E.V. Babcock replied to some of Royer's statements, he said, "Commissioner Royer is drunk with power. I am convinced that there is in the action of the State Health Department some ulterior purpose, something other than a desire to preserve public health. Unless forced by law I will not provide police service to make arrests for alleged violations of the influenza ban placed on this city by Acting Commissioner of Health Royer. In case arrests are made I will be responsible to the magistrates or judges."[46]

By November 8, the health bureau in Harrisburg had removed all restrictions, including those on the hours that businesses could be open, and left it to the retailers to suit themselves as to the hours they kept. One day later, Dr. Royer announced that the most extensive set of restrictions ever issued in Pennsylvania was lifted in every county in the state except in a "few isolated sections." It ended all the restrictions imposed on October 3.[47]

Members of the Harrisburg Health Bureau and the health commissioner, Dr. M.J. Raunick, held a meeting on December 10 with the city commissioners to consider the advisability of an ordinance quarantining houses where flu cases were located. Physicians present said it would be inadvisable for the present to enact such a measure "as too little is known about the length of contagion of influenza cases." They saw a quarantine as practical, but at present, it was not helpful to keep people in houses for 14 to 16 days. Doctors also argued that people faced with a quarantine but feeling ill would not contact doctors until the last possible moment and thus delay getting treatment. The meeting ended with the idea of quarantine being referred to the committee for future recommendation.[48]

Less than two weeks later, a report surfaced that there were flare-ups of the flu in a few places in the state: Erie, Allentown, Wilkes-Barre, Johnstown, and Uniontown. Boards of health in those cities had reimposed closing orders. Pittsburgh was also mentioned as having a flare-up, but nothing was done. Royer washed his hands of the matter when he stated that it was the policy of the Pennsylvania Health Department to leave closing orders and other restrictive measures to local health boards, which he had not done just six weeks earlier, unless conditions warranted otherwise.[49]

Physicians in Harrisburg reported new cases of influenza in late January 1919. Still, Raunick said it did not look like another epidemic similar to the previous fall. But nothing more happened in Harrisburg that was worthy of mention or the imposition of restrictions concerning the flu, and it remained free of restraint throughout 1919 and 1920.[50]

At the start of 1919, the Pennsylvania State Educational Association closed its

69th session in Harrisburg. The general session criticized the establishment of a statewide quarantine. The teachers declared, "We condemn statewide quarantine and indiscriminate closing of schools where adequate medical inspector and supervision are provided. We suggest rather a strict quarantine of individuals who are afflicted with a communicable disease."[51]

It took effect immediately. Schools of all kinds, public, private, and parochial, all had to close. Saloons, cafés, and all liquor concerns, including wholesalers and manufacturers, were closed on the evening of October 4 at 7 p.m., and Philadelphia, for the first time in its history, became bone dry as a means of combating the epidemic of influenza.[52]

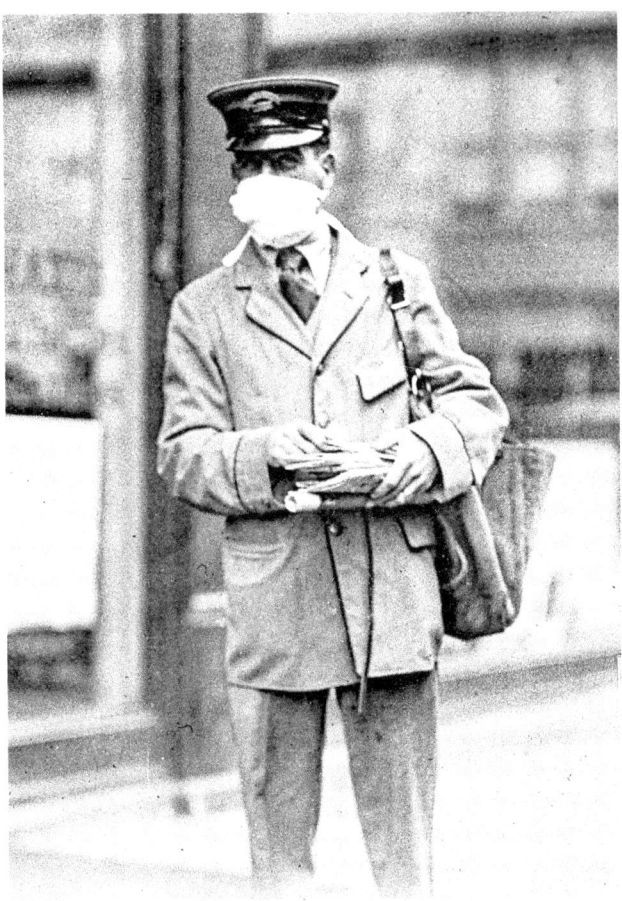

New York City letter carrier making his rounds, October 1918.

Schools in Philadelphia reopened on October 28, and all pupils and teachers had to undergo medical exams to attend. A warning was issued to Philadelphia residents not to indulge in an "orgy" similar to when the ban was lifted in Camden, New Jersey, just across the Delaware River. If such a thing happened in Philadelphia, saloons would have to close again. Theater managers held a meeting and decided to enter vigorous protests against the continuance of the ban on places of amusement in Philadelphia. Camden saloons were to remain closed until Philadelphia's influenza ban was lifted. Officials declared they would take no chance of repeating "the reign of terror that followed a rush of Philadelphia's undesirables across the river when the bars reopened yesterday." Churches were to reopen, along with the schools, but the rest of the restrictions remained in place. Conditions in Camden got so bad the day before that a reporter noted they "approached those of the Saturnalia of the ancients." Lawlessness reached such a height that Dr. H.H. Davis shut the saloons down in Camden again at 10:45 p.m. The saloons had been open since 11:30 a.m. that day. Migration from Philadelphia to Camden began early in the day and continued. Extra ticket sellers were added to the ferry company and to the trains. "Thousands of drunken men and youths" were

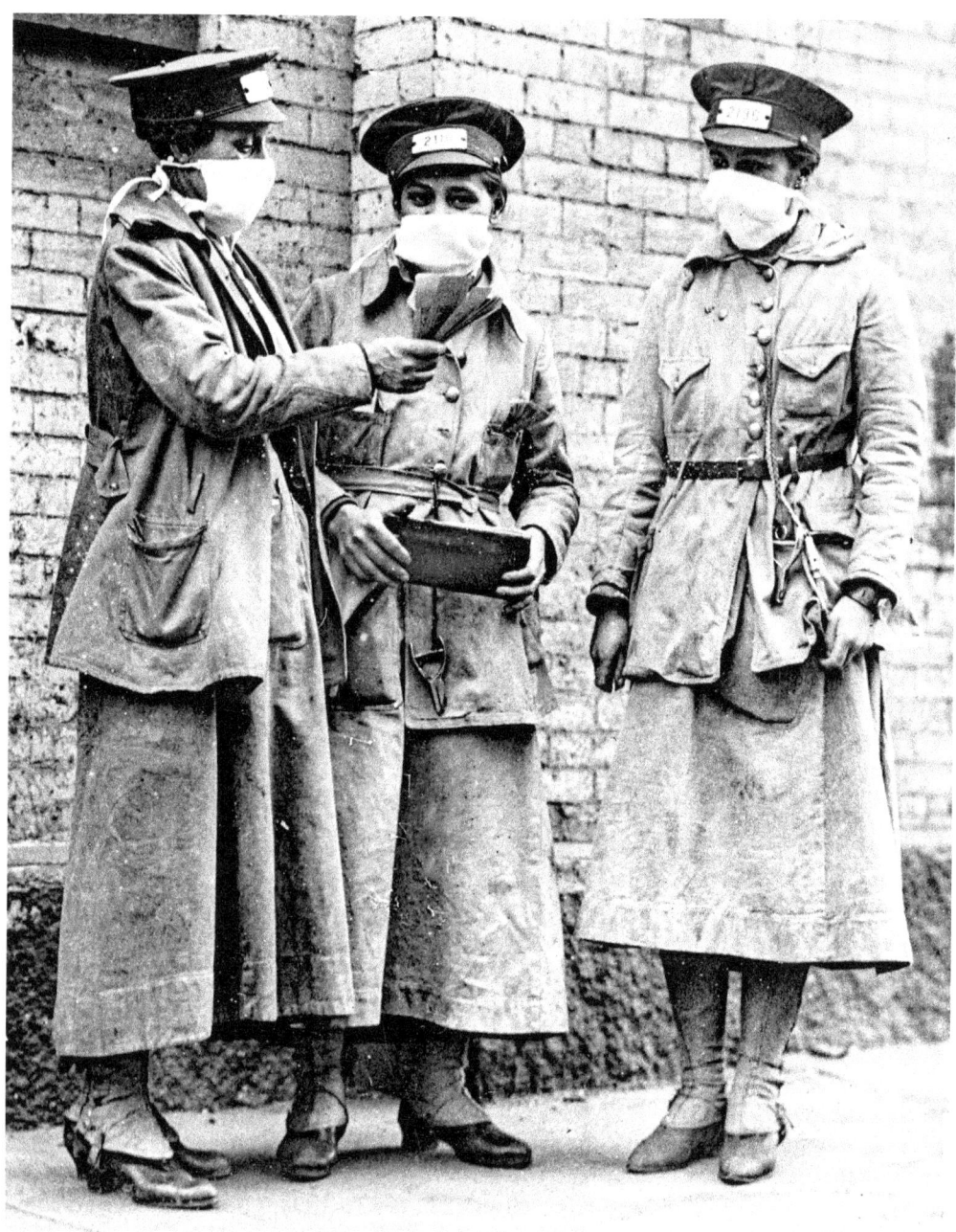

New York City transit conductors, 1918.

reported on the streets of Camden. Women on the sidewalks were subjected to "the grossest insults" by drunken men. By 9 p.m., at least 20,000 people from Philadelphia were in Camden.[53]

In Ellwood City, Pennsylvania, barbers were mandated to wear masks. Andy Weber, the Lawrence Avenue barber, was given a hearing on the evening of October 29 before Alderman Hancher and agreed to wear the influenza mask from that day onward. Weber claimed that he did not intend to expose anyone to the flu. He felt that if he was in good health and the customer was in the same condition, it was rather foolish to wear one of the "uncomfortable masks." However, after Hancher explained the situation to him, it was reported that Weber "cheerfully agreed" to wear the "flu preventor" in the future.[54]

In Scranton, later in October, the battle against influenza continued. A reporter wrote that the practice of wearing gauze and muslin masks to protect from the disease had become so general that "newsboys appeared upon the central city streets yesterday afternoon wearing them." Those newsboys obtained the masks at the Red Cross headquarters. In some barbershops in the central part of Scranton, the barbers were also said to wear face coverings while shaving and cutting hair. In an even more gruesome development, the Delaware, Lackawanna, and Western Coal Company had "men of experience" on duty at each mine. Before a worker was allowed to go to work, he was "looked over." If his appearance made him a suspected flu victim, he was sent to the hospital at the mine to have his temperature taken. And, if he had the flu, "close supervision [would] also be kept over the members of his families."[55]

When the authorities in Scranton presented their list of things to do to help control the epidemic, they did not mention masks, except that they should be worn when a person tended the sick. The article advised readers that if they had to cough or sneeze in public, to do so into a handkerchief. A mask was not suggested.[56]

One story in a Scranton newspaper on October 28 was almost certainly a plant. The headline read, "Newsboys plead for gauze masks." According to the story, the newsboys wanted masks, although the item admitted, "Nobody knows why they have such a fascination for them…. Now epidemic fighters are wearing masks, not because masks are a beautiful and comfortable thing, but because it is demanded that they wear them. And the small boys' greatest desire is to wear them, too." Reportedly, one day earlier, the newsboys crowded around the storefront of a place that stocked the masks. They became so unruly that police officers had to be called out to clear the area. And the window washer had to be called in to clear away all the grimy fingerprints the newsboys had left on the store's window. "And the boys had been gathering there for days, begging and pleading for masks. When asked why they want them no reason is ever given." This probably false, so-called story could be understood if the Scranton area of Pennsylvania, in general, was conducting a publicity campaign to attempt to coerce people to wear masks, but they were not. Authorities hardly bothered about masks, except to harass a few barbers.[57]

In Pittsburgh, the military authorities in the Pittsburgh district were entirely dependent on the Red Cross for hospital supplies such as sheets, pajamas, and face masks. From the University of Pittsburgh military officers, the Red Cross received a request for 7,000 face masks. According to the university authorities, all students there would wear those masks until the danger of the epidemic had passed.[58]

Although the state had imposed a blanket closure, it quickly abandoned responsibility for lifting the closures. At various times, the local boards of health in Pennsylvania lifted closures. By mid- to late November, many local areas, acting independently, had reimposed closure orders similar to, if not identical to, the original orders. Those communities included Erie, Johnstown, New Castle, Uniontown, and Wilkes-Barre. However, masks were not imposed or even recommended.[59]

Two Pittsburgh newspapers presented short items on December 13 about the American Public Health Association convention in Chicago, which had ended after four days of meetings on December 12. It stressed the differences that came to light at the convention. The *Pittsburgh Post-Gazette* stressed the difference between urban and rural, with rural health professionals favorable to the use of vaccines and masks while urban people opposed both. The other paper, the *Pittsburgh Post*, declared in its headline that "branding influenza mask as fake splits health conference." This paper presented the split as two factions: the pro-mask and pro-vaccine groups, against the anti-vaccine and anti-mask groups.[60]

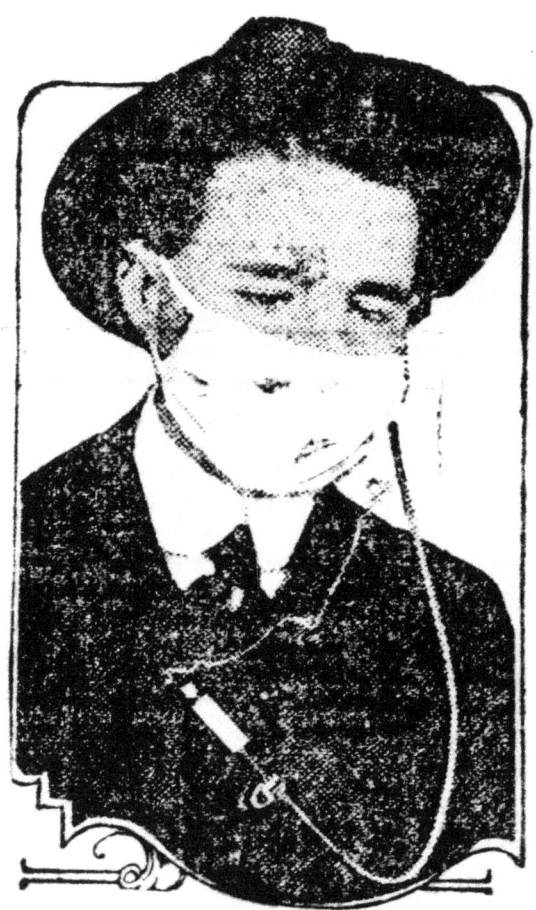

LADY NICOTINE BEATS MASK LAW.

A San Francisco ordinance requires every citizen to wear a mask during the influenza epidemic. This resourceful smoker attached a rubber tube to his cigaret holder, fastened the holder to his coat lapel with an ordinary paper clip and kept up his daily batting average in the cigaret league.

This photograph also appeared in many papers around America. It illustrated the problems people had trying to smoke while wearing a mask in a society where the percentage of smokers was much higher than it would be a century later.

5

South Atlantic

Delaware

At a special meeting, the Wilmington Board of Health and Dr. A.E. Frantz, secretary of the Delaware Board of Health, decided that the influenza situation was severe. If there were no change for the better in the 24 hours following October 1, it would exercise its authority and close all schools and "places of public gathering of every nature" until the epidemic was over. Dr. Robert E. Ellegood, president of the Wilmington Board of Health, ordered the action the next day. He claimed that 20 leading physicians and owners of theaters had requested that the board adopt such a rule. Two days later, on October 4, the Delaware Board of Health adopted a duplicate closing order to the one in force in Wilmington and imposed it on the entire State of Delaware.[1]

The liquor question occupied much of the Wilmington Board of Health's meeting a week later. The night before, there had been 36 arrests for drunkenness in Wilmington. The police force, working below strength due to flu absences, complained they could not handle all the drunkenness in addition to their regular duties. Wholesale liquor houses had been allowed to remain open and sell liquor. Complaints were also coming in from industrial plants that their work was severely hampered by absenteeism from alcohol consumption. Men who usually drank beer had turned to hard liquor as beer was unavailable. Wilmington authorities considered passing an order that no person could buy liquor at one of the wholesale places without presenting a doctor's prescription, as Philadelphia had already done.[2]

Satisfied that the influenza epidemic had abated to such a degree as to be much less dangerous, both the Delaware Board of Health and the Wilmington Board of Health decided, at special meetings held on October 24, to remove the closure orders they had imposed early that month. Effective Sunday, October 27, all restrictions were removed, with churches open and schools, theaters, saloons, and other public places returning to normal on October 28. Reportedly, the health authorities thought the churches should be the first to reopen.[3]

A liquor problem of a different sort hit the City of Wilmington a few weeks later. Authorities were determined to stop the surge of residents from Chester, Pennsylvania, and other places (all under lockdowns that included their saloons) to Wilmington saloons—then open regular hours. In four days at the end of October, 200 arrests for drunkenness had been made in Wilmington. The Wilmington Board of Police

Commissioners stepped in and limited saloon hours in Wilmington from 7 a.m. to 7 p.m.[4]

Late in November, the flu cases increased to such an extent that in Middleton, the local board of health closed the schools again on November 22, just a month after they had reopened. However, the use of masks was not discussed, nor were masks used or discussed during the first closure period that lasted close to one month.[5]

An editorial in a Wilmington newspaper on July 31, 1919, looked at the pandemic with the hope that the U.S. Congress would pass the Harding-Fess influenza bill. The bill would have appropriated $5 million to investigate influenza and allied diseases to determine their cause and prevention methods. The editorial summarized what little was known about the disease: "Nor could the wisest of health officials tell a frightened humanity how to avoid the germ, unknown and unexplainable. Preventive methods they advised were many, and mostly these were founded upon hope, built of good wishes, and to this day there is no exact indication of the success or failure of the flu mask, the thousand and one sprays, swabs and washes, nor even of the efficacy of the city-wide quarantine."[6]

Maryland

After a morning consultation on October 3, schools in Annapolis closed "for a few days." The meeting involved the Anne Arundel County Board of Education and the Annapolis health officer, Dr. William S. Welch. Less than a week later, all the other schools in Anne Arundel were closed. By order of the Maryland Health Department, based on recommendations from United States Surgeon General Rupert Blue, the closure was until further notice.[7]

More drastic action was taken less than a week later in Annapolis, when Dr. Welch closed all places of public assembly and virtually all public gatherings until further notice, under Rupert Blue's advice. A day or two after that, Dr. John D. Blake, Baltimore health commissioner, ordered all the churches in the city shuttered. It marked the first time in Baltimore history that such an official order had been given or that such drastic measures had been deemed necessary to safeguard public health. Blake also closed theaters and cinemas and prohibited all public gatherings.[8]

On October 23, the Maryland Health Department commissioner, Dr. Hampson Jones, was asked about lifting the restrictions in Annapolis and other communities and counties. Jones said he could not lift the quarantine until the doctors in Annapolis sent him a report on the conditions there. But one day later, Annapolis Health Officer Wellman officially announced the closure orders would be lifted on October 26, with theaters and cinemas reopening that day, churches the following day, and schools on Monday. However, schools were delayed until November 4 to coincide with Baltimore schools' reopening.[9]

The earliest suggestion for the face mask in Maryland came on September 30, 1918, in a letter written by Samuel Garner to the editor of an Annapolis newspaper. He pointed out that as soon as the Germans began using poisonous gas, the Allies found a counter in the form of masks that covered our soldiers' eyes, noses, and mouths. "It is strange that it was only a few days ago that some one in Baltimore suggested a mask to cover the nose and mouth as a protection against the Spanish influenza ... it would seem to be the most natural thing in the world for people to wear masks whenever grippish diseases are prevalent," wrote Garner. He said that he wasn't going to wait around for one, so he had made a mask for himself. He added that when he was in town, his nose and mouth would be "muffled up."[10]

An article in a Baltimore newspaper on October 2 declared that the Red Cross had an immediate need for 20,000 influenza masks for use at nearby military camps. Hundreds of women were needed to make them. All those women, of course, worked on a voluntary, unpaid basis. Such calls appeared in newspapers all over America in October. According to the story, "the faster they are supplied the more likelihood of checking the scourge, which is temporarily incapacitating thousands of Uncle Sam's fighting men ... the masks are being used not only for influenza sufferers, but also for experimental purposes as a means of preventing the spread of the infection."[11]

When the same Baltimore paper gave extensive directions to its readers on the prevention and treatment of the disease on October 8, face masks were not mentioned, except that they were to be used by people caring for the sick. Also mentioned was the frequent cleansing of the mouth and spraying the nose and throat with "simple" antiseptic solutions. Readers were advised not to talk directly in the face of others and to cover their nose and mouth with a handkerchief when coughing or sneezing.[12]

Two days later, Baltimore health commissioner, Dr. John D. Blake, ordered most department stores and other retail outlets to not open for business before 9:30 a.m. and to close by 4:30 p.m. He exempted dairies, grocery stores, drug stores, confectionery stores, cigar stores, and small stores in the outlying districts from the order. At the same time, he recommended that workers serving food, particularly in restaurants and hotels, wear gauze masks.[13]

Two additional days later, Blake clarified his order, saying that all wholesale businesses could stay open as long as they wished. That included wholesale dealers who sold liquor. He had thought about closing all saloons, hotel bars, and so on, but in the end, let them remain open with the same restricted hours that he had imposed on department stores—open only from 9:30 a.m. to 4:30 p.m. At this time, Blake issued another order requiring dentists to wear a gauze mask while working on patients. Dentists were forbidden by law from working on any patient without the "protection" of the mask. The order took effect at midnight on the same day it was issued.[14]

On November 6, Commissioner Blake lifted the last two restrictions that had been put in place in the City of Baltimore. All others had been removed by this time. One of them allowed merchants to send goods to customers "on approval" and exchange merchandise as was customary before the epidemic. The second and last restriction lifted was the one requiring dentists to wear masks, effective the following day.[15]

District of Columbia

In Washington, United States Surgeon General Dr. Rupert Blue issued a warning on September 13 regarding the Spanish flu in the United States. He cited an outbreak at Fort Morgan, near Mobile, Alabama, that occurred in August. At about the same time, a tramp steamer arrived in Newport News with almost the entire crew ill with the disease. Philadelphia and New York had reported a few cases four weeks earlier. The Boston epidemic was reported on September 11. Blue stated, "There is no such thing as an effective quarantine in the case of pandemic influenza, but preventive measures may be taken and should be taken."[16]

On September 25, the Potomac division of the Red Cross gave an order to the district chapter of the Red Cross to furnish 45,000 "so-called gas masks to be worn by soldiers in training here and by patients at Walter Reed Hospital." Those were the gauze flu masks. According to the account, this was the first instance in the history of the United States that "preventive measures in the form of a mask for general use to combat a disease has been known to be used. The orders for the masks are said to have been received by the District Chapter of the Red Cross from the War Department." However, no explanation was given as to why using masks to fight influenza was a good idea.[17]

A day later, a reporter remarked that the flu mask was "a modified form of the gas mask" and that "if the contrivance proves an effective preventive measure, it is believed it will be adopted at the various camps throughout the country where Spanish influenza has appeared." There was no attempt to verify the effectiveness of the device, and the mask went on, within days and a few weeks, to be used in all military installations across the country, always made by the Red Cross with unpaid labor, a volunteer force of women.[18]

Washington reached a height of hysteria on October 8 when it was determined that telephones needed to be masked. All telephones were therefore furnished with "gas masks" to safeguard against the spread of influenza among the thousands of war workers in the various departments, bureaus, boards, and commissions throughout the nation's capital. The sanitary corps of Washington inspected all the war work establishments and placed medicated gauze on all telephone mouthpieces.[19]

On October 9, the District of Columbia commissioners banned with immediate effect outdoor meetings, including church services, following recommendations from United States Public Health Service officers Dr. W.C. Fowler and Dr. Harry S. Mustard. Government officials had ordered 25,000 gauze masks for war workers in the departments who were "most generally exposed to danger of infection." The officials said that "other masks will be ordered later."[20]

An editorial in a Washington, D.C., newspaper disliked the shuttering of church services. The editorial argued that, for various reasons, the practice of church closures should end as the spiritual needs served by the church were especially needed in a time of world war and an influenza pandemic. "It should be assured that church services are short and so distributed through the day that no service is crowded; and that the church buildings are properly heated and thoroughly ventilated," wrote the editor. "If epidemic actually rages simple anti-influenza masks may be worn. With these precautions, the churches should be put on the footing of essential war industries and of factors which tend to check and not to promote an epidemic."[21]

The District of Columbia commissioners, as of October 12, considered ordering or suggesting the general use of gauze masks. It was believed that something official might be done along those lines before the close of business that day. The health authorities strongly recommended masks as a protection against contagion. Dr. Mustard, city health officer for Washington, stated that he believed those masks to be the best protection against the disease. "I am strongly in favor of masking every citizen of Washington," Mustard declared. "The plan seems to be the most practical one offered to check the spread of the epidemic." With hundreds of people wearing masks, the people of Washington would realize the seriousness of the situation, the authorities believed, and be willing to observe the "simple precautions" suggested by the health department. Those masks, said the story, protected not only the person wearing them but others as well. District of Columbia Commissioner Louis Brownlow was very much in favor of the general use of masks. "I strongly approve of the suggestion of the health officers and should like to see every citizen of the District wearing one of the masks," said Brownlow. The four relief stations established throughout the city had hundreds of those masks on hand for distribution to the public. A day earlier, a number of Washington's business concerns requested that the masks be distributed among their employees so they could wear them. One of the first business houses to advise people to wear masks was the Commercial National Bank. However, the account concluded that it was not likely that the authorities would issue orders requiring people to wear masks. Dr. Fowler stated that he believed the plan to order mask wearing was impractical, "and the habit must be established by the people themselves through their realization of the gravity and danger of the present crisis."[22]

Louis Brownlow, on January 26, 1915, as he took office as a new District of Columbia Commissioner.

On October 15, Dr. Mustard said the public health service was prepared to supply the entire population of Washington with gauze masks. It considered them to be the best of all preventive measures. It had 25,000 masks then, ready for distribution, and would obtain more if the demand was "created." Masks could be obtained at any of the emergency stations located in the city. Public health service inspectors notified barbers, dentists, and elevator operators to obtain masks. All people were advised to wear masks when they were riding on streetcars.[23]

That day, city post office employees in direct contact with the public appeared at their workstations wearing gauze masks. City Postmaster Merritt Chance appeared in one of the face coverings. All workers at windows serving the public were required to wear masks. Workers connected with the local draft board at the post office also wore masks. Health officials stated that it would not be necessary for letter carriers and workers on the mail room floor to wear masks. Clerks reportedly experienced difficulty with the masks at first. Many would take them off for a resting spell. One man said he now knew what a dog felt like when it was forced to wear its first muzzle.[24]

The public relations campaign waged by Washington authorities continued the next day when it was announced in the press that the "wearing of gauze masks promises to become general." Dr. Mustard's statement that 25,000 masks were ready for distribution, supplemented by Commissioner Brownlow's advice that masks should be worn by everyone coming into contact with "many persons," made it "practically certain [there would be] widespread adoption of this preventive measure." Reportedly, hundreds of people applied for masks at the emergency stations that morning, and "long lines of applicants formed outside the buildings." Dentists, barbers, and elevator operators generally were masked that day. "Many of Washington's army of young woman war workers appeared today on crowded street cars and at their desks with their faces muffled in gauze shields as a protection against influenza, a practice advocated by many bureau chiefs who feared utter demoralization of their war operations."[25]

On October 15, Washington health officials prescribed gauze masks for every person riding on the streetcars, along with the orders that barbers, dentists, and elevator operators also don the face coverings.[26]

The Washington department store of Lansburgh & Brother took advantage of the false story that Royal Copeland of New York City advocated using a chiffon veil by women to prevent the flu. He did not; it was a concocted story by a different department store selling chiffon veils. The Washington store was also flogging the chiffon veil and, in its ad, made another mistake when it called Copeland the health commissioner of Philadelphia.[27]

When a Brooklyn newspaper commented on the situation in Washington, it remarked that the employment of gauze masks was rapidly becoming common there. "It has even become frequent upon the street, particularly among young people who find a certain novelty in going about with the lower half of the face swathed in a white veil, covering the mouth and nose. Office boys and girl stenographers run errands with their masks on, if they happen to be wearing masks. In many of the restaurants the waiters are wearing them, under orders from the proprietors." In all the banks, the tellers and the clerks who dealt with the public wore masks. The

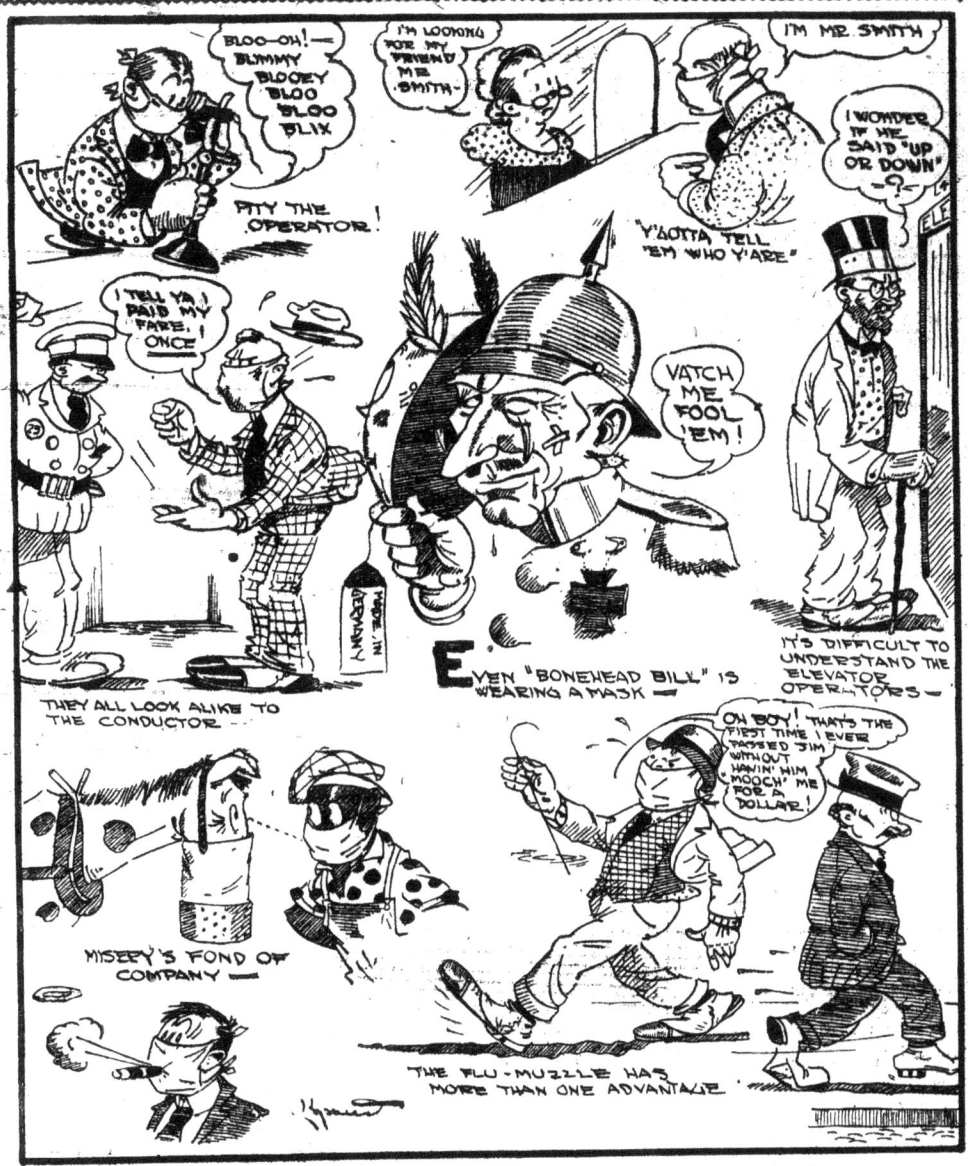

An editorial cartoon from the *Washington Post* all about the face mask.

use of masks was spreading rapidly in government departments, so it was reported. The authorities encouraged it. "Masked men and women may be seen riding in automobiles, until it seems as though Washington were receiving a visitation from the Ku-Klux-Klan." The journalist stated, "The masks are neither comfortable nor pretty, yet they are becoming quite popular among Washington people who think more of avoiding influenza than they do of their personal appearance."[28]

Virginia

At the request of Richmond, Virginia, Health Officer Roy K. Flannagan, to control the epidemic of Spanish influenza, city officials there ordered the closing of all churches, public and private schools, theaters, cinemas, dance halls, poolrooms, sideshows, "in fact, all indoor public gatherings." The order went into effect at 6 a.m. on October 6. On October 4, the Virginia Board of Health, through its commissioner, Dr. Ennion G. Williams, recommended closing all public gatherings except for schools. He advocated keeping schools open for educational purposes and regarded school closures as a "panicky extremity, since the school buildings are well ventilated, with not more than half the pupils in attendance." Flannagan believed that all schools should be closed on the grounds of public policy. Streetcars in Richmond were ordered to operate with windows open for ventilation. Motormen and conductors on the streetcars were instructed to keep the windows open.[29]

The orders left open the option to hold the Virginia State Fair, which was due to start later that week. However, three days later, the Virginia Board of Health executive committee issued orders to close all state fairs. It was also reported that the Richmond Health Department had been informed that certain citizens riding on the streetcars were "hostile" to open windows, noted a reporter, "some individuals going so far as to assault the conductor because he refused to shut down the windows." That caused the reporter to declare, "Unreasonable and unpatriotic people are to be found even in Richmond."[30]

As cases in Richmond did not decline, the next move came from the Virginia Council of Defense and not the board of health. The council ordered the closing of all tobacco warehouses in the state. It was the custom for great crowds to assemble around auction places.[31]

Quarantine restrictions were all lifted in Virginia at 6 a.m. on Sunday, November 3. The order came from the Virginia Board of Health and applied to virtually all communities in Virginia, including Richmond. Two days before the ban was lifted, the Richmond Academy of Medicine and Surgery passed a resolution expressing the opinion that it was the better part of prudence to postpone reopening until, in the opinion of Chief Health Officer Roy Flannagan, it was safe. The vote by the doctors was 20 to 4 in favor of postponement. Also speaking for the state board, Dr. Garnett said it did not recommend lifting any ban; the various conditions in the state made it appropriate to leave the matter up to local health officials.[32]

In Alexandria, Virginia, every church, cinema, poolroom, Sunday school, and other places where people congregated were closed as of October 4 until the Spanish influenza epidemic subsided. Dr. W.L. Wood of the United States Public Health Service announced the policy, acting under "special police authority." People congregating in the streets were also to be dispersed. Reportedly, it was the first time since the Civil War that places of public worship had to be closed.[33]

A couple of days later, Dr. W.L. Wood, "special state health officer," issued an order that from then onward, all the windows on the cars of the Washington-Virginia Railway Company had to be kept open. People who refused to leave the windows open were subject to arrest and the imposition of a fine.[34]

Dr. H.C. Robles, the acting medical officer in Alexandria, directed, on October 18, that all servers in lunchrooms, all barbers, and all employees of soda water fountains wear masks against influenza while they were serving the public. A total of 75 masks were distributed that day to such employees—all of them made by the local Red Cross. Barbers were said to have been among the first to comply with the edict.[35]

Restrictions were lifted in Alexandria in early November, along with all the other communities in Virginia. Sunday was the day initially picked for the reopening, based on the idea held by the authorities that Sunday was the least dangerous day, while Saturday was believed to be the most dangerous day.[36]

One account from Richmond on October 11 declared that "advice given to physicians that masks should be worn until the epidemic of influenza abates caused a rush on the workrooms that quickly depleted stock of thousands of the gauze protectors." Those were the Red Cross workrooms, wherein a single mask required six to ten minutes to make. It consisted of five thicknesses of gauze and was sold to the public at cost, three cents each.[37]

In Norfolk, when the statewide lockdown was imposed, the health commissioner distributed flu masks during the day and said that "all who desire them will be supplied. The mask is simply constructed of a double thickness of muslin, fastening behind the head with strings. A red mark on one side denotes the out thickness and serves to protect the wearer from using first one side and then the other next to the nostrils." The health officer, Dr. Schenck, declared that all dentists would be urged to wear masks while attending to patients. While he expected the dentists to take that precaution without his instructions, the request was issued as an extra precaution. On the same page of the paper, set off in its box, was the summary advice from Rupert Blue of the United States Public Health Service. No mention was made of masks.[38]

Dr. G.M. Converse was head of the local health district in Norfolk. On October 8, he ordered the barbers in his district to wear masks while attending to their customers for their shops to remain open.[39]

Dr. J. Fulmer Bright, described by a reporter as one of the best-known physicians of Richmond, contacted a local newspaper to make a statement: "I wish to enlist the aid of the *Times-Dispatch* in urging the extreme necessity of the universal wearing of nose and mouth masks during this epidemic of influenza ... The wearing of the little cheesecloth masks, which can be easily made or can be gotten from Red Cross headquarters at 3 cents apiece will do more than anything else to prevent the spread of the disease."[40]

In Richmond, the local military exemption board directed its members and employees to wear a gauze mask until the epidemic was "wiped out," by order of the U.S. Army surgeon general. The order stated that the various gargling agents on the market were of doubtful preventive quality, while the gauze mask (of four-ply thickness) "is a sure preventive." "Clerk of the Exemption Board Harry H. Hold stated that the offices employing any number of people might find it a good idea to accept the conditions laid down about the gauze masks by the Surgeon General [of the Army]."[41]

When a reporter with a Staunton, Virginia, paper noted the same rules for masking applied in his town at the local exemption board, he also noted that travelers from Richmond to his city wore, in some cases, that protection against the flu. He commented that "no laughs were produced by the strange appearance of the procession of travelers from the station, each wearing his face mask. Too much wisdom is shown by the adoption of the precaution to cause mirth."[42]

A year after the pandemic, in September 1919, the Virginia Health Officers Association held a meeting in Richmond. They appointed a special committee to prepare and report on definite plans for meeting any such repeat of a pandemic that might arise. Dr. Schenck, Dr. Emmet C. Levy of Richmond, and Mosby Parrow of Lynchburg were on the committee. During the meeting, it was revealed that most group members opposed the closing of schools, feeling children could be better supervised and given better access to health professionals if the schools were kept open. They also agreed that the virus had not been isolated. As a consequence, no positive preventive existed except the enforcement of rigid rules of sanitation and the avoidance of personal contact. Regarding a discussion of face masks, the news item drew on the conclusion put forward in a highly diplomatic fashion by Rupert Blue and the U.S. Public Health Service, which declared, "The use of face masks has not been attended with the success predicted for them."[43]

West Virginia

On the night of October 6, on the advice of the United States Public Health Service and the suggestion of West Virginia Governor John J. Cornwell, Health Commissioner S.L. Jepson called on local health authorities throughout West Virginia to close all schools, theaters, and other places where people congregated at the first appearance in their area of Spanish influenza.[44]

The following day, the Fairmont Board of Health acted on the request. It passed a resolution closing theaters, poolrooms, soda fountains, and other places of public congregation. It banned all public meetings until further notice. Dr. H.L. Criss, Fairmont health physician, explained that a single case of influenza in Fairmont was sufficient to make the situation "very serious" and justified taking stringent precautions against its further spread. Mayor Bowen reported that everywhere in his city where the drastic closing order was in place, it was met with "the heartiest cooperation."[45]

A few days later, Jepson issued an order requiring the quarantine of individuals for influenza. He sent the following to all health boards in his state: "To local Health Boards! You are hereby instructed that owing to the very wide prevalence of influenza in a virulent form, this department hereby issues instructions requiring all cases of the disease to be promptly reported and quarantined until entirely well. Local health officers are required when an outbreak appears in a community to close all theaters, poolrooms, soft drink places, schools, churches and Sunday schools. All public meetings must also be abandoned."[46]

At the end of October, city officials in Fairmont held a meeting to take stringent steps toward preventing the further spread of the flu. The action was to be taken to secure the cooperation of the public in that every effort would be put forth to prevent the assembling of people, to urge the people to avoid streetcars as much as possible, to stay at home, and "if possible stay well so that they not be on the public to care for, as the public is now overburdened with the care of those already afflicted." But then, on November 6, just a little over a week later, it was announced that all restrictions would be lifted entirely on Sunday, the 10th of November.[47]

According to a reporter's story, out of Charleston on October 17, there was something to celebrate. "At last, after all sorts of persuasion on the part of the City Health Commissioner and the Home Service Department of the American Red Cross, the people of Charleston are wearing gauze masks on the street and at duty where their work brings them in contact with many people." He added, "The boys and girls who carry messages for the telegraph companies, the auto drivers, and many others who are out on the streets constantly are wearing the masks. There was a request from the post office on Sunday night for 200 masks and the employees at the Federal building are wearing them—protecting the wearer from influenza and serving as a warning to those who come in contact with the post office employees that there is real danger of contagion." Willard Comstock, head of the Home Service Department of the Red Cross, tried to get the physicians of Charleston to wear masks on the streets, but they refused. Naively, the reporter asserted, "It is generally agreed that the wearing of the gauze will ward off the disease."[48]

In Shepherdstown, on October 17, the health authorities issued an order to close all stores and places of business where people assembled at 6 p.m. each evening. It was also ordered that barbers wear masks at work or close their places of business. According to this account, the barbers shut down their shops rather than wear masks and went off to pick apples for four dollars a day.[49]

North Carolina

Charlotte, North Carolina, implemented a quarantine at 6 p.m. on Friday, October 4. It involved shutting down the usual suspects—schools, churches, and places of public assembly. Soldiers from nearby Camp Greene were not allowed to visit the city, leaving the streets of Charlotte nearly deserted.[50]

On October 14, acting upon the advice of the Robeson County health officer, the town authorities of Lumberton lifted the travel quarantine it had in place barring travelers coming to Lumberton from Charlotte, Wilmington, Fayetteville, and all points in Bladen and Cumberland Counties. That particular quarantine had been in place for less than two weeks. The travel ban was a quarantine found to be unenforceable, admitted town officials, so it was removed. The town's other closures, such as against schools and churches, remained in force, as did a ban on public gatherings and congregation on the streets.[51]

Ordinance number 56 was passed on October 11, 1918, and signed by W.J. Lenoir, mayor of Lenoir, North Carolina. Under the order, any person returning to Lenoir or entering the community for the first time from districts where influenza was prevalent, and any person exposed to the disease, had to be quarantined in Lenoir for seven days. Any person who contracted the disease had to be quarantined until they received a certificate from an attending physician that stated they had completely recovered. Anyone who violated the ordinance was guilty of a misdemeanor and, upon conviction, would be fined $25 for each offense. Lenoir was in Caldwell County, and Dr. L.H. Coffey, the county physician, reminded residents of his county to wear gauze masks when attending any ill person or "when in the suspicious circumstances of influenza."[52]

More drastic was the step taken by Kings Mountain. The city council met on October 18 and enacted an ordinance requiring all stores to close on Saturday, October 19, at noon, and to remain closed for a week. Only drug stores were allowed to remain open and only to sell drugs and medicines; no other goods those stores stocked could be offered for sale. Food stores were allowed to take orders and deliver goods, but people could not enter the stores. People could go to the store door and pick up their order, which had been left outside. Barber shops could stay open, but inside the shop, the customer total could not be greater than the total number of barbers.[53]

At a meeting of the board of directors of the Retail Merchants Association at the end of October, a resolution was adopted calling upon the Health Committee of Winston-Salem to place a quarantine on all cases of influenza and people coming into contact with the disease. Said a journalist, "The board insists that those suffering with the disease should be isolated from well persons as far as possible." Business was pushing for more quarantines for the sick as a method to try to limit or remove restrictions placed on businesses.[54]

Restrictions in Charlotte were lifted at midnight on Thursday, November 7. The first case of Spanish influenza reported in Charlotte was on the 28th of September.[55]

An editorial in a Hendersonville newspaper on the day before Christmas 1918 remarked that the surgeon general of the United States, Rupert Blue, and the North Carolina Board of Health were advocating a quarantine for those sick with the flu instead of a quarantine of the well, as was the case with so many of the various restrictions. "Quite a number of cities have entered on this plan, the same as used against other contagious diseases," wrote the editor. "This sounds very sensible. This business of quarantining a well person and liberating the sick to spread disease among the masses appears quite insensible to us." If the sick were quarantined, reasoned the editor, the healthy could attend school, attend church, and hold social and business meetings.[56]

On the afternoon of January 11, 1919, Statesville's Board of Aldermen placed the influenza restrictions back in force again after having removed them only about ten days earlier. The reimposed restrictions allowed one-hour religious services in the town's churches on Sunday each week—the earlier quarantine had allowed no church services. Schools, theaters, and all public gatherings were banned as before. Also, the board passed an ordinance making it a violation of the law for people who had the disease or had been associated in any way with anyone who had had it to mingle with other people outside of their premises. At about the same time, the quarantine in Asheville was lifted in mid–February 1919, after having been in place for over a month, as a second round of restrictions. Again, Asheville was restored to normal conditions.[57]

When the Charlotte health officer, Dr. C.C. Hudson, reported on the flu cases to city officials on October 3, he said the use of gauze masks by nurses, doctors, and those attending the sick was "being generally adopted." A gauze mask made of four thicknesses of gauze would make it safe for anybody, claimed Dr. Hudson.[58]

An announcement from Greensboro, North Carolina, on October 10 observed that the local Red Cross chapter had agreed to make flu masks for physicians in Greensboro, implying that local doctors were not wearing masks at the time.[59]

As the caseload worsened in Albemarle, the local board of health considered taking stringent steps to control the spread of the disease. One step that was considered but not implemented was ordering all residents to wear masks outside their homes.[60]

In Charlotte, as was true across America, the fourth Liberty Loan committee had been in the midst of its canvassing campaign to raise money to finance World War I when influenza struck. The canvassing team captains met regularly, but attendance had been poor in Charlotte. Officials worried that the fear of contracting the flu kept attendance low. Thus, at the meeting held on October 15, flu masks were handed out to each of the captains as they arrived for the meeting.[61]

Around the same time, an article from Concord, North Carolina, declared that "quite a number" of influenza masks could be seen on the streets of Concord. And that the local chapter of the Red Cross had made up a supply of them and was furnishing them to anyone who wanted a covering.[62]

A report from Charlotte on October 16 claimed the use of masks was "becoming very general in the city." Many business firms and establishments had provided masks for employees that were "to be worn throughout the day." Many residents were said to be using masks to protect against contracting the malady. "This caution is accepted by physicians and those who have had experience with grip as the most reliable preventive that has been devised."[63]

The same type of report surfaced from Asheville at the same time. A reporter sarcastically noted that "certain sections of the downtown business districts yesterday seemed to harbor premature Halloween celebrators" until it dawned on the observers that "the adults whom he saw with faces masked were taking precautions against influenza." According to the journalist, that day was the first that people in Asheville generally appeared with face coverings. "There had been many masks worn heretofore but wearers have been careful to stay close to their houses. The precautionary masks have been discarded when visits to the business districts were necessary. But it was different yesterday." Some bank tellers were wearing them. And "wearers are expected to multiply now that the ice has been broken."[64]

When a Raleigh newspaper published its list of ten commandments for preventing the flu, it mentioned masks only once, in commandment number seven, "Use masks when taking care of the sick." Rule number one advised the reader to cover each cough and sneeze with a handkerchief and to cough and sneeze toward the floor or the ground, but did not advise the reader to wear a mask.[65]

Early in November, a Kinston, North Carolina, paper published a photo of a masked face with a full-frontal view and a side view—like police mug shots. It also included detailed instructions on what material to make a mask from and how to care for it by sterilizing it regularly and marking it with a dot so the outside did not accidentally get worn next to the face. The reader was assured, in all capitals, that "IN DOING THIS THE CHANCES OF INFECTION ARE PRACTICALLY NONE."[66]

South Carolina

Dr. James A. Hayne, secretary of the South Carolina Board of Health, ordered a general quarantine against public assemblies on the afternoon of October 8 "following orders" from Surgeon General Blue in Washington. Hayne called on all sheriffs and mayors throughout his state to act promptly, seeing that all schools, churches, theaters, and cinemas were closed and all public assemblies were forbidden. Caution was also observed in preventing the overcrowding of streetcars and other conveyances. Stores and hotel lobbies were to prevent assemblies.[67]

Greenville City and County in South Carolina were placed under that order the same afternoon the statewide order was issued. The order was communicated to Sheriff Rector and County Health Officer S.J. Taylor. The sheriff immediately notified the cinemas and other places of public gathering that they would have to close. A newspaper journalist was against the move, declaring, "The desirability of closing the public schools is of doubtful utility in the presence of an epidemic." He added, "To attempt to establish quarantine now would be like raising an umbrella to avoid getting wet when up to the ears in water."[68]

South Carolina lifted the quarantine on November 3, except in a few counties where it remained. Then, early in 1919, the restrictions were reimposed in certain places. The local health board in Marion, South Carolina, reimposed the quarantine—again, the usual suspects—in the middle of January. Children were barred from school and ordered to be kept in their own homes. Visiting between families was also prohibited. A quarantine that was reimposed in the community of Woodruff at about the same time was lifted just two weeks later, on February 3, with schools reopened and church services resumed, among other things.[69]

The Red Cross made an urgent request in Sumter, South Carolina. The organization had received an order for one thousand face masks to be used all over the state by the nurses caring for patients with influenza. Mrs. W.D. Boykin of the Red Cross told the press that she had appealed to the ladies to come and help, but she had practically no response. Some days, she explained, there was no one in the local workroom except herself. Boykin moaned, "I realize that there are a great many ladies who are now forced to do their work on account of the lack of servants, but I suppose there are some who still have servants and could help with this work; even those who have to do their house work should try and do it, at least with a part of their time and help with this work. If the ladies cease to help with these war activities, we had just as well notify the Kaiser that we are ready to surrender."[70]

When Dr. H.F. White, assistant health officer in Greenville, discussed the situation on October 11, he told the press that wearing a face mask to ward off infection was a good precaution. He declared that many people who came into contact with many others were wearing masks. White commended the wisdom of those who, having to deal with people at service windows, had put gauze screens over themselves. He suggested to banks that they screen their windows or cover them with glass so that nobody could talk directly to any of the employees. He further suggested placing explanations on such screens along with the slogan "Don't spit in my face."[71]

As the situation in Spartanburg worsened, Dr. H.D. Ward, from the United States Public Health Service in Spartanburg, was called in to oversee the situation. Immediately, he ordered all soda fountains to close on October 12. On October 14, the local board of health "requested" the residents of Spartanburg to provide themselves with face masks at once. On the following day, the local Red Cross issued hundreds of those masks to the people of that community.[72]

A newspaper in Rock Hill published a brief report from Dr. C.V. Reynolds, health officer of Asheville, North Carolina. Reynolds called attention to the correct way to wear a face mask "while attending those suffering from influenza." He stated that a person who put on a mask in the morning and wore it throughout the day without changing it had a better chance of contracting the disease than someone who went without the mask because the mask collected and held the germs. It was necessary, he said, that a mask be changed several times during the day and that it should also be sprayed with a disinfectant, which was recommended by a physician.[73]

An editor with an Abbeville newspaper noted that the movie theaters were closed in his town. That meant that residents had been deprived of several installments of a serial called the *Hooded Terror*, which caused the editor to say, "There were plenty of Hooded Terrors on the streets Wednesday however after the face masks were given out and people put them on."[74]

On October 19, Secretary of the South Carolina Board of Health, Dr. J.A. Hayne, urged people who worked in groups to protect themselves from infection as much as possible by wearing gauze masks. He insisted that the masks were quickly and cheaply made and were "effective." "Clerks in stores where customers in all stages of health are constantly coming and going, and employees in public offices can easily take this step to protect themselves." According to Hayne, "A strip of gauze about six inches wide and some ten or twelve inches long can be fastened over the nose and mouth by a string or rubber band around the head, and a person is thus rendered practically safe from the germ."[75]

In mid–October, an editor noted that the local authorities of Walhalla asked the town's citizens to adopt the nose and mouth mask to stop the spread of the flu. The request "was readily complied with by a possible majority of our citizens, yet many prefer to take their chances unmasked rather than to go about looking, possibly, a bit ridiculous. We understand that the authorities have since, in co-operation with the local board of health, taken more stringent measures, substituting for their very sensible and democratic request a command in the shape of an ordinance in usual form, with penalties attaching for non-compliance on the part of citizens." The editor thought the mandating measure was appropriate.[76]

When the editor of a Greenville newspaper assessed the situation in the eastern part of the United States on December 7, he reprinted an article from the *American Journal of Public Health*. The article concluded that the prophylactic measures employed in the East were the conventional precautionary ones against infection, the face mask, and the anti-influenza vaccine. Among the curative measures advocated were open-air treatment, serum from convalescent patients, and, again, the anti-influenza vaccine. In reducing contact infection, the face mask, the staggered-hour system of transportation, education about public hygiene, and the closing of schools, assemblies, and so on have probably helped somewhat. However, he felt there was little hope of controlling the epidemic along those lines since the disease was so highly communicable. This piece offered no solutions to the problem. It concluded by saying, "Regrettable and discouraging as it is, we must nevertheless admit that in this specific catastrophe, the ambulance possibly will help more than the fence."[77]

A Columbia paper published a lengthy article on what made the Spanish flu epidemic so deadly. The article appeared in mid–December 1918, when many lockdowns and restrictions were, and would be, reimposed for a second time, or even the first time, in various parts of the nation. The article discussed the abnormal social conditions of the time—meaning world war. It featured a sketch illustration of people wearing masks. It claimed that since air infection was probably the most common method of spreading influenza, "the use of masks is based upon rational principles." However, nowhere in the article were masks mentioned as a solution.[78]

In Columbia, near the end of January 1919, Dr. Clarence Smith, a city health officer, was busy carrying out instructions from the city board of health about measures to check the further spread of the epidemic. That day alone, between 75 and 100 homes placed under quarantine were placarded. Smith said, "The Red Cross has furnished us with masks which are being provided for homes that are placarded. The attendant on the patient is to wear a mask whenever in the room with the patient; if this order is not carried out, it will become necessary to quarantine the home, prohibiting anybody from entering or exiting."[79]

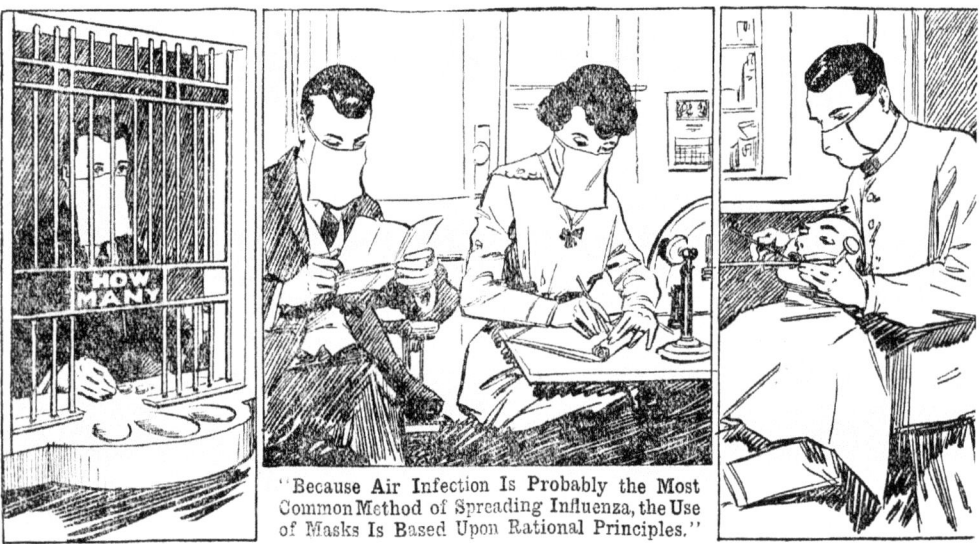

"Because Air Infection Is Probably the Most Common Method of Spreading Influenza, the Use of Masks Is Based Upon Rational Principles."

An illustration from a Columbia, South Carolina, newspaper stated that "the use of masks is based upon rational principles."

Georgia

On October 7, it was announced that for the next two months, unless otherwise ordered, churches, schools, cinemas, theaters, poolrooms, billiard halls, and dance halls in Atlanta were to remain closed to the people. Also, all vehicles carrying passengers in the city must run with the windows open "notwithstanding the temperature, except in cases of a downpour of rain." The Atlanta City Council passed the order as a precautionary measure against the further spread of influenza. The city council's action was in addition to a previous order issued earlier in the day by the health board to close all the above-listed facilities. The story claimed that Atlanta theater businesspeople expressed a "perfect willingness" to abide by the ruling. The Atlanta health officer, Dr. J.P. Kennedy, declared the disease was increasing. After consulting with Dr. Abercrombie of the Georgia Board of Health and other health officials, they deemed it best to close "such gathering places as would serve to further spread the malady." Dr. Kennedy also produced a telegram he had received from U.S. Surgeon General Rupert Blue, which asked that public gathering places be closed.[80]

On Friday, October 18, various health and public officials met. They passed a resolution that empowered the Georgia Board of Health, led by Dr. T.F. Abercrombie, to take complete charge of the situation and to issue and remove whatever regulations were needed in the various towns and counties of the state. Gainesville, Georgia, not only closed the schools and banned public gatherings but it also made a rule that crowds on streetcars had to be limited to the number of seats in the car. The College Park, Georgia, Board of Health had passed a regulation for residential quarantine that mandated "every patient with influenza must be isolated, the residence quarantined and the house fumigated at the termination of the disease." On the recommendation of Dr. C.M. Curtis, chair of the College Park Board of Health, a resolution was passed to call the attention of the state board of health "to the fact that a number of physicians consider whiskey the best remedy to be given to influenza patients, in a prostrated condition, to prevent the developing of pneumonia."[81]

As of 5 p.m. on Saturday, October 26, practically all the cinemas in Atlanta were at least two-thirds full. The movie theaters were allowed complete operation in Atlanta. Still, there were enforced restrictions on their hours of operation.[82]

Soon after that, restrictions were removed everywhere in the State of Georgia. Then, shortly after that, Georgia subjected itself to a second round of quarantines in some places. In Augusta, the city health board reestablished a quarantine closing churches, schools, cinemas, theaters, and all other public gatherings. That was done on January 11, 1919. Then, on January 31, those same authorities in Augusta ordered the quarantine to be lifted as of Saturday, February 1. All restrictions were lifted except for the schools, which were to remain closed for a time. According to the account, it had been decided to end the quarantine on the previous Saturday, "but many citizens urged that this not be done, and their counsel prevailed."[83]

When D.W. Tiedeman, a federal health officer assigned to Americus, Georgia, recommended that all residents wear flu masks during the epidemic, a news item remarked, "It is expected there will be a general patriotic compliance with the request." The recommendation was made after Dr. C.J. Williams, who was in charge of public health conditions in Macon, Georgia, stated that masks were "the best preventative" of influenza. Stephen Pace, chair of the Americus Red Cross chapter, stated that his chapter stood ready to make the masks for all who would wear them. The journalist said, "Don't be alarmed when you see your neighbor tomorrow with a gauze mask over his or her nose and mouth.... Little discomfort, it is stated, is experienced by wearers of the masks, and as soon as the custom becomes general no attention will be attracted by the wearers." The journalist added that the health authorities recommended wearing the masks as a precautionary measure and indicated that unusual precautions were being taken to try to control the spread of the disease. Helpfully for the readers, the usual instructions were provided for those who wanted to make their own. In conclusion, the reporter asserted that the authorities "have no authority to compel the people to wear gauze masks, but they strongly recommend it. Since the people want to escape influenza and live, there would seem to be no necessity for compulsion."[84]

On October 18, the Columbus, Georgia, Board of Health took stringent measures to deal with the flu. One measure was to bar carnival attractions and other amusements from the Chattahoochee Valley Fair, if it was held. Another was to order mask wearing in all stores, offices, and manufacturing plants employing more than five workers and to request that all people entering those places and the general public do likewise. A reporter remarked, "The matter of wearing masks generally is put up to the public as a matter of citizenship, and loyalty to the city, and on that grounds it is expected that a goodly portion of the local population will co-operate with the health authorities." Note that store, office, and plant workers were "ordered" to wear the masks; customers were only "requested" to do so. J.K. Hoskins, acting health officer and sanitary engineer for the U.S. Public Health Service, signed those orders.[85]

The order in Columbus took effect on October 21. The day before, an editorial appeared in one of the local papers that urged people to wear masks. Pointing out how serious the epidemic was, the reporter declared that "the board of health has issued orders in the hope that obeying them will result in the prevention of the spread of the disease. These orders make it mandatory that in certain instances persons wear gauze masks. In addition to these orders, the request is made that all persons wear them." The editor then observed that since the health board took the step because it believed that it would result in positive results for the people, "it is the duty of the people to respond uncomplainingly, and gladly. It matters not what your individual opinion may be concerning the efficacy of these masks, you should remember that you do not know everything, and that it is at least possible that this is one of the things that you do not know, and it is your duty to do whatever you are called upon to do to prevent the further spread of this disease." He acknowledged that there were differences among authorities as to what to do concerning the disease, "and the opinion is well nigh unanimous that these gauze masks will prevent the germs which are flying in the air, from being taken into the system. If they will do so, then no one should object to wearing a mask." The editor concluded, "The order concerning the wearing of masks becomes effective tomorrow morning, and it is to be hoped that everyone will comply with it immediately. Already a large number of people in the city are wearing masks, and it is to be hoped that by tomorrow morning, compliance with the order and request will become general."[86]

In College Park (GA), a similar order, but a little more drastic, was imposed around the same time. In that community, all people working in or visiting stores or public places were required to wear "medicated masks." The order meant that some antiseptic had to be applied to the face covering.[87]

It was expected on October 14 that within the coming 24 or 48 hours, the Georgia Board of Health might take "radical action" in the operation of fairs all over the state. The board of health considered the advisability of issuing an order that all people attending fairs or other gatherings in the state, not already covered by the general order of the board, be required to wear anti-influenza masks. Secretary Harry Robert of the State Fair Association called on Dr. T.F. Abercrombie, secretary of the state board of health, regarding the state fair in Macon, due to open in less than a week. "Protective measures for the safeguarding of the public, which at the same time will not preclude the operation of these fairs, were discussed" at the meeting. The state health board advised Robert to proceed based on an order to be issued requiring all people entering the fairgrounds to wear a mask. The same question was considered for the Southeastern Fair in Atlanta, which had opened a few days earlier. When Atlanta shut down all the usual suspects earlier in October, the Southeastern Fair was exempt. That had produced a good deal of adverse publicity and complaints to "higher-ups." Later the same day, October 14, the Georgia Board of Health ordered that every person entering the grounds of the Southeastern Fair wear a mask. Police officers were stationed at each gate to enforce the order.[88]

Another account in the same paper on the same day claimed that there was talk of wearing flu masks in Macon, and "several were seen on the streets yesterday. These are a piece of gauze large enough to cover the mouth and nostrils. They have been used successfully in some places." The Macon Public Health Service held a meeting, and Dr. C.L. Williams, public health officer, said, "The gauze face mask is about the best preventive we can secure and they should immediately be made."[89]

In compliance with the request of the Georgia Board of Health and the U.S. Public Health Service, Melts' Bakery, beginning on October 15, required all salespeople who came into contact with the public to wear flu masks. Proprietor J. Melts said, "I have already tried to take every precaution to protect the public from coming in contact with diseases of any kind through this bakery or through its employees and in having the young ladies who sell bread wear these masks, I feel that I am only doing my duty to them and to my customers." Melts added, "Flu masks have already proven a great preventive toward the spreading of this disease and I want to be absolutely certain that no one catches it by coming to this bakery."[90]

Gauze masks, as a preventive of Spanish influenza, along with plenty of fresh air and suitable clothing, were the edict of the Macon public health officer and city Mayor Glen Toole. In a statement given to the public and the Macon mayor, it was announced that no public places would be closed. Still, beginning on October 21, every person entering the theaters must wear a "regulation" face mask. The same regulation would govern the patrons of the state fair when it opened. Reportedly, the Macon officials were firmly of the opinion that closing places of amusement and the public schools would do nothing toward counteracting the spread of the disease, but on the other hand, they felt that keeping those places open would make it possible to enforce patrons' use of face masks. Surgical gauze was considered the best for this purpose, though cheesecloth folded twice would "answer fairly well." The face mask would affect theater employees, restaurant workers, and employees at all public gatherings. Concerning closing theaters, churches, and schools, the Macon health officials stated, "Closure of all such places have been carried out in many places attacked with influenza, apparently without appreciable modification of the epidemic. It is believed that closing would cause severe hardship upon the city without any commensurate benefit."[91]

Although the compulsory wearing of flu masks—by employees of public eating places, theaters, soda fountains, and railroad stations—did not become effective until October 21, many people in Macon were reportedly wearing them on October 18. A reporter said, "Where the masked face was a novelty a day or two ago, it is now almost as frequently encountered as the unmasked."[92]

As part of Macon's masking order to take effect on October 21, all children attending public schools in Macon were required to wear flu masks. Failure to do so would result in their being refused admission to the schools.[93]

As part of the public relations blitz of Macon newspapers to hype masks around the middle of October, it was also noted that all the telephone operators at the Macon Telephone Exchange were wearing masks and had been doing so for two weeks. "Seated at their respective posts in long lines wearing the necessary headpiece plus a white gauze mask tied around the face, they give a 'harem' impression, the veil covering all the face but the eyes and topped off by an elaborate headdress." The rest of the piece praised the phone company for the excellent care and concern they displayed to their operators regarding training, working conditions, et cetera. It was likely a paid piece inserted by the Macon phone company.[94]

When the Macon City Council met on the night of October 22, the council members wore no flu masks. Just before calling the meeting, Mayor Glen Toole observed that two newspaper reporters in attendance wore masks. A reporter said, "Not a cough or sneeze was heard throughout the session, so it is probably safe to say that no germs drifted down the throat of any city law-maker."[95]

Near the end of October, the Macon public health officer, Dr. C.L. Williams, was emphatic in his statement that the epidemic was not yet entirely under control and that the same care and vigilance had to be displayed by the citizens. Williams declared, "Stay out in the open air, avoid contact with people suffering with the malady, wear the influenza mask whenever in crowded places and keep the body suitably and comfortably clothed."[96]

In a Macon courtroom on November 6, Recorder Maynard and Health Inspector Gibson discussed whether the health department's ordinance governing flu masks required that cooks wear the masks in restaurants. The inspector asked that the sentences imposed on Jesse Stubbs and Mary Rose in police court a day earlier for not wearing the masks in a restaurant be suspended. He said he told them and several other restaurant cooks that the ordinance did not require them to wear masks in the kitchen. Recorder Maynard held that because employees at soda fountains were required to wear masks while preparing drinks, he believed it was just as necessary that the cooks wear the masks while preparing food. He agreed to suspend the sentences since the defendants had been advised not to wear the masks.[97]

The argument in the Macon court was largely moot since, on the same day, the masking rule was lifted. A reporter wrote, "Macon discarded flu masks Wednesday. The bits of medicated gauze have been so much in evidence for weeks they were decidedly 'conspicuous by their absence,' as Macon people went to work Wednesday morning." C.L. Williams, head of the health department, had lifted the order the day before. The rule had required wearing face coverings by people at public gatherings, by people serving food and drinks, and by employees of barber shops and similar places. In the future, only soldiers and those serving them must wear masks. As far as the City of Macon was concerned, the order was revoked entirely. Motion picture theaters reopened on the same day as well. They had not been subjected to a closure rule but were closed due to the inability to obtain films from the distributors.[98]

Restrictions in various parts of Georgia continued to be lifted at various times. At the end of December, Camilla, Georgia, removed the ban on church services after a closure of about two months. In Sandersville, Georgia, at the same time, the community's public schools reopened after also being subjected to a closure order for some two months.[99]

In Atlanta, Georgia, the chief surgeon at the military installation Camp Gordon wanted, on October 4, 100,000 influenza masks at once and before midnight that day, if possible. He asked the Atlanta chapter of the Red Cross to make them. Mrs. Eugene R. Black, head of the women's workrooms at the Atlanta Red Cross, said the organization had sufficient material to manufacture the masks, "so it is merely a question of securing sufficient labor," she concluded. Thus, this chapter of the Red Cross urged every woman who could help in the emergency to report for work. She explained that making the masks did not require skilled or experienced workers and that any woman would be welcome.[100]

On October 10, the Atlanta health officer, Dr. J.P. Kennedy, spoke of crowded downtown stores and suggested that those would be good places to wear the flu mask. People working in factories or shops where ventilation was not perfect were the ones who needed to exercise the most care.[101]

Although public gatherings had been shut down in Atlanta, the Southeastern Fair had been granted an exemption. However, patrons of the event had to wear masks to enter the grounds and while on the fairgrounds. Because Dr. T.F. Abercrombie's order that all visitors to the fair had to wear masks "had apparently not been understood by everybody," fair officials did not rigidly enforce the order on Tuesday. It was stated, though, that the order would be mandatory and enforced for everyone on Wednesday and for the few remaining days of the fair. Nobody would be allowed to enter the grounds or remain inside without a mask "in proper place." The Red Cross had agreed to supply the fair with 10,000 masks a day—40,000 for the remaining four days. Still, whether the organization could accomplish such a task was yet to be known. Therefore, patrons were advised to bring their masks rather than hope the Red Cross could fulfill its vast order. Helpfully, Dr. Abercrombie gave instructions on how to make a mask yourself. "Take a piece of gauze the size of a sheet of typewriter paper. Fold it twice, so that it will fit an envelope. Then attach strings to the four corners and tie these strings at the back of the neck. The mask covers the nose and mouth so that the wearer breathes through four thicknesses of gauze. A clean handkerchief is just as good as the gauze."[102]

While the fall term of the Thomas Superior Court was not held due to the flu pandemic, Judge W.E. Thomas decided to hold a grand jury session in Thomasville to clear up some cases. The grand jury was to hold its sessions in the courtroom, and all panel members were to wear flu masks. The city and county health authorities had consented to the session.[103]

Following an ordinance passed by the Manchester, Georgia, city council on October 26 that required all people in the city to wear masks until further notice, almost every person employed by the AB&A Railway walked out on strike the following morning. The workers stated they would return to work once the ordinance was repealed, declaring they could not wear the masks while at work.[104]

Florida

Beginning on October 8 and for the following ten days, the Orlando Board of Health closed all the usual suspects in Orlando, Florida. The city health officer, Dr. Sylvan McElroy, said all people with colds should remain at home. All employers were told to see that their employees with colds remained at home. The order had an immediate effect. In Orlando, it meant the cancellation of a Liberty Loan drive (these events took place all over America and were designed to have people buy government paper with the money raised by the government used to finance the war).[105]

Dr. McElroy urged residents of Orlando not to visit any of their neighbors who were ill with the flu.

He advised people to avoid overcrowding, and on Saturdays, families should let just one household member do the weekly shopping. At a city council meeting, Mayor James Giles proposed a resolution that the rest of the council unanimously accepted—that all businesses and stores had to close no later than 5 p.m. each day, except for Saturday, when they could be open until 6 p.m. Those stores and businesses could not open before 7 a.m. each morning.[106]

Effective October 9 in Tampa, the Tampa Board of Health closed down the usual suspects. There were to be no public gatherings indoors. The order came as a suggestion from the Florida Board of Health. People were requested not to congregate in buildings in "large numbers." In a city council session in which Tampa physicians debated the closure order, Dr. Bartlett emphatically declared himself against the partial shutdown, contending that stores, cigar factories, and all public eating places afforded as many opportunities for transmission of the disease as did the places specified to be shut down. Dr. Atlee agreed. But their appeals went unheeded, with only the usual suspects of schools, churches, and all places of public amusement being ordered to close.[107]

As part of the measures to control the spread of the flu, the Tampa Fire Department, in cooperation with the city's board of health, on the afternoon of October

19, sprinkled two downtown streets, Franklin Street and Seventh Avenue, with disinfectants, said to be a "carbolic acid mixture." As chair of the city health board, Mayor Donald McKay proclaimed that cigar factories were not to open before 7 a.m. and to close no later than 4 p.m. Restrictions were lifted not long after, with Tampa schools reopening on Monday, the 11th of November.[108]

Dr. J.W. Shisler, Miami health officer, and Dr. H.C. Babcock, president of the Miami Board of Health, announced on October 9 that schools, theaters, and other amusement places would remain closed for the present. Members of the city's ministerial association voted to close the local churches on Sunday and to close all church services during the remainder of the week. Shisler advised that all nurses handling flu cases should wear gauze masks, or "helmets."[109]

Shisler ordered all churches, schools, theaters, the YMCA, lodges, and dance halls to close and forbid any mass meetings on October 9 as a preventive measure in the fight against influenza. The theaters and schools had previously been closed at the request of the city's board of health. Still, the order of October 9 was mandatory and affected other gatherings not included in the request. The mandatory order also included funerals and weddings. Other Florida cities that had imposed the standard "[Rupert] Blue Public Gathering Protocols" at about the same time included Jacksonville, Pensacola, St. Augustine, West Palm Beach, St. Petersburg, and "many other communities."[110]

In Miami, Mayor John W. Watson issued a more drastic order on October 23, shortening business hours and closing down all businesses overnight except drugstores. Under the order, no store or business establishment could open before 9 a.m. and had to close no later than 4 p.m. Restaurants could open at 6 a.m. and had to close no later than 6 p.m. Also exempted were the ice plants and the offices of professional men. Even pressed into service were the Boy Scouts of Miami. One or more scouts were placed in each restaurant to ensure that all dishes and utensils were adequately cleaned and sterilized. They also saw that none of the dining rooms were "crowded." The scouts were tasked with asking crowds they might see on the streets and elsewhere to disperse.[111]

Then, beginning on October 28, business hours, with a few exceptions, returned to normal. The Miami Board of Health took action to that effect at its meeting on October 26. Soda fountains had to remain closed, pool rooms had to close at 6 p.m., and theaters and amusement places had to remain shuttered. The board of health learned and decided at the meeting that the compressed business hours did little except lead to store congestion—something the board of health sought to avoid. Dr. Shisler was empowered to enforce the no loitering rule in stores and was told to call in the police and the Boy Scouts. "Loafing" in cigar stores and other places would not be tolerated, and Shisler was empowered to close any premises that allowed loitering.[112]

On the evening of October 30, another dramatic change in Miami occurred when the city board of health decided that, beginning November 1, business in Miami could return to normal. They removed all restrictions except in the "colored town," where everything remained closed until further notice, thanks to the health board. The reason for that decision, said the board of health, lay in the fact that the epidemic did not hit the black part of town until about a week after it hit the white part of town.[113]

Winter Park, Florida, Mayor Walter H. Schultz proclaimed on October 10 at the direction of the Florida Board of Health to immediately close all public meetings for ten days—that included the usual suspects. Schultz also requested that all parents prevent their children from "promiscuous visiting from house to house." He suggested that, while each family remained as much as possible in the open air, they be prevented from congregating in groups. The churches of Winter Park had also decided to close for one Sunday, at least, to show their willingness to aid in any way possible. The other establishments were mandated to close, while churches were requested to shut down.[114]

Jacksonville, Florida, reported on October 24 that all restrictions that were in place in the city, mainly the closure of the usual suspects, would be lifted as of Sunday, October 27.[115]

A Miami newspaper published a photo of a Boston police officer wearing a mask. It was a well-used shot that appeared in newspapers around America, mainly in October. The caption told of the 1,700 masks issued to the Boston police force. The photo was always the same, but the caption differed from place to place. The caption in Miami, as in virtually all the captions used in America, left the distinct impression that every officer in Boston wore a mask during every hour of every shift. In reality, the Boston officer was only required to wear it when doing ambulance work or dealing directly with a person ill with influenza.[116]

The Tampa Electric Company provided their employees with bottles of antiseptics such as glyco thymoline, pinoleum, and Lysol soap. Two female workers in the office had been kept busy making gauze face masks that were being furnished to all the firm's employees and to a few outside friends, together with an antiseptic solution for the masks. Bottles of antiseptic gargle were also distributed to the staff.[117]

Among the new restrictions to take effect in Tampa cigar factories on October 21 was one mandating that windows in plants be kept open, with the cigar workers being cautioned against coughing, sneezing, and spitting on the floor. Members of the Rotary Club were to be placed as inspectors in the factories and were given police powers to see that the regulations were enforced. The idea of forcing the cigar workers to wear gauze masks had temporarily been abandoned. Still, all cigar makers were advised to take that precaution during their work. Tampa Mayor McKay said he would get an opinion from City Attorney Wall. If it could be done, orders would be issued for all people to wear masks on the streets, in stores, or in public places.[118]

According to an account in a Tampa newspaper on October 21, "Gauze masks made their appearance in large numbers today. Street car conductors, clerks, city officials, and persons whose work brings them in contact with the public were particularly prominent with this protection."[119]

A couple of days after the Rotarians were appointed special sanitary officers with police powers to enforce regulations concerning the cigar factories, the group made its first report to Tampa Mayor McKay. "It has also seemed to us that if some plan could be devised for getting the employees to wear masks a considerable amount of danger would be eliminated," said the report. "We understand that this matter has been under consideration by the health authorities possibly, from the practical standpoint, it could not be worked out. This, too, would have to be a general order to be at all effective."[120]

A small ad in a Tampa newspaper on November 5 for the Elks' Barber Shop under the headline "Safety First!" declared, "The Elks' Barber Shop is the place where you can get your work done in perfect safety. All Barbers are wearing the up-to-date Sanitary Masks used and suggested by the National Red Cross Association."[121]

At the end of the American Public Health Association convention in Chicago on December 12, a Tampa paper reported that the organization expected to develop measures to control the disease if it should return. This summary stated, "Not all the health officers attending the meeting favor the face mask or vaccination, but there are said to be among the measures likely to receive approval. The question of whether it is best, or even necessary, to close schools and public assemblies to prevent the spread of influenza is to be decided and wide differences of opinion have been expressed regarding these subjects."[122]

When a different Tampa newspaper presented its summary of the event, it noted that the group could not develop a definite plan for fighting influenza because of divergent views. The paper also noted that the divergent views tended to pit urban health professionals against rural ones. Its headline for the piece was "Quarantine and use of masks ridiculed as flu preventives."[123]

The Florida Board of Health was represented at the Chicago convention, held from December 9 to 12. On January 17, 1919, it presented its summary of the American Public Health Association gathering. Concerning masks, the report declared, "The wearing of proper masks in a proper manner should be made compulsory in hospitals and for all who are directly exposed to infection. It should be made compulsory for barbers, dentists, etc." It continued by observing, "The evidence before the committee as to beneficial results consequent upon the enforced wearing of masks by the entire population at all times was contradictory, and it has not encouraged the committee to suggest the general adoption of the practice. Persons who desire to wear masks, however, in their own interests, should be instructed as to how to make and wear proper masks, and encouraged to do so."[124]

6

East South Central

Alabama

At a full meeting, the Dallas County Medical Society ruled to close all public gatherings indefinitely, which involved all the usual places shuttered under the Rupert Blue Protocols throughout the county, including in the county seat of Selma, Alabama. The shutdown was effective on October 10, including the schools. Two weeks later, Spright Dowell, Alabama state superintendent of education, stated that the attorney general's department had ruled that school boards could pay teachers locked out of their classrooms.[1]

The first fine in Montgomery police court for violating one of the restrictive rules came on October 29, when John Service was found guilty of violating the rule against selling soft drinks during the flu epidemic and called on to pay a fine of one dollar.[2]

Following an executive session on October 29 in Birmingham involving the county board of health and the Birmingham city commissioners, the restrictions placed on the city in early October were removed. As of October 31, Birmingham theaters and cinemas could open, department stores could advertise bargain sales, religious services could be held on Sunday, November 3, and public gatherings could once again take place.[3]

As November began, Selma debated whether to remove its quarantine in light of Birmingham's reopening. There was a split among the doctors of Selma, with some in favor of retaining the restrictions and others ready to remove them. Practically all the schools in the state, which had been closed for several weeks, reopened on November 4. Only a few schools in isolated communities remained closed.[4]

At a meeting of the Montgomery County Health Bureau on December 6, a call was made for a referendum to hold a mass meeting on reimposing the quarantine in Montgomery. Some doctors at the meeting argued in favor of a reimposition, while others opposed such a move. A suggestion was also made that a rigid quarantine for individuals suffering from the disease might be a better way to proceed. A few days later, it was expected that further agitation for the reimposition of the flu quarantine in Montgomery would cease following Rupert Blue's statement, "The country need not fear that the influenza epidemic will return. It has come and gone for good."[5]

When "milder measures" failed to check the spread of the disease in Roanoke, Alabama, the city council, after two sessions on October 21, decided to require all people living in the city to wear anti-influenza masks when away from their premises. "This precautionary measure is considered one of the best known and at the same time one that interferes least with the freedom of the citizens and the on-going of regular business," wrote a journalist. "While the new regulation is objectionable in the respects that it obscures the smiles of the fair sex and interferes with the chewing and smoking proclivities of 'mere men,' yet it is being cheerfully adopted for the most part." Failure to comply with the ordinance subjected the violator to a fine of up to $100.[6]

Dr. Carl A. Grote, the Huntsville health officer, was one of the many health professionals who attended the American Public Health Association convention in Chicago from December 9 to 12. Grote said he was one of over one thousand other health officers in attendance. The only thing they agreed upon at the convention was that no one knew much about the disease. Two conclusions were reached: the cause was unknown, and no effective measures for prevention were available. Concerning closures, Grote noted that data at the convention indicated that, in large cities, there was just as much influenza where they closed the usual suspects as where they did not close them. And Grote added, "Masks are theoretically good, but of little practical value."[7]

Dr. J.D. Dowling was the health officer for Birmingham, Alabama, as well as the county health officer for surrounding Jefferson County. Reportedly, several people were seen on the streets that day wearing masks made of gauze over their mouths and noses, which Dr. Dowling said was a very good thing for them to do.[8]

"Wear a gauze mask. This is the request health authorities are making of every one for co-operation in eliminating influenza from Birmingham." That's how a reporter started his article for the December 6 issue of a Birmingham newspaper. Dr. J.D. Dowling, city and county health officer, was convinced that with the "hearty co-operation of every citizen," Birmingham's influenza could soon be reduced "to a minimum." Dowling said, "We are convinced that the wearing of a simple gauze face mask is the most practical and efficient general method to limit the spread of influenza." He noted that "some cities have undertaken to enforce this by law, but we feel that the people of this district need only to be called upon to wear these masks and it will be done more thoroughly than if an effort were made to enforce such a regulation by police methods." And he added, "A person wearing one of these masks not only enjoys almost absolute protection, but the added satisfaction of knowing that he is not dangerous to his neighbor. It is suggested that the masks be exchanged for fresh ones at intervals of several hours, but a soiled mask is far better than none at all." Dowling concluded, "If enough people will wear face coverings during the next few days there will be no occasion to interfere with the normal activities of life."[9]

A day later, it was acknowledged that Dowling and other authorities were under pressure in Birmingham to close the schools. Those authorities' position was that the benefits obtained from closing the schools would not justify the cost. Dowling continued to argue that the most productive method in the fight against the epidemic was the gauze mask, a practical and effective safeguard. The health department believed masks should be worn in all places of public assembly, on streetcars, and elsewhere.[10]

BOUND AND GAGGED?–NO, SHE IS WARDING OFF INFLUENZA GERMS

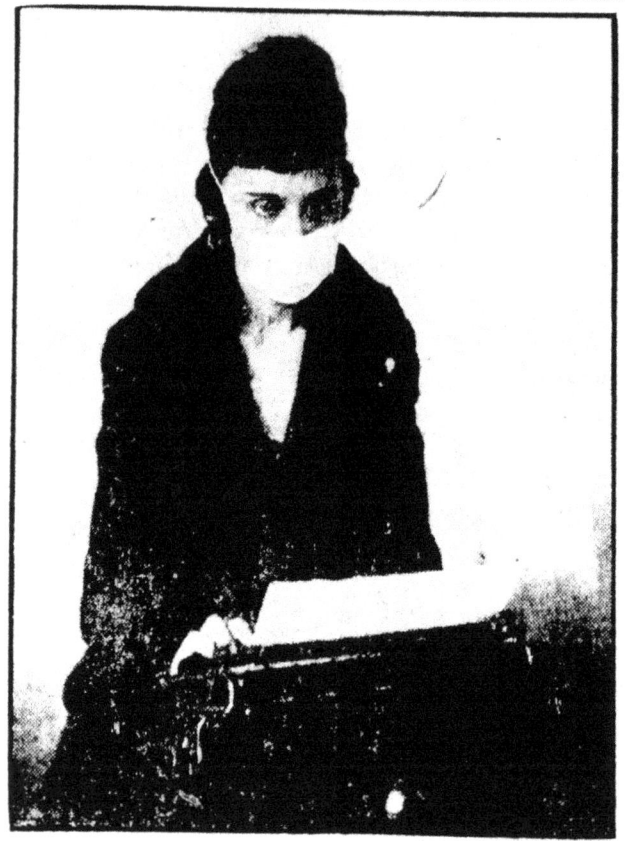

This Birmingham girl is an advocate of preparedness and is wearing the gauze mask suggested by health authorities to help ward off influenza as she goes about her daily duties. It looks rather "haremesque," but an influenza germ is said to grow frightened, to duck and to run every time it sees one of these masks.

A Birmingham, Alabama, woman models a mask for her fellow residents to set an example and show that she had prepared herself for any possible attack by an influenza bug. Health officials in her city urged people to don masks, although the caption on the photograph admitted the young woman looked "haremesque."

One more day later, and the same Birmingham paper published on page one a photo of an unnamed Birmingham woman at work with her typewriter—masked. The tongue-in-cheek caption declared she looked "rather haremesque, but an influenza germ is said to grow frightened, to duck and to run every time it sees one of these masks."[11]

As December dragged on, rumors continued to make the rounds that Birmingham might have to adopt a law mandating wearing face masks. Dowling told a meeting that he had received a telegram from San Francisco authorities advising him that officials there had made wearing masks compulsory and that it was believed the measure was better "than closing up business."[12]

At another meeting, Dowling again argued that wearing gauze masks could accomplish more in combating influenza than a closing order. When he made that pitch before the Jefferson County Medical Society, it endorsed a resolution by the board of health to keep the city open during the second wave of the disease.[13]

On December 15, J.R. Hornady, Birmingham commissioner of health and education, in discussing precautions taken against the flu, asserted, "To enter a room where someone is ill with influenza without wearing a mask is like jumping overboard at sea without putting on a life preserver."[14]

Mississippi

Following the Rupert Blue Protocols, Jackson, Mississippi, closed down the usual suspects on October 8. Jackson Health Officer H.F. Magee issued the order, acting under the instructions of Dr. W.S. Leathers, executive officer of the Mississippi Board of Health. And he was acting on the instructions "recommended" to him by U.S. Public Health Service Surgeon General Blue.[15]

Dr. C.F. Carter, Attala County health officer, ordered the closure of several small communities' business houses and all county stores on October 17. They were to remain closed until further notice from him. He also prohibited all public gatherings. It came to the reporter's attention that the neighbors were neglecting people in the county who had influenza. He felt that was wrong: "People should wait upon each other even at the risk of being infected themselves, because it is their Christian duty to do so." He urged his readers to use masks when in the sick room.[16]

Speculation circulated on October 21 that restrictions would be lifted in Mississippi, probably within ten days, except in a few communities, according to Dr. W.S. Leathers, executive officer of the Mississippi Board of Health. Meridian had passed an ordinance that all businesses close at 6 p.m. The only exception was drugstores. Loitering on the streets in Meridian had also "almost been forbidden."[17]

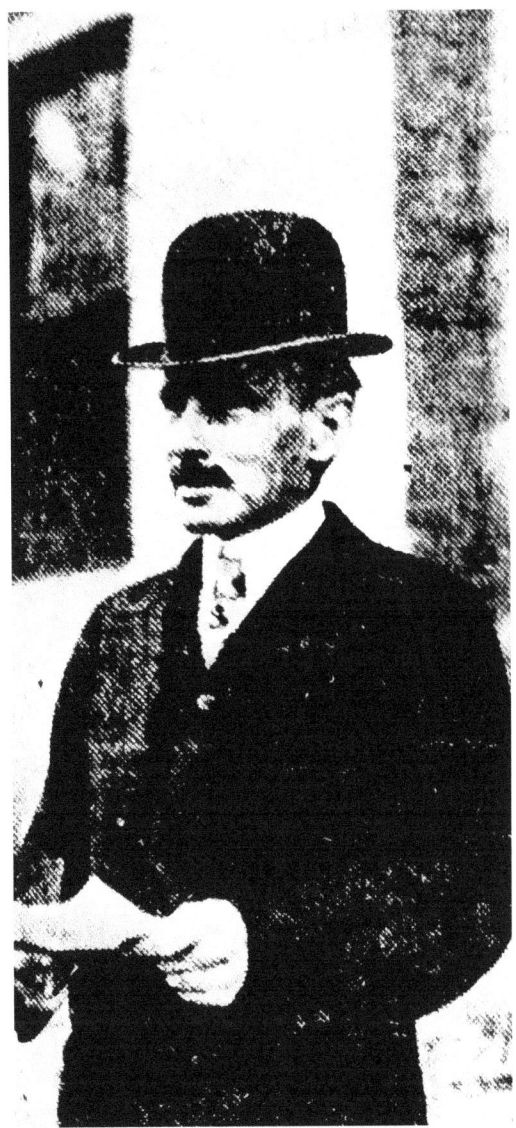

J.R. Hornady, Birmingham, Alabama Commissioner of Health and Education, was a big advocate of masks. He compared entering a flu patient's room unmasked to being "like jumping overboard at sea without putting on a life preserver."

Following a state and city health authority conference on the morning of October 25, the quarantine in Jackson was extended for at least another week. It was a decision said to be almost unanimous. In the end, the restrictions were lifted entirely in Hinds County (of which Jackson was the county seat) on November 8.[18]

After 6 a.m. on Monday, October 21, no person was allowed to appear on the streets of Vidalia, Mississippi, or in the stores or saloons without wearing a flu mask.

The penalty for violation of the law was a fine of ten dollars or a 30-day jail sentence. The Vidalia town council passed the order on the evening of October 18. The ordinance also provided that the conductors of all trains would be notified, as well as the Natchez and Vidalia Ferry Company, so that passengers whose destination was Vidalia could be warned. Guards were to be posted at entry points to the city to see that the order was obeyed. According to the article, "The passage of this ordinance is in accordance with the recommendation of Surgeon General Blue and is only a matter of precaution." That statement was false. Blue never advocated using face masks, except for attendants in the sick room.[19]

On October 15, a Biloxi newspaper published an article that outlined the U.S. Public Health Service's thoughts, as many newspapers across America did. It contained no advice about masks, and people were advised to wear them only in the sick room while attending to one of the victims of the Spanish influenza epidemic. Even then, the advice was hardly dramatic: "Nurses and attendants will do well to guard against breathing in dangerous disease germs by wearing a simple fold of gauze or mask while near the patient."[20]

In December, an editor with a Jackson paper remarked that there was "no cause for alarm." He stated that "the *Daily News* is inclined to agree with a majority of the business and professional men of the city that the municipal authorities acted rather hastily in issuing a closing order to check the spread of Spanish influenza." The type of disease was mild, the death rate was low, and he said it "does not appear that the situation is of sufficient gravity to warrant drastic action." He concluded that "since one radical step has already been taken [first closure order], and others are contemplated, it is to be hoped that the health authorities will quit guessing and base future actions on actual knowledge of conditions." He made no mention of masks whatsoever.[21]

Tennessee

The Tennessee Board of Health, on the morning of October 7, advised all cities and towns "where influenza is prevalent" to close cinemas, theaters, and all nonessential places of public gathering and to close schools and churches if the situation called for such action.[22]

Knoxville imposed its closure orders at midnight on October 9. Dr. W.R. Cochrane, Knoxville director of health, said orders would not affect public meetings solely for "patriotic purposes," such as Liberty Loan drives and Red Cross meetings, all in furtherance of the war effort. Cochrane also requested the Knoxville Railway and Light Company open a window at the front and rear ends of streetcars to increase the ventilation, and said, "an occasional laxative is also suggested."[23]

Chattanooga imposed its shutdown on October 8. H.D. Huffaker, commissioner of education and health, issued a statement in which he warned the parents of the schoolchildren to keep them off the street, or they would be taken into custody. Police divided the city into five areas and assigned an officer to each district. Those police officers were tasked with doing an inspection tour of all the department stores, hotels, restaurants, and other public places. Each of those establishments was ordered to have all the windows kept open during the day and to have floors and cuspidors properly fumigated twice daily. Businesses violating that rule would be ordered to close their stores until after the epidemic was over.[24]

City, county, and state health authorities in Nashville decided to lift the imposed restrictions on Friday, November 2. One month later, speaking at a Nashville Engineering Association meeting, C.A. Derivaux of the U.S. Public Health Service addressed the association on the flu epidemic in Nashville and pointed out that "the recent results showed that the much practiced system of quarantining had proved a failure."[25]

Tennessee, like many other states, found itself reimposing closure orders after the first wave of the disease passed through. By then, the local health authorities, such as the city or county, usually imposed closure orders here and there, rather than the state stepping in for statewide restrictions. Charleston, Tennessee, imposed a second wave quarantine on itself on January 21, 1919, and then removed all the restrictions on February 3.[26]

Reportedly, Tuesday, October 15, was the first day flu masks appeared on Knoxville streets. However, reports from other cities claimed that they had been widely adopted. Red Cross nurses and nurses' aides had used masks when caring for sick soldiers quartered in the city, as had members of households where cases of the flu were being nursed. A reporter described the scene this way: "They're wearing 'em! At first the general public wasn't quite sure that they'd guessed right, but after seeing one elderly lady and two or three young girls on Gay Street peeping as demurely over gauze flu masks as an Oriental maiden peeps over her veil, they remembered that flu masks had been prescribed as a preventative for Spanish influenza."[27]

In mid–March 1919, when health authorities were worried about the number of cases then observed, the Tennessee Board of Health appealed to its citizens to follow four simple rules in combating the disease. Only rule number three mentioned masks, and that was only in the context that physicians should wear one when they attended flu patients.[28]

A Knoxville paper got into the celebrity game when it published a photo of a famous American woman wearing a flu mask and invited the reader to identify her. The text talked about the problems of identifying masked family and friends and said that "wearing of the epidemic masks in hundreds of cities provided a national test of the sharpness of the American's perceptions. And in unnumbered cases, it proved that, with the concealment of but one feature, intimate friends might pass one another unrecognized." At the end of the brief article, it was revealed that the woman in the mask was acting superstar of the era Mary Pickford.[29]

In Chattanooga, just after the lockdown was imposed, a brief report observed that soldiers coming into town from the nearby military installation wore white masks over their mouths and noses by order from their superiors. The journalist said, "Strangers getting on the [street]cars, especially at the terminal station, are made to wonder what is the matter with the soldier boys, as the long rows of khaki-clad boys present a rather peculiar sight with their noses and mouths covered up." The title of the piece was "Looks like gas masks."[30]

Before noon on Friday, October 11, white gauze masks by the thousands appeared in Chattanooga. Hotel clerks, servers, bellhops, employees in soft drink establishments, drug stores, public eating places, restaurants, elevator operators, clerks in the stores, and all people coming into contact with the public were wearing gauze masks. City and federal health officials took the step Friday morning. Everyone from the graduate druggist to the hotel bellhop was ordered to wear Red Cross masks. The order came after a conference with Dr. Ben Brown, the health director; Health Commissioner H.D. Huffaker; and Dr. C.P. Knight. Brown recommended that the step be taken at once. The local health officials immediately approved it, and the inspectors started at once in automobiles and on foot through the city's business section, warning all managers of public places to obtain face coverings for their workers. In speaking of that precaution, Brown stated that it

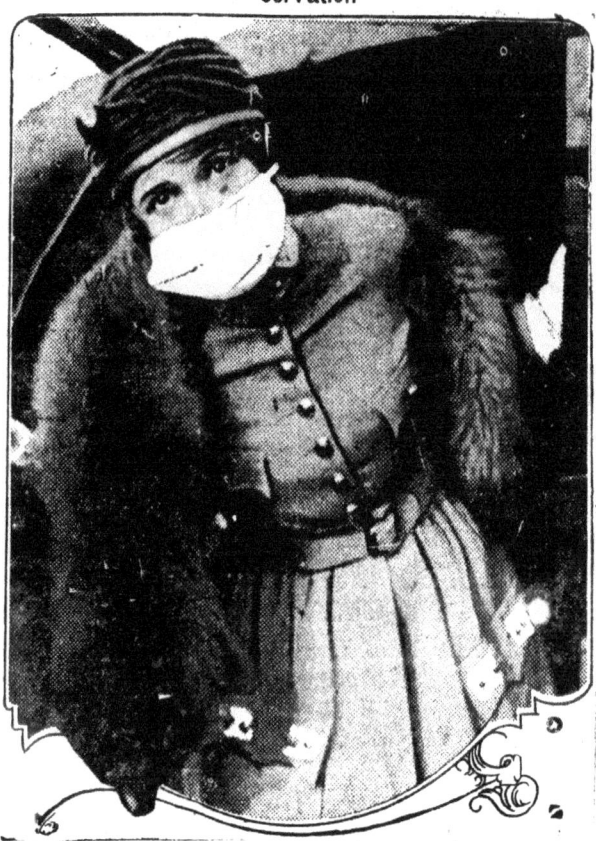

One of America's most widely known women, wearing "flu" mask. Do you recognize her? See last paragraph of story for her identity.

This newspaper featured a quiz for its readers. The goal was to guess which celebrity was hidden behind the mask—and, of course, to sell the public on the idea of masking up. The celebrity was a superstar actor of the era, Mary Pickford.

was being carried out throughout the East and that many southern cities had taken it up. Brown even supplied instructions on how to wear the mask, noting that it should be put on perfectly dry and without any medical solution. "The mask when used properly prevents any germ from passing through it to the nose or mouth."[31]

With virtually no lead time from the issuance of the order to its implementation, the situation was hopeless for those in Chattanooga looking for a mask. Many businesspeople came into the health authority offices to get masks for their employees, only to be told they would have to get the women in their employ to make them. All department stores were advised they would have to make the face coverings they needed in their stores. However, the health authorities promised to give them a sample copy of a face mask to use as a model if they needed one. The Red Cross workroom was inadequate, although they made as many as possible. According to the press, elevator operators and Western Union messengers wore masks even at that early date, and "most everybody on the streets were masked."[32]

Every barber shop in Chattanooga was ordered to close for the day on Saturday, October 12. When they reopened on Monday, they were still required to wear masks. Reportedly, people were "eagerly availing themselves of the opportunity to wear the gauze masks." The previous day, a hundred people waited within the walls of the Red Cross workrooms, asking for masks. "The crowd became so dense that it was necessary to call a policeman to disperse them." A police officer was later sent to the establishment, where he limited the number of people admitted to the workroom to no more than five or six people. "The wearers and the would-be wearers are not confined to the waiters and other classes named by the health authorities, but masked persons are seen everywhere on the streets, in the elevators, and the stores, and many who have no masks, constantly carry their handkerchiefs before their mouths as a protection."[33]

As many other newspapers did, a Chattanooga paper published the Rupert Blue advice on the flu from the U.S. Public Health Service. The Chattanooga Railway & Light Company paid for the ad, which made this one different.[34]

Dr. Brown requested that Chattanooga merchants mask clerks. Health officials scheduled a later meeting to explain the reasons for the request to the merchants, and the health officials were optimistic the merchants would cooperate with the authorities to defeat the epidemic. A journalist noted, "The mask question is still eliciting some comment from local physicians, one of whom quotes the medical journal as saying that masks made of gauze are more dangerous than protective." Dr. Knight advised against medicating the masks. A practice said to be increasing in popularity. "One man appeared on Market Street yesterday wearing a mask that bore unmistakable evidence of having been thoroughly soaked with Vick's croup salve. The odor was noticeable at some distance, and the mask presented a distinctly unsanitary appearance."[35]

On October 18, patrons at the Chattanooga Market House found the stall operators there to be devoid of face coverings, although they had previously worn masks for days. Many stall operators declared the masks were much worse than the flu. Market master Andy Ware was the first to appear masked and then the first to appear without a mask. Ware said the mask gave him a terrible headache.[36]

When a Chattanooga paper covered the end of the Chicago convention of the American Public Health Association in December, it gave a more biased account than most. It featured the fact that Dr. E.C. Rosenow of the Mayo Brothers lab in Minnesota declared that 90 percent of all flu deaths were preventable if they had just used his vaccine, which was worthless. Nobody ever got good results using it except him, and he was selling it on that basis and making money for himself and the Mayo Brothers. This news account also featured Dr. Woods Hutchinson, a syndicated columnist who insisted that the pandemic would vanish from America if everybody wore a mask for seven days.[37]

Kentucky

The Kentucky Board of Health, on the evening of October 6, issued a proclamation closing all the establishments mentioned in the Rupert Blue Protocols. Gatherings of all kinds were banned, including gatherings on street corners. People were also prohibited from visiting each other's homes. The health board "discouraged" all unnecessary travel and social visiting. Dr. John G. South, president of the Kentucky Board of Health, and Dr. J.N. McCormack, secretary of the Kentucky Board of Health, signed the order.[38]

One month later, the statewide restrictions were modified, to some extent, in some areas. Church services were permitted in Jefferson and Warren counties and Mayfield in Graves County. Theaters and schools in those same areas could reopen. Restrictions in all other counties remained in place. As the flu conditions in their areas improved, upon the application of county health authorities to the state board of health, they would be modified. The restrictions of enforced closure against soda fountains and saloons, which had to close at 6:30 p.m., remained in force.[39]

Most of those restrictions disappeared over the first few weeks of November in Kentucky. However, like other states in America, Kentucky found itself reimposing the rules in some cases. Due to the reappearance of influenza in Kirksville (Madison County) and its vicinity, health officials on December 1 ordered an immediate reimposition of the closure orders, shutting down the usual suspects of schools and churches.[40]

Richmond, also in Madison County, reimposed its quarantine at the start of 1919. Those rules were rigidly observed at the city's Opera House on January 6, when Hugh Dargavel was appointed special usher with the responsibility to see that every other seat was left unoccupied. Patrons were there to see the latest Douglas Fairbanks film, and, it was said, all who attended had read the regulations in the newspaper and seemed desirous of cooperating.[41]

In Murray, Kentucky, six of the town's citizens found a man guilty of violating public health ordinances on January 29, 1919, and fined him $100. He defended himself by declaring the law had no right to close the church, and he intended to defy it. The prosecutor noted that all the other churches in Murray had complied with the closing order. The trial, while public, was held before only the officials and witnesses—no public gatherings were allowed under the rules.[42]

On October 19, the Kentucky Board of Health in Paris, Kentucky, issued an order requiring all barbers to wear influenza masks while serving their customers and all soft drink outlets to close from 6:30 p.m. Saturday until 6:30 a.m. Sunday, and every day thereafter.[43]

Dr. J.S. Locke was the health officer for Mason County. Near the end of October, he advised the public about the flu epidemic. Locke stressed that it was a crowd disease and that crowds should be avoided. He did not comment on masks except to say, "Wear a well adjusted mask if you must go into possibly infected places, and wash the hands and face and cleanse the nose and throat with a warm salt solution as soon as you get home. Physicians and nurses should be even more exacting about these precautions, changing and boiling the mask every two or three hours."[44]

In the wake of the American Public Health Association convention ending on December 12 in Chicago, the editor of an Owensboro, Kentucky, paper published his thoughts. He noted that it was a stormy convention, with the doctors not agreeing, even among themselves, as to what, if anything, could and should be done to stop the epidemic. "The health commissioner of Detroit said that closing public schools, theatres, and schools was useless and that the wearing of masks was an evidence of foolishness. Others took the opposite view, and said that there was no way to stop it except by commingling of crowds." Thus, some favored closures, while others opposed them. Given such confusion and disagreement among the medical profession, this editor concluded, "In view of this disagreement of those supposed to be experts in matters of health, would it not be a good idea for the people to take the matter into their own hands. Quit talking and thinking about influenza, and it will not reach you."[45]

A Louisville editor expressed skepticism over face coverings in an October 29 editorial. He observed that no accurate comparisons had been made concerning masks; thus, their efficacy was unknown. In particular, he cited San Francisco, which was in the news all around America due to its harsh and vindictive policies about masking. The editor said, "Assuredly the compulsory wearing of masks involves hardships and inconvenience hardly warrantable unless it can be shown that definite results are obtainable." Louisville had no mask ordinance, nor did they push the idea onto the public.[46]

A very early newspaper account that appeared on October 1 featured a reporter who remarked that in Lexington, thousands of people that day donned "anti-influenza 'gas' masks" as the epidemic began to appear and spread in Kentucky.[47]

Lexington Health Officer Furlong gave permission at the beginning of November for a football game to be played at the city's Stoll Field between Lexington High School and Somerset High School, on condition that all the spectators wore influenza masks. The game drew 3,000 fans. Police were on hand to see that no one without a mask was admitted.[48]

7

West South Central

Louisiana

As of midnight on October 9, New Orleans was placed under the usual restrictions when the city and state health authorities imposed the Rupert Blue Protocols. Churches, theaters, business colleges, schools, and poolrooms were all shut down as of the next day. Public meetings were also forbidden. Streetcars were limited to a carrying capacity of two people per seat. No sporting events, concerts, or street crowds were to be permitted. The original program provided for saloons and soda fountains to close. However, the health board granted a respite to those businesses on the grounds that closing all other amusement places would reduce the number of people frequenting saloons and soft drink parlors. Streetlights were turned off early in the downtown section to prevent the gathering of crowds. "Move on" commands were freely given by police officers. Retail merchants agreed to release employees in three groups, staggering hours to help reduce crowding. A similar quarantine was imposed on the Louisiana communities of Pineville and Alexandria on October 7.[1]

A brief editorial appeared in a Shreveport paper near the start of November. The journalist pointed out that the city and state health authorities disagreed about responsibility for the flu restrictions imposed. Disagreements "show pretty clearly that some are ashamed of it. But, who is to pay the losses." The reporter pointed out what few others ever mentioned: the pervasive arguments between state and local health authorities as each tried to push any blame onto the other. It was pretty standard for the state to step in at the start of October and impose statewide restrictions (where the state had such power) but then back away in a week or so, leaving the restrictions in place but leaving it to county or city and local authorities to decide about when to remove them or reimpose them. If the state was all-knowing regarding blanket impositions, why was it not all-knowing when removing such quarantines?[2]

Health authorities set the reopening date for cinemas, theaters, schools, and all other places of amusement for Saturday, November 16. After a conference between Dr. G.M. Corput of the United States Public Health Service, Dr. Oscar Dowling of the Louisiana Board of Health, and Dr. W.H. Robin, superintendent of New Orleans City Health, as well as about 20 city and parish health officers from many parts of Louisiana, the reopening was announced. Many of the health officers were opposed to allowing indoor places to reopen as long as one percent of the population was suffering from influenza.³

On the morning of October 23, every Bell Telephone Company operator in Shreveport was presented with a gauze mask and instructed to always wear it while on duty. It was compulsory. Also, some post office employees in the city had been equipped with masks. Then, claimed a reporter, "Experiments have proven this method of precaution a great aid in avoiding the disease, and in some of the larger cities, as many as 3,000 employees of a single concern are compelled to wear them at all times. Boards of health have recommended the flu masks, and their use has already become almost universal."⁴

Also, in Shreveport, to prevent contagion among workers, members of the Home Health Volunteers, Mrs. J.E. Hews and Mrs. J.A. Lupa, advised all group members and their helpers that they should wear masks while they went about their duties. Dr. G.C. Chandler, president of the board of health, advocated the measure and saw it as a valuable precaution that people wear masks when on downtown duties in stores and streetcars.⁵

After being in force for one day, Monroe, Louisiana, modified the order closing businesses except from 9 a.m. to noon and from 2 p.m. to 5 p.m. After that, business hours were from 8 a.m. to 5 p.m. The parish council of defense, the mayor of Monroe, and the city board of health also requested that people in stores who served the public wear masks.⁶

"Flu masks are doomed" was the headline of a New Orleans article on October 29, based on the statement of Dr. G.M. Corput of the United States Public Health Service. He had said that masks "are harmful to the wearers, in that they prevent the free breathing of fresh air, essential at this time, and that they do not keep out the germs." Servers and other employees in most New Orleans restaurants and soda fountain establishments set aside the masks they had been wearing when they became aware of the remarks made by Corput. He also said that no orders had come from his agency regarding the use of masks. Captain P.H. Bingham, who oversaw sanitation for the U.S. Army in New Orleans, had issued the order. He arrived in person at the U.S. Public Health Service office in New Orleans and announced that he would put the order into effect. All establishments with a sanitary card in the city were affected. Bingham's order compelled every employee of such a place to wear a mask at all times while on duty. In the case of a violation, an establishment stood to lose its sanitary card, which meant a shutdown of the business. Very shortly after that disagreement, Bingham was "reassigned." It was then understood that all health measures would be placed under Corput's direction. Dr. Oscar Dowling said the Louisiana Board of Health had not ordered flu masks. Given the evidence, the doctor declared he did not see why the masks had ever been worn.⁷

On the eve of November 16, when all restrictions in Louisiana were lifted, a reporter gleefully said, "A new relic may be placed on the uppermost shelf of the family 'what-not.' The article is a folded strip of gauze, and a careful examination will prove it to be an influenza mask."⁸

Arkansas

In Arkansas, a drastic quarantine became effective wherever Spanish influenza "has appeared." The Arkansas Board of Health issued the standard Rupert Blue Protocols at noon on October 7. Among other items was a prohibition on the congregation of people in private homes. Enforcement of the order began that day in Pulaski and Lonoke Counties. In Lonoke, Dr. J.C. Geiger, who was in charge of the United States Public Health Service, and his assistants enforced the order. In other counties, local health officials enforced the order. Another restriction applied to streetcars: no one was allowed on streetcars unless a seat was available. Retail establishments could hold no special sales—nothing that would increase crowding. It was also unlawful for individuals to congregate in groups in department stores, lodges, or private residences. Whenever the order became effective in any county, no child under 18 was permitted to be on the streets except when "absolutely necessary," unless the child was over 14 and regularly employed. The Arkansas Board of Health officer was Dr. J.C. Garrison.[9]

The Fayetteville Board of Health held a special meeting on October 8 and issued an order prohibiting all public gatherings. The order embraced the usual suspects and included "home gatherings." It was effective October 9 at noon. They even closed a Red Cross meeting that had been planned for October 10.[10]

J.C. Geiger announced on October 30 that restrictions in Pulaski City would be lifted on November 4. Little Rock removed the same restrictions. The flu situation was said to have improved to such an extent that the opening of the cities was moved forward one day to November 3. Only one restriction was left in place—there was to be no dancing permitted in Little Rock.[11]

When a second wave of influenza moved through Arkansas, Dr. C.W. Garrison, health officer, gave his opinion in January 1919 that it would not be necessary to place another quarantine on the state, despite the rising number of flu cases. The health department did, however, urge the use of flu masks to prevent the spread of the disease, especially in the case of those who came into contact with victims of the disease. Garrison also spoke harshly about the practice of handshaking.[12]

Two-thirds of the way through October, the epidemic in North Little Rock was reportedly under the control of health authorities, who were optimistic the quarantine would soon be lifted. It had been suggested that the barbers be forced to wear masks, as in Chicago, "as the disease is given every opportunity to spread if the barber is suffering from the ailment."[13]

The Arkansas health officer, Dr. C.W. Garrison, when worried over the possible return of influenza late in November, said that if it were to be kept out of Little Rock, people should exercise care in making needless trips. If a quarantine should be reestablished in Little Rock, said Garrison, the health department would probably issue an order compelling people to wear masks.[14]

Two months later, Garrison was again worried about a rise in flu cases and appealed for more nurses to come forward to help tend to the sick. It was reiterated that Garrison favored wearing masks to prevent the spread of the disease and that masks should have been worn by people who cared for those ill with the malady. While Garrison threatened mask compulsion on occasion, nothing was ever done.[15]

Oklahoma

Spanish influenza was added to the list of quarantinable diseases in Oklahoma. Local health officers throughout the state were given full authority to close the usual suspects when, in their judgment, conditions warranted such action being taken. Dr. John W. Duke, Oklahoma health commissioner, issued the order on the afternoon of October.[16]

One day later, in Ardmore, all theaters and cinemas were closed. However, all city schools were kept open for the present. At one of their regular meetings, the mayor of Ardmore and the city commissioners made the decision. Much debate at the meeting centered on the idea of school closures. Three doctors at the meeting told the city school superintendent, C.W. Richards, that closing schools was unnecessary.[17]

It was announced that Chickasha and Grady County teachers were to receive full payment for their enforced idleness due to school closures. It was also ruled that the teachers had to remain in the city or county to receive the benefit. There were 270 teachers in total in the city and county.[18]

Things changed somewhat in Oklahoma when Duke imposed a statewide quarantine. A week later, under pressure to remove the restrictions, Duke warned that a too-early removal would require the state to reimpose restrictions shortly thereafter. One feature of the order was the ban on public gatherings with over 12 people assembled. All restrictions were eventually lifted at midnight on Saturday, November 9.[19]

In Muskogee, Oklahoma, hyping the mask was left to the local Red Cross chapter. An article in the local press declared, "Wear ward masks! They are Dame Fashion's latest addition to men's and women's attire. But they are not a thing of beauty but the latest and one of the most effective means of preventing the spreading of the influenza epidemic." Every woman connected with the local Red Cross was said to be wearing those ward masks, "a strip of gauze folded two or three times and tied about the head so as to protect the nose and mouth. In this manner the wearers not only protect themselves from inhaling the flu germs but if the wearer should have the disease, they protect others from catching the germs which they might otherwise spread." Mrs. Grant Foreman, head of women's work at the Red Cross, said, "You can't urge the wearing of these masks too strongly. The other evening going home on the car I was most glad that I had the mask on for sitting close to me was a man who unmistakably had the influenza. He continually sneezed and coughed and made no pretense of covering his mouth to prevent the spreading of germs." The article concluded with two brief sentences. "Get busy! Wear a mask!"[20]

Just one week later, the same newspaper in Muskogee published Rupert Blue's summary article on behalf of the United States Public Health Service. Many papers across America did so. Virtually no mention was made of masks except for tending to sick people. Even there, the warning was weak: "Nurses and attendants will do well to guard against breathing in dangerous disease germs by wearing a simple fold of gauze or mask while near the patient." Blue also addressed the situation the Red Cross woman brought up in the previous paragraph. Blue noted that where crowding was unavoidable, as in streetcars, care should be taken to keep the face so turned as not to directly inhale the air breathed out by another person. Blue said, "It is especially important to beware of the person who coughs or sneezes without covering his mouth and nose." But there was no mention of a mask.[21]

Dr. Fred S. Clinton advocated using masks to prevent the spread of the flu in Tulsa, and he wrote a letter to the mayor in support of masking. He said, "It discourages smoking, chewing, eating, drinking, and spitting in public except under such conditions when the individual is not a menace to his companions." He believed masks should be changed every three or four hours and then sterilized by washing and boiling.[22]

When Tulsa looked at the possibility of the usual closures in mid–December as part of a second wave, Mayor Charles H. Hubbard of Tulsa sought advice from Dr. B.A. Wilkes, acting assistant surgeon of the United States Public Health Service, who had been sent to Kansas City to take charge of the situation there. He discouraged letting the disease interfere with the usual operation of places of business. Wilkes said, "A general ban is not necessary by any means, nor is it necessary to hamper the city's business life while conducting a health campaign. Most effective health campaigns have been conducted in other cities without any sort of ban. That is the first thing, called for by excitable persons, but experience has proved it a failure." Wilkes favored the home quarantine as the most crucial step to take. In refusing to close his city again, Hubbard urged businesses to use fumigation and other hygienic practices on their businesses but mentioned nothing about the mask. Wilkes also said nothing about masks.[23]

The city commissioner in charge of the Oklahoma City Health Department urged, on November 21, that all people wear flu masks when in crowds, including in theaters, churches, and so on. If one did not want to wear a mask, Mr. Donnelly said, the next best thing was to spray and gargle the throat after returning home from a crowd.[24]

A public service ad appeared in a Custer County, Oklahoma, newspaper on December 5, signed by Ellis Lamb, Custer County superintendent of health. It explained that masks were compulsory everywhere. Lamb suggested two thicknesses of ordinary bed linen or six layers of cheesecloth as an option to make a mask. He falsely argued that masks effectively saved thousands of lives, "of which Government statistics will bear out." Of course, none of those statistics were presented. Lamb generously allowed an exemption to mask wearing for people eating in restaurants "owing to the impossibility of wearing them at such places."[25]

One week later, it was reported that every citizen in Clinton had been wearing gauze, linen, or handkerchief masks to comply with Lamb's order. A reporter said, "This is a necessary health measure, as by that means only can the deadly menace of this disease be averted. Those who do not voluntarily conform to the rule will be prosecuted."[26]

Then suddenly, on December 19, two weeks after the compulsory mask order was implemented, it was annulled. No explanation for the cancellation of the order was reported in the press.[27]

Texas

On October 13, in a pitch to the State of Texas from acting Governor R.M. Johnston (during the absence of Governor W.P. Hobby, who was in Washington, D.C.), he explained that he clearly understood that influenza was a crowd disease. "Therefore I, R.M. Johnston, Acting Governor of the State of Texas, without assuming to this office the authority of dictating to or prescribing a specific course of action for the municipal authorities of the state, make the suggestion that the local authorities give their careful consideration to the recommendation of Federal and State health authorities with a view to discontinue public assemblies, closing public schools and places of public amusements in localities where the prevalence and severity of the disease renders such a course of action necessary and admissible." Austin, Texas, had already taken action on October 9, when it imposed the Rupert Blue Protocols on the city.[28]

Other cities in Texas followed suit around the same time, with Beaumont imposing similar restrictions to Austin's. Another city where the city health board took steps was El Paso. Dr. George Smart, Travis County (containing Austin) physician, held a conference with health officials on October 11, and they decided to close schools, churches, lodges, all amusement places, and so on. He urged parents to keep their children at home and told them to "insist your neighbors do the same." He wanted the children to get as much fresh air as possible, which did not mean they must be shut up, but he said, "Keep them at home." Smart also urged people to avoid neighborhood visits and advised them to "transact as much of your business as possible over the telephone." His advice was easier said than done because just 35 percent of housing units had a telephone in 1920.[29]

When El Paso imposed its quarantine, it did so for one week. Then it extended the order for another week. In the first week, public schools were closed, but high schools were open. In the second week, both were closed. El Paso's chief of police ordered his men to wear flu masks when they were called on to deal with dead bodies.[30]

Mayor W.D. Davis lifted the quarantine imposed in Fort Worth, Texas, effective at midnight on October 26. A couple of days later, attendance at Fort Worth schools was reported to be 10 percent lower than before the quarantine order. Such numbers were common in America. The children were not necessarily sick but healthy. Fearful parents kept them home, primarily due to the panic instilled in them by many health authorities in many jurisdictions.[31]

In Amarillo, the health board and the city commissioners quarantined their city against all travelers in the influenza-infected territory, explaining that "they will be kept in detention camps until proven healthy."[32]

In San Antonio, the city health officer was Dr. William King. After Rupert Blue's Protocols were issued as a recommendation, King declined to impose them in San Antonio. On October 16, King met with the San Antonio Board of Health, and suddenly they decided to impose the Blue Protocols. They became effective on October 17, but the restrictions were lifted on November 11. King and the board of health met again on December 5, and dealing with an increase in cases, a second quarantine was imposed, but milder since schools and churches were left open. But then, on December 10, King again ordered everything closed in the original Blue Protocols. The San Antonio Board of Health voted to rescind the order on December 21 with immediate effect, which led to looming lawsuits from cinema owners and others.[33]

A report in a brief news item on October 6 from El Paso observed that nurses handling flu cases at private hospitals were beginning to wear masks "especially prepared" to keep out influenza germs. The article was titled "They're wearing gas masks in El Paso."[34]

In Dallas, just before Christmas 1918, it was reported that Dallas barbers, dentists, nurses, and others who might come into contact with influenza sufferers would be forced to wear masks if the recommendation made by Dallas City Physician A.W. Carnes with Mayor Lawther was approved by the city commissioners. However, it was not approved.[35]

When a Fort Worth newspaper covered part of the American Public Health Association convention in Chicago in December 1918, it featured the comments of one of the over 1,000 health professionals in attendance, Dr. Woods Hutchinson, a nationally syndicated columnist. The article said that Hutchinson had brought about the compulsory wearing of masks in San Francisco. He was described as being so confident that masking was 100 percent effective in breaking flu epidemics that he offered, while at the convention, to go to Kansas City and give his services if the city would provide an ordinance requiring every person to wear a gauze mask. When he spoke at the convention, a reporter said, "He followed other health experts who have scoffed at the mask as a preventive measure." Another speaker at the convention was Dr. S.J. Crumbine, secretary of the Kansas Board of Health. He said just two slender hopes had been developed in the fight against the epidemic: "the prophylactic inoculation brought about by Dr. E.C. Rosenow of the Mayo Foundation, in which he has considerable faith and the wearing of masks."[36]

8

East North Central

Michigan

It was reported on October 13 that the Michigan Health Board would issue an order closing the usual suspects. The state board met in Lansing a day earlier and decided to permit each municipality to work out its problems and to issue orders as local conditions warranted. Governor Albert Sleeper approved the decision. However, his ban on public gatherings was to stand. Several Michigan cities had by then closed the usual suspects. Those cities included Alma and St. Joseph. However, each of them allowed their schools to remain open.[1]

The Detroit health commissioner, Dr. James W. Inches, and the Detroit Health Board decided not to close public places in the city, calling the measure "valueless." The Detroit transit company told Inches that it would comply with his mandate to remove the two upper windows of every streetcar to aid in ventilation.[2]

Then, on October 18 in Lansing, Governor Sleeper reversed his decision and ordered all the usual suspects in the Rupert Blue Protocols to be shuttered. The mandate applied statewide, but most of the communities in Michigan had by then implemented their own closures. Some communities, such as Detroit and Grand Rapids, opposed the order, while others favored it. Detroit officials stated the order would not affect Detroit schools; they would remain open.[3]

Three days later, Detroit health authorities said strict compliance with the statewide closing order was observed throughout the city on the first day. On the same day, the health authorities and other city officials said that all public, private, and parochial schools would be closed as of October 24.[4]

Detroit extended its closing order a couple of days later by banning all outdoor meetings and ordering all stores to close at 4:30 p.m. beginning Wednesday, October 23. Stores had been closing under an order at 5:30 p.m.; later, on October 26, the closing time changed again to 5:00 p.m., supposedly to ease streetcar congestion. The ban on outdoor activities came from Dr. R.M. Olin, secretary of the Michigan Board of Health, because the board had learned that several cities were planning outdoor gatherings to avoid the ban on indoor meetings. Detroit schools reopened on November 4, and a large organization of schoolteachers, all of whom had been idle due to the shutdown and who the authorities had put to work as aides and investigators during the flu epidemic, was disbanded. Stores in Detroit could resume usual hours as of November 2.[5]

Public schools closed at noon on October 24 in Port Huron by order of the board of education. Streets that were heavily used were to be sprinkled continuously during the day and flushed at night. All stores had to close at 4 p.m., except on Saturday, when they all had to close by 6 p.m. Under the order, signed by Dr. W.J. Duff, Port Huron health officer, all parents "must insist" their children remain in their yards or enclosures. Children congregating for play or any purpose at any time or place were not permitted. Before the order was issued, about 50 of the mayors and health officers from the state's main cities attended a meeting in the governor's office in Lansing, where they unanimously decided not to include public schools in the closing order issued by the governor. It was felt that if the schools were closed, the kids would congregate in other places but be unsupervised. The doctors at the meeting opposed school closure. However, Port Huron officials decided to ignore that advice and force kids to stay home. By doing so, they argued that they had overcome the objections.[6]

Dr. Olin, secretary of the Michigan Board of Health, issued a statewide order on December 10. It took effect immediately and mandated that only doctors and nurses could enter or leave the premises of an influenza victim. Every house with a case of influenza was to be placed under strict quarantine. The order was sent to every health officer in the state. At the same time, Kalamazoo banned public meetings for a second time and shuttered schools once again. Bangor closed the schools until the new year and banned all church services and public meetings for the second time.[7]

On January 10, 1919, Crystal Falls rescinded the influenza quarantine that had gone into effect on December 9. The cinemas reopened, the skating rink flooded and readied for skaters, the dance halls reopened, and life returned to normal.[8]

In Detroit, on October 22, a reporter declared that the day had brought a "marked increase" in the use of masks in downtown Detroit. Elevator operators, newsagents, telephone operators in business exchanges, information clerks, and the like "all were wearing them." Dr. Inches was the Detroit health commissioner, and he was no fan of the face coverings. He asserted, "Many of the masks now being used are worthless and the wearers would be better off without them. They should be 8 and 12 play and then should be used only by medical men and nurses who are in the sick room." It was also reported that Flint had supposedly ordered people to wear masks. On the same day, Port Huron Health Officer Duff ordered that clerks wear flu masks, although not the customers served by those clerks.[9]

In Lansing, it was reported on October 18 that the women employed at the local draft board office wore gauze masks. The reporter said, "Here the exposure to the public is great as the work of the draft board must go on. Even the novelty of such masks did not bother the young women and they went about their work in the usual manner."[10]

As Lansing health officials debated what steps to take, Dr. Wright stated, "In view of the fact that clerks in the stores are brought face to face with a large number of people each day it is advisable for them to wear the gauze masks. Every man, woman and child is requested and urged to do everything possible to assist in stopping the spread of influenza."[11]

Escanaba had a drastic mask ordinance in place as of early December. On the evening of December 7, four men were arrested for failing to wear flu masks. One store was forced to close its doors because the proprietor was found serving customers while not wearing a mask. Members of the community's board of health were reportedly determined on rigid enforcement of the rule requiring all people appearing outside of their homes to wear a mask, and all violators of the provision were to be promptly arrested. Dr. A.J. Carlson, Escanaba health officer, issued an order stating that stores where rules were "flagrantly violated" would be closed and not allowed to open for a specified period. Suddenly, though, just two days after the mass arrests, Carlson ordered the mask rule rescinded, effective on December 10.[12]

As of mid–December, Kalamazoo had imposed the influenza shutdown for the second time. A journalist claimed that "hundreds of workers" in stores were wearing flu masks. It was the same situation in the Flint and Bay City communities. Dr. Olin of the Michigan Board of Health recommended that residents of all "influenza ridden" towns wear masks.[13]

A Battle Creek, Michigan, newspaper reported the end of the American Public Health Association in Chicago on December 12. This paper observed that some physicians at the convention regarded masks as "poppycock" and the closing of churches and amusement places as "entirely unnecessary." In contrast, others contended such measures were "most efficacious." The piece also noted that the group referred the questions to a committee of five to study the situation and develop recommendations based on the evidence presented at the convention.[14]

Detroit was another city that published the fake story in which Dr. Royal Copeland recommended that the chiffon veil for women to use as a flu mask was just as good as the real thing. The Detroit paper featured the brief story on page one. Copeland never recommended the real flu mask, let alone a veil, outside of people tending the sick.[15]

In Detroit, on October 18, it was reported that draft board officials, stenographers, and clerks formed an interesting group of "masked marvels" due to an order requiring them to wear muslin masks as a sanitary precaution against the flu. "It was a hard blow for the women for it rendered the usual effectiveness of face powder impotent." However, the report added, "As novelty the masks had a good effect so far as genial spirits were concerned. They were likened to harem veils, mosquito screens, and mole covers. For the men these masks are a distinct inconvenience inasmuch as no provision has been made for pipes, cigars or cigarettes."[16]

As in other cities, the Red Cross in Detroit was charged with making masks. The health board was thinking about giving the coverings to nurses, war workers, factory women, and others who might need them. Mrs. Russell Alger was in charge of the Red Cross workroom, and she urged women to come out and do volunteer work making the masks. She said, "They need not be afraid of the influenza themselves for the workroom is sprayed thoroughly twice a day with disinfectant and practically all of the women who come do wear face masks while they work." Alger explained that the Red Cross was then making an improved mask over the original. The new ones were eight-ply thick compared to the four-ply thickness of the old ones. Alger declared, "Persons using the old masks should wear two together, or double one."[17]

Dr. Inches, as Detroit superintendent of health, had published a public service advertisement that tried to clear up some confusion regarding wearing masks in Detroit, with no blanket orders in place. While he advised that people use masks in some cases, he was against "indiscriminate" use and wearing them in the open. Likely, he created as much confusion as he cleared up.[18]

If the technical aspects of the mask were confusing in Detroit, it only got worse a few days later. Major Victor G. Heiser of the United States Public Health Service announced from Lansing that "masks must be 250 strands to the inch to be effective. You may have three thicknesses of 40 by 44, or eight strands of 20 by 18. The masks should not be worn over two hours without sterilizing and must always be worn with the same side front. This can be arranged by a mark on the outside."[19]

Two days before Dr. Inches left Detroit for Chicago and the American Public Health Association convention, he explained to a reporter why he opposed the use of masks and the closure of schools. He said those methods "tend to unnecessarily frighten the public and weaken their resistance to the malady."[20]

Ohio

On October 7, Mansfield, Ohio, ordered that all places of public gatherings must close—it was the cast of usual suspects. The city's board of health made the decision at 2:30 p.m. that day, and the closures were to last for an indefinite period. Schools, churches, lodges, dance halls, and bowling alleys all had to close that day. Theaters could remain open until midnight the following day, when they would be shuttered. No congregating was permitted in saloons, cigar stores, and poolrooms. Those places could remain open, at least for the present. Still, purchases in such places had to be made "promptly," and the purchaser had to refrain from lingering in the store. Dr. Guy T. Goodman was the Mansfield Health Officer. The residential quarantine was also established and described as "rigid," with no one allowed in or out of the residence. Ashland, Ohio, was about 13 miles away from Mansfield, and the latter community was worried about the number of cases in Ashland, so the Mansfield Board of Health passed a resolution that forbade any resident of Ashland from entering Mansfield

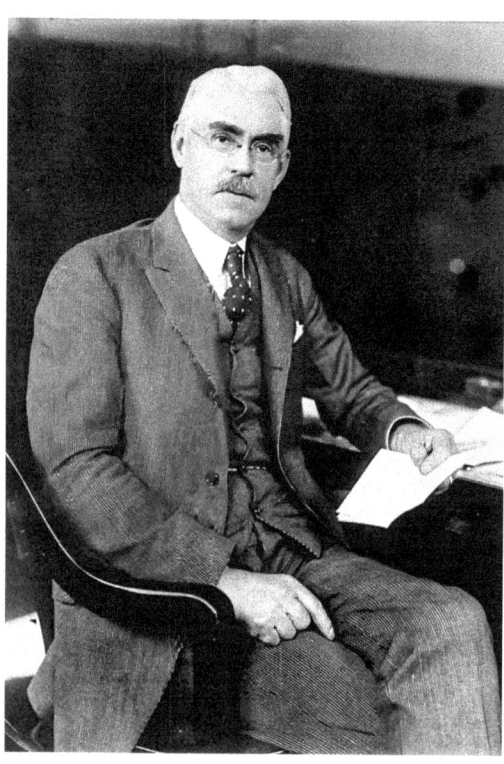

Health Commissioner James W. Inches of Detroit at his desk, 1919.

unless the visitor had a written declaration as to good health that had been received from the health officials in both places.[21]

One day later, the Steubenville Chamber of Commerce demanded that the city's health board close the usual suspects as a precaution against the flu. The health board refused the demand because no disease cases had been reported in the city. However, they agreed they would impose a lockdown "at the first time of danger." Meanwhile, Ohio health officials urged vigilance on the part of its residents, but not hysteria, in dealing with the epidemic.[22]

One day after that, the health authorities in Marion, Ohio, refused to close the saloons in town, as demanded by the community ministers, whose churches had been ordered closed for at least two weeks. The board refused their demand to close the saloons because closing them would require closing ice cream parlors and other stores.[23]

On October 11, the Ohio Board of Health stepped in and ordered the imposition of Rupert Blue Protocols statewide. In all communities not affected by the disease, the closure order would become effective just as soon as the local health officials "discover[ed] cases of influenza." Ohio Governor James M. Cox, acting state health commissioner James E. Bauman, and officials representing cities with populations of over 3,000 met and reached that decision.[24]

Cleveland entered an at least two-week shutdown on October 14. All churches, theaters, and public meetings came under the ban. The question of closing schools was to be decided in the following day or two, and they closed on October 15. All Liberty Loan community meetings scheduled for the week, which numbered over 100, were to be held outdoors.[25]

An order was issued on October 19 to the City of East Liverpool's traction company that limited the carrying capacity of its streetcars to the seating capacity of each car. The city health officer was Dr. J.W. Chetwynd. At a hearing on October 19, three saloon keepers in East Liverpool were ordered to pay fines on charges of violating the health board's closing order. The liquor dealers charged and fined were I.J. Allen, Joseph Vorndran and Jess Yoemans.[26]

Akron Health Officer Charles Nesbitt forwarded a communication to Gordon Davies, the police court prosecutor, calling on him to take action against individuals he named as participating in the Firestone Park gathering on October 18, violating the influenza regulations that barred such gatherings. Twenty-four people, along with "others," were named in the communication as having gathered at the park in violation of board of health regulations prohibiting indoor or outdoor public or private assemblies. The Akron health officer had issued the order on October 12.[27]

A general tightening of the restrictions imposed by the Ohio Board of Health on Ohio communities was noticeable throughout the state on October 24. Acting Health Commissioner James E. Bauman had declared a day earlier that no lifting of closing regulations would be countenanced without the authority of the state health department. In Columbus, where theaters, churches, and schools had been closed for the past ten days, orders were issued closing all eating places, saloons, and clubs after 8:20 p.m. It was claimed that action was taken not because the situation was worsening but to prevent such an outcome. As part of Bauman's new orders, local health officers throughout Ohio who annulled closing orders "made necessary" by the influenza epidemic without permission from the Ohio Board of Health would be removed from office. Bauman's no-nonsense approach was evident in Bellaire and Kingston. Physicians and nurses regarded the situation in Bellaire as serious; however, Dr. D.W. Boone, Bellaire's health officer, did not. In response, Bauman ordered Boone's removal from office. Bauman also suggested that the superintendent of schools at Kingston, Ross County, be arrested for opening his schools in "illegal defiance" of a closing order.[28]

Health authorities and Mayor Schreiber issued orders on November 2 to lift the influenza quarantine in Toledo. Churches would open on November 7, saloons on November 8, churches and theaters on November 7, and public schools on November 11. The quarantine was also lifted on November 7 in Urbana. However, Mayor Talbot retained the ban on church services, standing in cinemas, and all other congested gatherings. In Wilmington, Ohio, the city health board met and voted to let the churches open on November 7 after four weeks of closure. However, night services remained under the ban. The board planned to meet in a few days to decide on the advisability of opening theaters and schools. In all these cases, the Ohio Board of Health granted authority to local health boards to lift the quarantines.[29]

Effective at midnight on Saturday, November 2, Springfield lifted all bans, except for those on cinemas and theaters. The original closing order had gone into effect on October 14. Springfield Health Commissioner E.B. Starr had issued the orders.[30]

As of November 5, downtown businesses in Cleveland could remain open until 6 p.m. instead of closing by 4 p.m., as had been the practice for the previous two weeks. Churches could hold services from November 10 onward. Local health officials in Columbus lifted the ban on outdoor gatherings around the same time. Cinemas could reopen, but they could not admit children under 15. Saloons, restaurants, and other public places, then closing at 8:30 p.m., could resume their regular hours. Marion, Ohio, removed all restrictions on November 10 and 11. Youngstown lifted their bans at noon on November 14. However, theaters were limited to 80 percent capacity, while poolrooms were limited to playing and seating capacity. Saloons could not have people congregating or crowding.[31]

Mansfield lifted its influenza quarantine in gradual steps, starting in early November, based on a decision reached at a meeting of health board members. Churches and public gathering places could open. Still, attendance was limited to "adults over 16 years of age." Children could attend church and return to regular school a week or so later. The no later than 7 p.m. closing ban was also removed. While theaters could reopen, the health board passed a resolution in which theater managers and employees were compelled to refuse admittance to anyone "showing signs of illness…. Those who are suffering from colds, who cough or sneeze cannot be admitted and should they gain entrance, must be promptly ejected when the condition is noted." Two Ohio communities, Galion and Ashland, reopened everything at once around this time.[32]

All schools in Marion, Ohio, were closed on December 2. The city board of health was expected to reimpose the original closing orders and restore the quarantine later that day. Later, the board empowered Marion Health Officer Charles A. Tobin to take measures to stamp out influenza. Tobin suggested he might require all people doing business in downtown stores to wear masks. He had reimposed bans on all theaters, churches, and public gatherings. Stores and saloons were forced to close no later than 6 p.m. daily. On December 20, Marion closed all churches, lodges, and saloons. At that time, both local newspapers suggested editorially that all members of the city's board of health hand in their resignations because of the off-and-on bans, regulations, and so on. A day earlier, Dr. J.S. Lunger had resigned from the board of health, although he gave no reason.[33]

Dr. McCrory was the Bucyrus health officer. He said on December 18 that the flu ban in his community might be lifted in the next week, depending on developments in the influenza situation over the coming days. One hundred six deputies were sworn in to enforce their flu regulations on the same day in Marion. Saloons, churches, cinemas, theaters, lodges, and soft drink fountains were closed tight. All people riding on streetcars, clerks, and store customers were required to wear masks. All business houses not entirely closed had to close by 6 p.m. The action taken by the board of health in hiring the extra deputies followed the refusal of cinema managers to close their venues, as required by law, on December 16 and 17. One day later, after the harsh response from the health board, cinema owners, saloon keepers, and merchants refused to close their businesses on the grounds that the city's mayor had failed to sign the order. Reportedly, nobody wore flu masks, but the police made no arrests.[34]

Lima, Ohio's health board instituted new rules that took effect at 6 a.m. on December 19. In cinemas, every other seat was to be left vacant. The same rule applied to all theaters, lodge rooms, churches, and assembly rooms of other kinds. All schools were closed until further notice. Children under 12 were banned from streetcars, theaters, stores, and other business places. Kids were allowed in restaurants and hotels only when accompanied by their parents. Clerks, employees, and customers were not to congregate—50 square feet of floor space had to be allowed for each individual. Special sales of all kinds were banned, while "loiterers and loafers" were to be arrested. Streetcars in Marion had to have four windows "wide open" and be fumigated every hour. All other public gathering places were to be fumigated every three hours. Concerts, lectures, sports, public and private dances, and similar assemblies were prohibited. The mask law stayed on the books in Marion. Still, officials declared the police would not enforce it, and wearing the masks was "left to the option of the individual."[35]

As the number of cases increased in Coshocton, so did the fear level. Officials in Ohio were particularly frantic, spreading panic around the disease. One of the town's newspapers printed a story on page one of a November edition with a rumor that the disease then prevalent in the city and county was not the Spanish flu but was rather "a pulmonary form of the black death which decimated the population of Europe several centuries ago." In Coshocton that day, it was remarked that the American Art Works Company cooperated vigorously with local health officials to stamp out the epidemic. The firm had prepared several hundred flu masks, enough to meet the needs of both its factory and office staff. The "properly sterilized and disinfected" masks would be ready for distribution to the employees in a couple of days.

A reporter said, "While in Coshocton there is nothing compulsory about the wearing of the masks, they have proved such an efficient aid in stamping out the epidemic in other places that it is anticipated they will be generally adopted here."[36]

The next day, it was announced in Coshocton that clerks at the post office who transacted business with the public through the service windows had started to wear influenza masks.[37]

Cases continued to increase in Coshocton, and a reporter wrote on November 19 that the "wearing of influenza masks is becoming more general each day. Drivers of laundry wagons and other delivery wagons were wearing masks Tuesday."[38]

Early in the pandemic, at the start of October, a Cincinnati newspaper reprinted an editorial that originally appeared in an Indianapolis paper. He argued it was the responsibility of each to safeguard themselves and others from disease. He thought people coughed and sneezed all too often with no regard for others. The cougher and spitter had no business and no right to be at public gatherings of any sort. "If necessity takes him away from his home he should wear a surgeon's mask. This simple device will protect his neighbors from infection, and while it may be neither pleasant to wear nor especially attractive to behold, it is at least the badge of a man who has a sincere desire to do his duty."[39]

According to Dr. E.G. Burton, Lima health officer, there was no immediate prospect, on November 5, of lifting the ban on public meetings or seeing the resumption

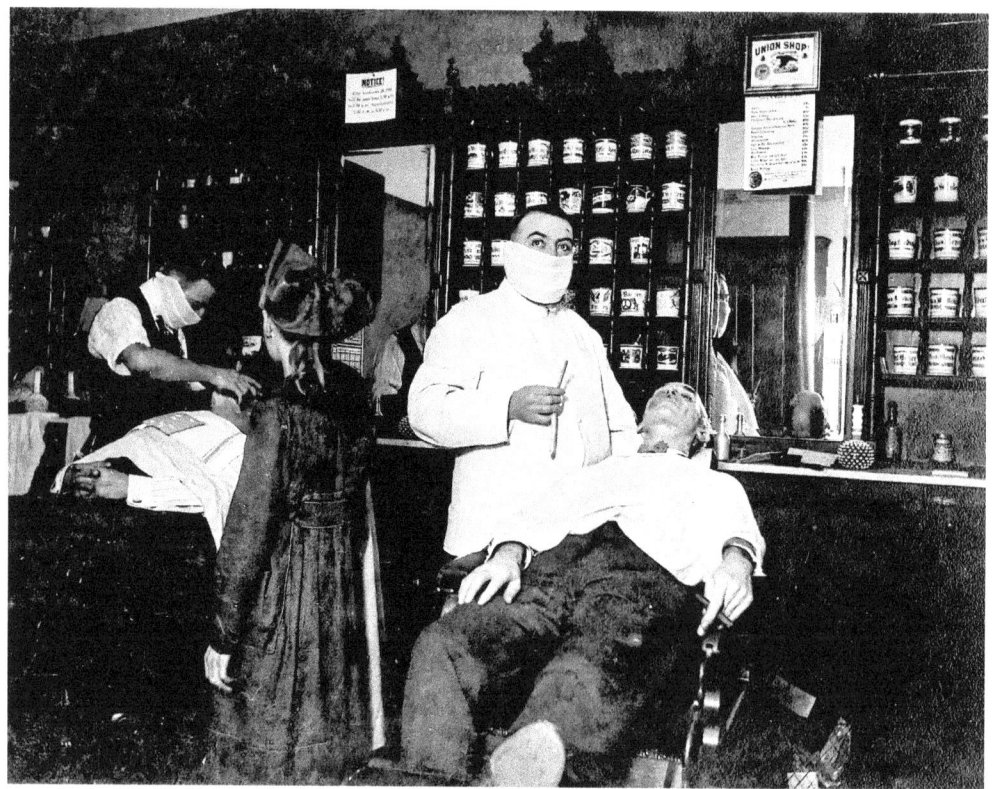

Cincinnati barbers.

of business as usual. Burton said he was sorry that a meeting at Memorial Hall had been scheduled for that night. He explained that the board of health had authorized it in his absence. Burton said he would not like to cancel the gathering as it was a war project, so he exclaimed, "My suggestion to all who attend that meeting tonight is to wear masks to guard against influenza."[40]

When a Lima newspaper covered the American Public Health Association in Chicago, which ran from December 9 to 12, it featured the comments of Dr. Woods Hutchinson, a syndicated medical columnist of some fame but far less intelligence. He was an outlier at the convention when he insisted that gauze masks and vaccines were the only successful methods to fight the influenza epidemic. Hutchinson commented that hospital doctors protected themselves with masks but would not insist on them for civilians. Giving Hutchinson as much coverage as this paper did left the reader with the impression that his opinion was popular at the convention. It was not.[41]

On December 12, it was reported that flu masks were to be worn in Lima by order of the city health bureau. They were to be made of gauze or cloth of not less than twenty or more than forty meshes per inch. The cloth was to be folded into six thicknesses, five inches wide and nine inches long. A tape had to be attached to each corner and tied behind the head, with the mask covering the nose and mouth when used. Masks had to be worn in cinemas, theaters, streetcars, club rooms, churches, retail stores and business houses, railroad interurban ticket offices, and "any other place where ten or more persons publicly assembled." The order took effect at 6 p.m. that very day. A journalist said, "The alert will be sounded at Lima at 6 o'clock tonight, and influenza 'gas masks' will be in order." Also, that day, it was reported that 700 high school girls began turning out masks for themselves, their relatives, and other schoolchildren. The order for mandatory masking came from the city health board, which found the city detention hospital was full and that influenza cases were not admitted to the city hospital. Dr. Burton, the city health officer, informed J.E. Collins, the superintendent of education, that the mask rule "did not necessarily apply to the schools," but Collins decided whether the rule was good enough for the rest of the city, the schools should follow it too.[42]

When a Lima journalist described the scene in his city that evening when the masking rule went into effect, he started by writing, "Lima stalked the streets in disguise last night when scores appeared with the first flu masks. Self-conscious customers, faces muffled in white, mumbled through their swathings to equally self-conscious clerks, similarly muzzled, in downtown stores." And he added, "In the theaters and movie shows the possession of a proper mask was as important as the purchase of a ticket in gaining admittance. The unmasked were strictly taboo. Performers at the Orpheum appeared on the stage masked." Police Chief Rausch issued orders requiring the strict enforcement of wearing masks in all public places. Thousands of handouts bearing the text of the order and a warning from the police were distributed throughout the day. The penalty for violating the ordinance was a fine ranging from $25 to $100. However, the police made no arrests as they allowed a grace period, as there was very little time between the passage of the order and the time it went into effect.[43]

The Pastors' Union of Lima urged its followers to comply with the rule. Speaking on behalf of the group, the Rev. G.W. Lilly declared that while they were preaching, pastors could remove their masks, and church singers could do the same. In his statement, Lilly said, "There may be no deviation of church services. We ask our people to co-operate with us at this time, comply with the order of the health board regarding the wearing of masks, but come."[44]

The editor of a Lima paper issued an editorial in which he went even further than the health board. He argued that "if there is any need of wearing masks in the stores of Lima and in the street cars and theatres, there is need of wearing them on the streets.... That is the almost universal opinion of the people of Lima, as near as it can be gathered.... But the board has adopted only half-measures, has gone only half the way." He urged his city's health board to order the schools closed and to "require masks to be worn everywhere."[45]

A day later, the mask rules became even harsher. Schools, saloons, barber shops, lodge rooms, and wholesale establishments were added to the places where masks had to be worn. The health board adopted the new order on December 13, and it became effective at 6 a.m. on December 14. According to the new order, all schoolchildren were to be provided with two masks to be replaced or sterilized every three hours. Students who arrived at school not wearing a mask were to be denied admission. On December 13, "nearly 50 per cent" of the schoolchildren wore masks. Upon entering the shop, patrons of barbershops had to don masks and keep them on until they sat themselves down in the barber's chair. Patrons of restaurants had to wear masks while waiting to be served. They had to put them back on immediately upon leaving their tables. The most sweeping change in the new order was that masks had to be worn everywhere where one or more people congregated (annulling the former rule of ten or more). Fines for violating the mask order remained as they had been, ranging from $25 to $100.[46]

Businesspeople meeting for a smoker at the upper-class Lima Club on the evening of December 13 sipped drinks through straws and smoked cigars through holes punctured in their masks. Over a dozen men attended the smoker, all wearing masks throughout the evening. The meeting was called for the Lima stockholders of the Turnbull Motor Truck Company. One of those present was the mayor of Lima.[47]

Forty-six citizens of Lima, drawn from all strata of society, pleaded guilty in the city's police court on December 16 to charges of having been caught in business houses without flu masks on Saturday afternoon and evening, December 14. They were caught by uniformed officers and one plainclothes officer. Each admitted a violation of the order, and Judge Botkin fined each one dollar. Botkin warned them from the bench that the police would continue inspections of business establishments until the board of health rescinded the order. Another twenty people charged with the same violation did not appear in court. The article listed all 66 people by name and address.[48]

On December 16, the Lima Board of Health decided that the flu mask order would stand and remain on the books. The public was asked to cooperate with the board. However, the reality was far different. Police enforcement of the masking law was "not expected." None of the people in attendance that night at the city council meeting or the Lima Board of Health meeting wore masks. Forty-seven more people were arrested on the weekend for violating the mask order. When they appeared before a judge on Monday, December 16, they were each fined one dollar. Seventy had been arrested, but the other 23 did not attend their court appearance.[49]

A more rigid quarantine was rumored to supersede the mask as a means of helping to stamp out the flu in Lima if the board of health followed the opinion of the Allen County Hospital meeting on the night of December 17. Following the discussion, the society passed a motion condemning the promiscuous use of the gauze mask as impracticable. The physicians, though, were unanimous in their opinion that people in direct contact with the disease should use masks.[50]

When F.S. Laux, proprietor of a dancing academy, appealed for permission to conduct Christmas parties, the board of health ruled on December 21 that dancing in Lima, even when the dancers wore masks, remained banned. The mask law still had not been repealed, but it was not enforced anywhere, and everybody ignored it. Still, it was the board's opinion that because dancing came under the new ban, it could not be allowed even when masks were used.[51]

Indiana

Indianapolis schools, churches, theaters, and cinemas were ordered closed. The city's health board ordered a ban on all public gatherings on the afternoon of October 6. The order was effective the following day and was to run indefinitely. Several hours after the board acted, the Indiana Board of Health received a telegram from Rupert Blue in Washington directing a similar move in every city and town in Indiana. It was a telegram received all over America by state officials everywhere. By 9 p.m., Indiana health officials had sent telegrams to every county health official in the state, asking for the usual suspects to be closed and for all public gatherings to be closed. The Indianapolis health officer, Dr. Morgan, had already agreed to allow a "small" number to hold meetings involving gatherings at which Liberty Loan bonds were flogged to the public. Morgan declared there must be no letup in the sale of Liberty bonds.[52]

A couple of days later, Morgan extended the closing order in his city. It then applied to poolrooms, bowling alleys, and lodges. Dr. Morgan then attempted to restrict loitering around cigar stores.[53]

The Indiana Board of Health banned all public gatherings until midnight on October 20. This order compelled streetcars to operate with all windows kept open, however, only when the temperature was 50 degrees or higher and it was not raining. Meetings could be held outdoors, but only if the meeting was to take place in a territory where there were no cases of the disease. A second condition was that the meeting could only be held if a permit had been obtained from the state health board. The order applied to all of Indiana.[54]

The next restriction in Indianapolis was applied to retail stores on October 14. An order issued on October 12 by Morgan mandated that all stores, except for grocery and drug stores (but only those within a specified downtown area), had to open no earlier than 9:45 a.m. and close no later than 6:15 p.m., effective on October 14. The purpose was to eliminate crowding on streetcars during rush hour and to allow factory workers an opportunity to arrive and leave work before store employees and shoppers.[55]

Just as suddenly, the order was removed. The influenza quarantine in Indianapolis was lifted on the last day of October. Businesses could resume their normal course with only a few minor health rules enforced. State officials added that about half of Indiana counties would be relieved of their restrictions by midnight on November 2. Schools in Indianapolis reopened on November 4. The only restrictions that were to be retained were those requiring streetcars to keep their windows open and that people suffering from colds or suspected of having symptoms of the flu be excluded from theaters.[56]

Then, according to Dr. J.N. Hurty, secretary of the Indiana Board of Health, the restrictions on the entire state were to be lifted. Hurty left it up to each local jurisdiction, county, or city to continue any restrictions if they saw fit.[57]

The Bedford health officer, Dr. H. Voyles, issued a signed proclamation on November 21 stating that from that day onward, a strict residential influenza quarantine was imposed on every family within the city limits of Bedford in which there was a case of influenza. That meant all family members, except the breadwinner, had to stay on the premises for at least five days after the last case on the quarantined premises was free from fever. To be allowed to go to work, the breadwinner had to stay out of the patient's room. All houses quarantined were to be placarded. City physicians were legally required to report daily to the city the names and addresses of influenza cases.[58]

In Terre Haute, managers of 14 theaters were arrested on November 29 when they opened their doors in violation of an order from the city board of health officials. They were charged with conduct endangering public health. After being released on bail, six of the men again opened their venues and were then rearrested and taken to jail.[59]

The Clay County health commissioner, G.W. Finley, stated on November 19 that streetcar conductors, servers, store clerks, barbers, and other people serving the public had to wear flu masks. The order went into effect within 24 hours. Nurses and physicians were also ordered to wear them. Finley remarked that "this order will be issued in the hopes that wearing of masks will eliminate the possibility of placing the ban back on all of Clay County." Brazil is the county seat of Clay County. Finley made evident what many left unsaid. The first restrictions were lifted all over America, only to find they had had no effect. Many places reimposed the bans. However, the first set of restrictions had led to much protesting by business interests and others, often unreported. That made health officials squeamish about reimposition. Turning to an impossible hope, some decided to impose a new rule—masking—since it involved no business shutdowns and no reduction of hours. Thus, they hoped it would mean less pressure on them for the measures they had imposed.[60]

When George Finley's order took effect on November 20, people in stores, businesses, theaters, and cinemas also had to wear masks. All schoolteachers and pupils also had to wear masks. It was observed that cinema patrons did not need to have "regulation" gauze masks, and, a reporter said, "a handkerchief placed about the nose and mouth will serve the purpose equally as well as a gauze mask."[61]

Clay County changed its mask rules on November 25. Health Commissioner George Finley and the committee on public health (appointed that same morning by Finley) adopted the new rules that day. People in the open air did not need to wear masks, but people did in all other situations, stores, and businesses. All people coming from homes where cases of flu existed had to wear masks, even on the street. All people neglecting or refusing to wear masks when entering stores or other public places were subject to arrest and prosecution.[62]

At noon on November 26, the Finley health committee met and voted to rescind the city's flu mask order, except for families with flu in their homes, where all were required to wear face masks of butter cloth or equally fine mesh material. No reason was given for the order rescinding masking. Still, the committee said it "especially recommends that clerks protect themselves by wearing them while waiting on customers."[63]

Dr. E.G. Freyermuth, secretary of the South Bend Board of Health, responded to the masking order in effect in Indianapolis imposed by the state. He was strongly opposed to such a practice, believing it to be injurious to the wearer's health, except in the case of a nurse attending to an influenza patient. He said, "Of my own accord I would never order the wearing of these masks here, only when persons are with influenza patients."[64]

In Columbus, the ban against public gatherings (the second one) took effect at 6 p.m. on November 19. The local health board reinstated the regulations but did not order wearing flu masks. For now, the board said it would issue no such compulsory mask-wearing order. Reportedly, some of the barbers in the city were wearing them. A reporter noted that he had seen two men on the street wearing masks, or, he reasoned, it might have been one man he saw twice.[65]

Under orders of the Newcastle Board of Health, city residents had to don masks as of November 21. People needed to wear masks everywhere except in their homes and on the streets. Cinema owners and store managers were expected to police the rule on their premises and ensure no one entered without a face covering.[66]

The Evansville health officer, Dr. Linthicum, said on November 22 that the city's health board would not issue an order to make masking mandatory or an order to close any place. However, it did advise everybody to avoid crowds and to wear masks. He said, "Closing down plants would mean starvation to many people." During a time when nobody, owner or worker, was compensated for forced time away from work (except teachers, to some extent), Linthicum was one of the few officials who considered that factor.[67]

At the meeting where Linthicum gave the above remarks, representatives of the manufacturers and the merchants who attended protested wearing masks and placing bans on businesses, as during the first wave. School physician Hartloff told the board that wearing masks was an efficient preventive. Merchants complained that wearing masks would frighten women from their stores, but Hartloff countered that the shoppers would soon get used to them.[68]

In Seymour, Indiana, in keeping with an order issued by the local health authorities, when a specified number of people were employed in a room of specific dimensions, they had to wear flu masks (numbers not given). As a result of that rule, the accountants at the Baltimore and Ohio Railway donned masks on November 23.[69]

During the first wave in Indianapolis, the capitalist class of Fort Wayne, in conjunction with city health officials, published a full-page ad in the local newspaper designed to strike fear and terror into the readers' hearts. Officials had often said they wanted to avoid panic, but this ad belied such nonsense. Panic was something they wanted to induce and did, as witnessed by this ad.[70]

The Fort Wayne Board of Health enacted an order on December 3 that everyone had to wear a mask everywhere except at home and in the open air. It had to be worn in all public places and in offices employing three or more people. The order went into effect the very next morning.[71]

On December 4, the newly appointed influenza committee held a special meeting. The committee members were Arthur F. Hall of the Lincoln National Life Insurance Company, Walter S. Goll of the General Electric Company, J.L. Sessler of the Fort Wayne Typographical Union, E.M. Steele of the Steele-Myers Company, and the Rev. Arthur J. Folsom. The committee was to act as an advisory board to the city's health board. They declared, "If the board of health has the universal co-operation of the people during the next few days, it will not be necessary to close the places of business during the Christmas season. If all the people will kindly suffer a few slight inconveniences for a few days in unselfish devotion, not only will the city be saved from the horrors that have visited other cities, but all business houses and public places may continue uninterrupted." The board of health appointed Charles Spillner, formerly of the Fort Wayne Police Department, as captain of a force of 25 special police officers who would see that the rules regarding wearing masks were rigidly enforced. The board of health also appointed John Swaidner, lieutenant of a force of ten special officers, to patrol the downtown district during the evening. Those men would visit all places where the public congregated and see that no one went unmasked. The General Electric Company took that initiative, masking its entire force a day earlier. No employee could work without a mask. The Reverend Folsom declared that "the influenza mask is a badge of patriotism.... Now the public faces a scourge that can be met by the exercising of personal care. The mask does the trick, and the man who does not wear a mask is exposing not only himself and his family to the possible ravages of a highly contagious disease.... It's a patriotic, a humanitarian duty for everyone to wear a mask until the danger point has been passed."[72]

On December 9, Dr. D.F. Frost, deputy county health commissioner of Huntington County, signed an order compelling the public to wear masks in all public places, including customers in restaurants when they were not eating and employees in all offices where more than five people congregated. Masks did not have to be worn in the open air. The secretary of the Huntington Board of Health and Frost also issued orders to close all schools in the city, churches, theaters, cinemas, and stores. All other establishments could remain open, but eating places were warned their patrons needed masks. Special police officers were to be appointed to see that the rules were "carried out to the letter" and to police the stores, forbidding more than 25 people to assemble in a store at one time. A residential quarantine was to be enforced, with houses placarded, barring the public with the warning "stay out." The decision to wear masks reportedly came after "considerable discussion." Those working in factories were not asked to wear masks at work. Health officials said that if those steps did not work to curb the disease, "more drastic steps [would] have to be taken."[73]

In Muncie, Indiana, Mayor Rollin H. Bunch proclaimed an edict on October 24 and had it published in the local newspaper. In it, he announced that, in effect, Halloween was being canceled that year. Masks, when used in the context of Halloween, were dangerous, and when passed in the store from person to person (passed in the Red Cross workroom from person to person), they might infect many.[74]

Muncie, Indiana, did not adopt a mask mandate during the influenza epidemic, going against the tide of the state. An editor with a newspaper there, speaking in particular about the masking mandate in Indianapolis, said, "And the peculiar point of the situation is that nobody is certain that wearing a mask has anything to do with keeping away the deadly germ. One medical authority says that ten million of these pesky little creatures could cluster on the head of a pin and there hold a court ball. If so one can readily see that the perforations in gauze masks probably look like arches of triumph to a flu germ that wished to enter the mouth of nasal passages of any wearer." And of course, he was correct. But the media hardly ever mentioned this. This editor concluded, though, "And if wearing a mask upon the thoroughfares or in crowds makes the wearer happier, gives him a sense of security that he would not otherwise have, by all means wear the mask."[75]

A few weeks later, an editor with the same Muncie newspaper, probably the same one, had this to say: "If a microscope is truthful and pathology is a true science, you may as well use poultry wire netting on your screen doors to keep out the flies as to wear gauze masks to keep out the influenza germs."[76]

A paper in Logansport summarized the American Public Health Association meeting held in Chicago from December 9 to 12 with more detail than most newspapers. The paper stressed the lack of agreement on what to do about the flu. The health officers generally avoided deciding by vote, but a few informal votes were taken. Did the attending physicians favor closing schools in big cities to fight the disease? "On the showing of hands, only a few went up for closing, while a great many went up against the proposition. The health officers present were plainly against closing in such cases." Dr. W.H. Hill of Minneapolis and president of the Minnesota Public Health Department, chair of the meeting, summarized the situation by commenting, "The consensus I have met with here and elsewhere is that the advisability of closing the schools for the influenza does not exist." Relative to the use of the face mask, a doctor from Cook County (Chicago) hospital declared that it seemed to him that the medical professionals had lost all control of its reason: "If this influenza organism is so small as some claim it is, that you can not see it with a microscope, I can not see why it can not go through any mask. It would be like expecting the bars in the jail window to keep out the flies." Also mentioned in this summary piece was the opinion of Dr. James W. Inches, Detroit health commissioner. He said that masks were "pure fakes" as a means of halting the flu and declared that the closing of cinemas, churches and so forth had not proved to be of benefit.[77]

In Indianapolis, Dr. Herman G. Morgan, secretary of the Indianapolis Board of Health, was already working toward masking the entire city as early as September 29. In response to "many" inquiries the board had received regarding the gauze masks people were advised to use when tending sick flu patients, Morgan published instructions on page one of the local paper, telling readers how to make a mask. He also got the cooperation of theater and cinema managers to eject any patrons they found in their venues who were coughing or sneezing. A notice to that effect was to be seen at the box office, and it was also to be displayed on the screen. Morgan assured those managers that if they cooperated, there would be no need to close their venues.[78]

Then, in December, the Indianapolis Board of Health ordered masks to be worn in the city, essentially everywhere the public could and did gather—everywhere except at home and in the open air. The masking mandate took effect the next day. Officials said that masks should cost no more than ten cents, and enough material to make five to six masks could be bought for 25 cents. Given the sudden onset of the order, people were given an extra day before police enforcement of the mandate began. A subhead of the article declared, "precaution is taken by local health instead of general ban." By then, all public schools and the public library had been closed. Public meetings "except those of vital importance" were "discouraged by the board of health." Public gathering places would not be closed (except the schools, which were closed indefinitely) unless such places permitted violations of the masking order. The board of health had considered reimposing the original quarantine. Still, it felt it would be disastrous to business, especially as the Christmas shopping season was arriving. Schools were closed because it was difficult to impose masking on children and impractical in the case of small children. The problem of enforcement was left to the places affected. If they failed to monitor customers and allowed them to enter their outlet unmasked or move about unmasked in the store, the store would be closed. Regarding the disposal of masks, Morgan said, "The public is instructed not to throw used masks about in public buildings or in the streets. Masks may be used repeatedly if they are cleaned and sterilized. After use they should be rendered sterile by boiling them for a half hour, rinsing and drying. Carry an extra supply of masks with you and change them three or four times each day. After wearing the mask wrap it in paper and take it home to be cleaned. Be very particular that the same side of the mask is worn next to the mouth and nose each time." He did admit that, in some cases, common sense would have to be used. For example, in restaurants, diners would have remove their masks. Actors, ministers, and public speakers would find it almost impossible to wear masks while talking, so the coverings could be removed temporarily and replaced as soon as possible.[79]

Mandatory masking in Indianapolis became effective the next day. According to a reporter, the city board of health had placed the matter of deciding whether business should continue in Indianapolis on the individual and, to a greater extent, the employer. According to Morgan, if there was a tendency on the part of the public to disregard the health regulations, the only resort was to close all the business houses and public gathering places. Thus, Morgan had it both ways. If flu cases dropped, he could claim credit for it. However, if they did not drop, or if they even increased, Morgan could blame the general public. Smugly, Morgan said, "We will give the mask a trial as has been done in other large cities. If there is an unwillingness to abide by the order, the only thing left is to close up business generally. The protective mask has been used with excellent results in many other places."[80]

On the same day, Herman Morgan explained the efficacy of the gauze mask. He began by saying the impression prevailed that viruses (germs) travel singly, and he went on to say, "while this occasionally may be true, they are carried on mucous and dust." Wearing a gauze mask prevented the passage of germs into the respiratory tract. Viruses traveled in large groups, riding on mucous and dust balls. Thus, not a few tiny viruses but a big gang of them all riding on a ball of snot hit somebody wearing a mask. That argument was nonsense in 1918 and would be nonsense one hundred years later. It was a desperate attempt by scientists to explain how the huge holes of, in effect, chicken wire blocked the tiny virus. Not everyone bothered to try to present any proof or experimental evidence of such a claim. Morgan added that "surgeons for years have used gauze masks over the nose and mouth when operating to prevent moisture from the mouth and nose from entering the wound." While that was true, it was not to prevent infectious diseases from being transmitted. Theoretically, in a surgical setting, everyone was healthy (excluding the reason the patient was being operated on). If one of the participants in a surgical procedure turned up with a bad cold or a case of the flu, the surgery would be postponed, at least in theory. When Morgan was asked whether church singers should remove masks while singing, Morgan asserted that the masks could be removed.[81]

The dubious distinction of being the first person in Indianapolis arrested for not wearing a flu mask was Louis Reston, 24. Police Officer Healaco took him into custody in a poolroom. Reston was charged with profanity. While the charge was not explained, perhaps it was due to Reston taking offense at being arrested in the first place. No disposition of his case was reported.[82]

After a day of masking in Indianapolis, a report declared that "everybody" was wearing a mask in the city and that there were almost no exceptions. There were even many people wearing them in the street. Morgan was confident that if the public would comply with the spirit and letter of the regulations, "the epidemic [could] be broken up within a few days." Morgan again "explained" the idea that the germs did not travel singly but were carried on particles of dust or mucous, "and that being the case a gauze mask of wide mesh offers little or no protection to the wearer." But because dust or mucous carried the germs, the mask almost entirely intercepted them. He also reiterated that the mask had been used with "great success" in other cities to forestall the spread of the malady.[83]

An Indianapolis editor commented on the masking rule and complained about those complaining about the face coverings. "There are always some who know more than experts on every subject and who are ready to oppose authority on any proposition. Those who are convinced that the masks are doing no good, that the wearing of them is a needless inconvenience, should stop to realize that at most it is only an inconvenience. It certainly is doing no harm and the logical conclusion is that it is accomplishing very important results." According to the editor, those responsible for public health were not "ordering the people to go about wearing masks because

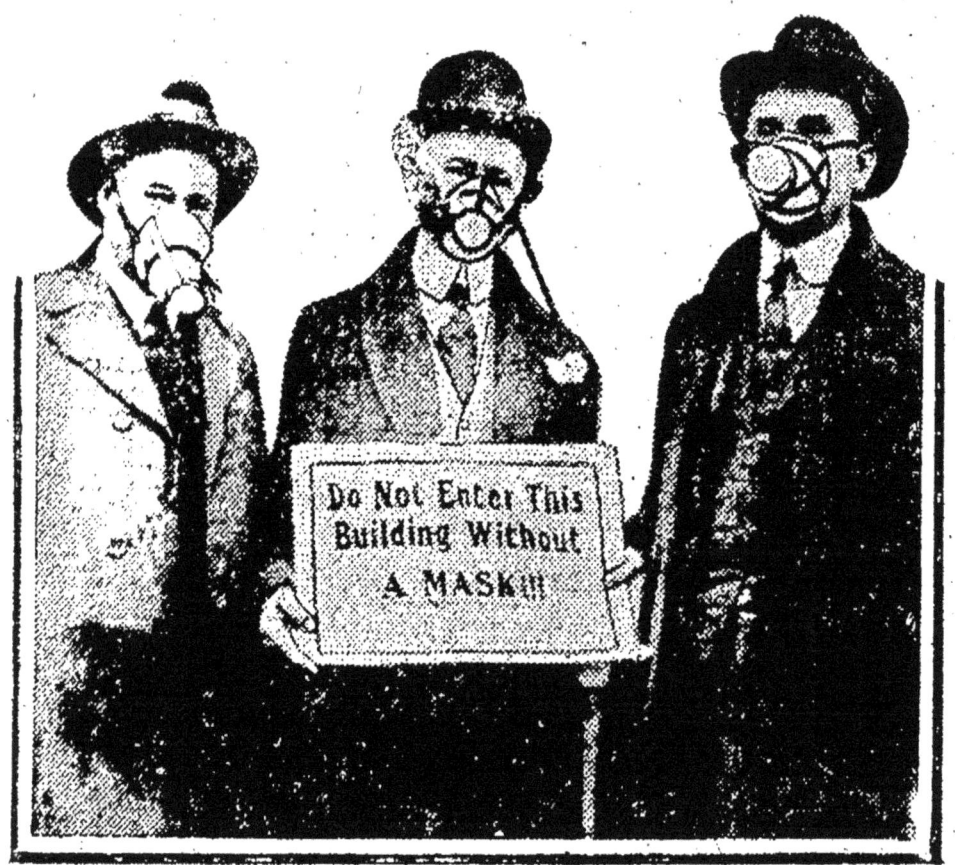

LEFT TO RIGHT—M. DROHLICH, KANSAS CITY, MO.; V. W. BROWN, CHICAGO, AND FRED C. VASICEK, KANSAS CITY.

Three men in Indianapolis appeared in front of a building in a sarcastic protest over the masking mandate.

those are ornamental nor, as some seem to think, to show authority." In conclusion, he declared, "The flu mask was not invented in Indianapolis. It has been used with very satisfactory results in some other communities. Those who should know believe it will be effective in stamping out the influenza in this city. Our masks are designed to protect us personally to protect us personally and the least we can do is to co-operate in an attempt that is made to safeguard our own health."[84]

On the first Sunday after the masking rule came into effect in Indianapolis, although the city board of health had not forbidden church services, few of the churches were expected to hold services. That was due to the pastors thinking it was inadvisable because the congregations were compelled to wear flu masks.[85]

While the editor favored compliance and obedience with the masking rule, the public grew increasingly restive. The Indianapolis Board of Health said it "deplores the obstructive criticism that is being hurled against the mask-wearing order." An angry Dr. Morgan fumed, "This method of preventing cross-infection has been successfully used in a number of cities and has been used by surgeons for years to prevent droplet infection from reaching the field of operation.... Medical literature is full of data which proves conclusively the efficacy of this method." He added, "This is not a time for destructive criticism, petty jealousies or knockers, but an occasion for every individual to aid in the enforcement of the preventive measures."[86]

The city board of health met at a special meeting on the gravity of the flu and determined that their rule to close schools and mandate masking would remain in effect. Part of its statement declared, "The wearing of a mask is a scientific precautionary measure which will aid in the suppression of influenza and contagious pneumonia; therefore, every citizen is requested to co-operate with the board by wearing the mask in public, both for the protection of himself and fellow citizens." Despite the brave words, the board was not getting any cooperation and desperately sought a way to get out of the problem. They would, of course, never admit they had made a mistake. So the board said, "The public is advised that judgment and discretion may be used in adopting this measure; that for example, a clerk in a store not waiting on a customer or an individual in an office or factory where ventilation is adequate and there are no crowds, the wearing of the mask is optional."[87]

At the meeting, Morgan reiterated that when the board adopted the mask-wearing regulation, it had put into effect an order designed to permit the business and social activities of the city to continue with as little hindrance as possible. He argued further that the board members were unanimous in declaring the efficacy of the gauze. He denied the validity of the many criticisms that the mask was an unsanitary device that did not prevent the transmission of influenza germs. When the board of health presented "options" where the mask need not be worn, many people in Indianapolis took that as permission to discard the face coverings completely, according to a reporter. Last night, "on street cars and in many public places fewer wearers of masks were visible."[88]

A day later, the Indianapolis Board of Health capitulated completely and rescinded the order requiring gauze masks to be worn everywhere except the home and the street. However, the order that closed all the schools remained in place. With a straight face, Dr. Morgan declared the influenza situation "seems to be markedly improved." Although he presented no evidence for that contention, "the board is of the opinion that the recommendation of wearing gauze masks as a preventive measure against influenza can with safety be rescinded. This measure enabled the board to bridge over a very alarming influenza situation and to reduce the chances of cross-infection." He added, "While the mask recommendation met with some opposition, the spirit of co-operation in the beginning was all that could have been expected and enabled the board to cut short the present epidemic." Never willing to admit a mistake or defeat, Morgan thundered that if the epidemic again reached an "alarming stage, the board necessarily [would] be compelled to consider either the recommendation of the mask or a rigid ban on all forms of business and public assemblies."[89]

An editor dealt with the subject on the day the masking order was rescinded. First, he pointed out that members of the Indiana Board of Health disapproved of the Indianapolis Board of Health's mask order. The state board members, meeting in Indianapolis while the law was in effect, did not wear masks. Those members also let it be known that the local health officers had, "in the opinion of the state authorities, made fools of themselves. It was an incitement to revolt against the authority of the city health board. The health department was divided against itself." In conclusion, the editor asserted that due to that conflict, "we have a great weakening of public authority as far as it is concerned with the preservation of health. And the law was struck by men charged with that duty. The masks, all agree, are uncomfortable; certainly, they are not decorative. It is by no means certain that they are not to some extent efficacious."[90]

Other cities in Indiana mandated masks and then rescinded the order. Resistance was everywhere in the state. The city and county health boards in Lawrence County mandated a strict ban on all public gatherings. Merchants were told to ventilate their establishments and to keep their windows and doors open during business hours. They were also instructed to see that everyone entering their outlet wore a mask. Businesspeople and manufacturers met with city health officers Thursday concerning the influenza situation. As a result, a day later, on Friday, the masking order was rescinded. On November 23, the city board of health in Martinsville canceled the mask mandate, explaining that all flu cases in the community were under quarantine.[91]

Illinois

On September 30, Dr. John Dill Robertson, Chicago health commissioner, ordered a virtual quarantine of every case of influenza in Chicago. Every victim of the disease was commanded to go home and stay there. No visitors were allowed on the premises.[92]

Two weeks later, on October 14, the recently created executive committee of the emergency commission ordered all theaters and cinemas to close in Illinois to combat the flu outbreak, starting on October 15 and continuing indefinitely. It was to be promulgated as a legally binding Illinois Department of Health order. Local authorities would enforce it throughout the state. Also closed were lodge meetings and night schools. Public schools with a medical inspection system, such as in Chicago, would not be closed. A decision on churches was put off. One type of public gathering allowed was the Liberty Loan rallies to finance America's participation in the war. Also to be closed were "all other places of public amusement." However, no action was taken at that time because the phrase "amusement places" needed additional definitions and rulings.[93]

Shortly thereafter, other Illinois establishments fell victim to closing orders. Dr. St. Clair Drake, director of the Illinois Public Health Department, explained that all public dances had been suppressed and skating rinks closed. Many schools throughout the state without adequate medical inspections had also been shuttered. In explaining the term "other amusement places" in the closing order, Dr. Drake said it was a matter of local action and applied to all places where crowds congregated.[94]

Those Chicago theaters and cinemas closed by the epidemic reopened on Friday, November 1. Illinois health officials warned cities downstate against taking similar action before Monday, November 4. The warning resulted from reports that Springfield, Bloomington, and Danville had made arrangements for reopening their theaters on November 1, three days before the official date.[95]

Dr. John Dill Robertson of Chicago announced that on November 4, the flu restriction lid would practically come off, and Chicago would return to normal. On November 2, Dr. Drake issued the order for 14 other Illinois communities to have their flu restrictions lifted on November 3. That number included the cities of Evanston, Rockford, and Wilmette. The quarantine in the central part of the state was expected to be removed later that week. Still, other parts of Illinois were expected to remain under restrictions for longer.[96]

Decatur was to be released from its quarantine on November 8. According to Dr. Drake, it was one of several central Illinois communities to have restrictions lifted at that time. However, some rules remained in place. Medical examinations of teachers and pupils would continue. Enforcement would be made of sanitary conditions in churches, and people who sneezed, coughed, or showed "symptoms of influenza" were barred from churches, theaters, and other public gatherings.[97]

In the Illinois community of Streator, some restrictions remained in effect in December. Quarantines in residential homes were partially lifted, with people placed on their "honor" to isolate all patients. The head of a family could attend work, but no one else from the household could. But the head of the household was forbidden from attending private gatherings. Poolrooms were opened, and churches could hold one service on Sundays. Lodges and clubs were still closed. Stores were open, but they could not hold any special sales. Saloons could open from 5 a.m. until 8 p.m., except on Saturdays, when they could stay open until 10 p.m. Dr. Drake of the state health board formatted those regulations. All chairs had to be removed or turned to the wall in the saloons; no chairs or card tables were to be used; and no card playing was allowed. The number of patrons permitted in saloons was not to exceed five people (not counting staff). They were to remain inside the saloon for no longer than it took them to transact their business. Funeral services were allowed but with no more than 15 people in attendance. Undertakers were required to report all funerals to the police so there could be "police supervision." All windows had to be kept open during the one "brief" service a church was allowed on a Sunday. Worshippers were to be seated "widely apart," and the minister conducting the service was required to "eject any person who coughs."

Barbers were compelled to wear masks and had to use a fresh one every hour.[98]

Dr. John Dill Robertson, the Chicago health commissioner, was early in his suggestions about the mask. He suggested, on September 26, that all people carry a mask made of gauze soaked in an odorless disinfectant. When anyone coughed or sneezed, the commissioner said the mask should be donned, as in that way, the spread of the disease would be frustrated.[99]

When at least some people in Chicago wore them as October began, a newspaper in Oshkosh, Wisconsin, mocked them by writing that "harem veils" were affected today by Chicago's "white wings." In plain language, the reporter observed that those people were wearing the anti–Spanish influenza masks recommended by city health authorities.[100]

Chicago passed no mandates concerning wearing masks but did use a little persuasion. On October 2, a Chicago newspaper published a composite photo that featured three people wearing masks: a city street sweeper, a county hospital nurse, and an intern. A few days later, it featured a brief piece on page one that gave the reader instructions on making a mask. Most newspapers in America published such material, but Chicago illustrated its piece, unlike most other papers.[101]

A piece in a Chicago newspaper favoring face masks by Dr. A.R. Reynolds, a former city health commissioner, presumably of Chicago, but it was not specified, said, "A new, simple, cheap and successful device has been developed. It is called a face mask…. If such a mask is promptly applied in the early stages of every case of influenza there will be little or no spread of the disease." He added that if the general public "can be made to use them there will be no need to restrict public assemblages or impede in any way the usual habits of the public. As there are and will be mild undetected cases of the disease, and those who may have recovered from it who may be carriers, prudence demands that everybody should wear the mask in crowded rooms, on the street, on windy days, or when engaged in dusty occupations."[102]

When the American Public Health Association met at a convention in Chicago from December 9 to 12, most large or relatively large newspapers in the United States covered it to some extent. Perhaps because it was the host city, Chicago covered the meeting more thoroughly than most other cities. A piece published in Chicago headlined it as the nation's scientists starting a war on influenza. President of the association was Dr. Charles J. Hastings of Toronto, who spoke of the over 800 physicians assembled: "This is the greatest life saving crew in the civilized world." Committees were appointed to report on preventive and relief measures. Dr. W.O. Sherman of Pittsburgh noted that the disease continued despite all preventive measures, such as face masks and closing public places. Dr. W.H. Kellogg of San Francisco said he had started with great confidence in the face mask. Still, in his city where this was tried, he did not find that the death rate was lowered appreciably over cities where it was not tried. Hastings remarked that Toronto, where the mask was not used and people were warned that the vaccine was only an experiment, had the lowest death rate of any city in North America.[103]

A piece that appeared after the final day of the convention reported that following a heated debate during which masks were called "poppycock" and the closing of theaters and churches as "entirely unnecessary," the public health group decided it was not ready to go on record with any recommendations and appointed a committee of five to "fight it out." The committee comprised Drs. W.A. Evans, D.H. Armstrong, W.C. Woodward, W.H. Davis, and E.F. Kolf. They were to take up the flu situation where the association left off, consider the mass of flu evidence presented at the sessions, and make recommendations to be applied in fighting the epidemic. Members of the committee refused to comment directly on the statements made the day before by Dr. James W. Inches, Detroit health commissioner, that flu masks were "pure fake" and "poppycock."[104]

What was unusual about the *Chicago Tribune*'s coverage of the convention was that they published what the committee had to say and their conclusion. Almost no other newspaper in America did so. The report from the committee was delivered on the evening of December 13. The report said, "Vaccines are not looked upon

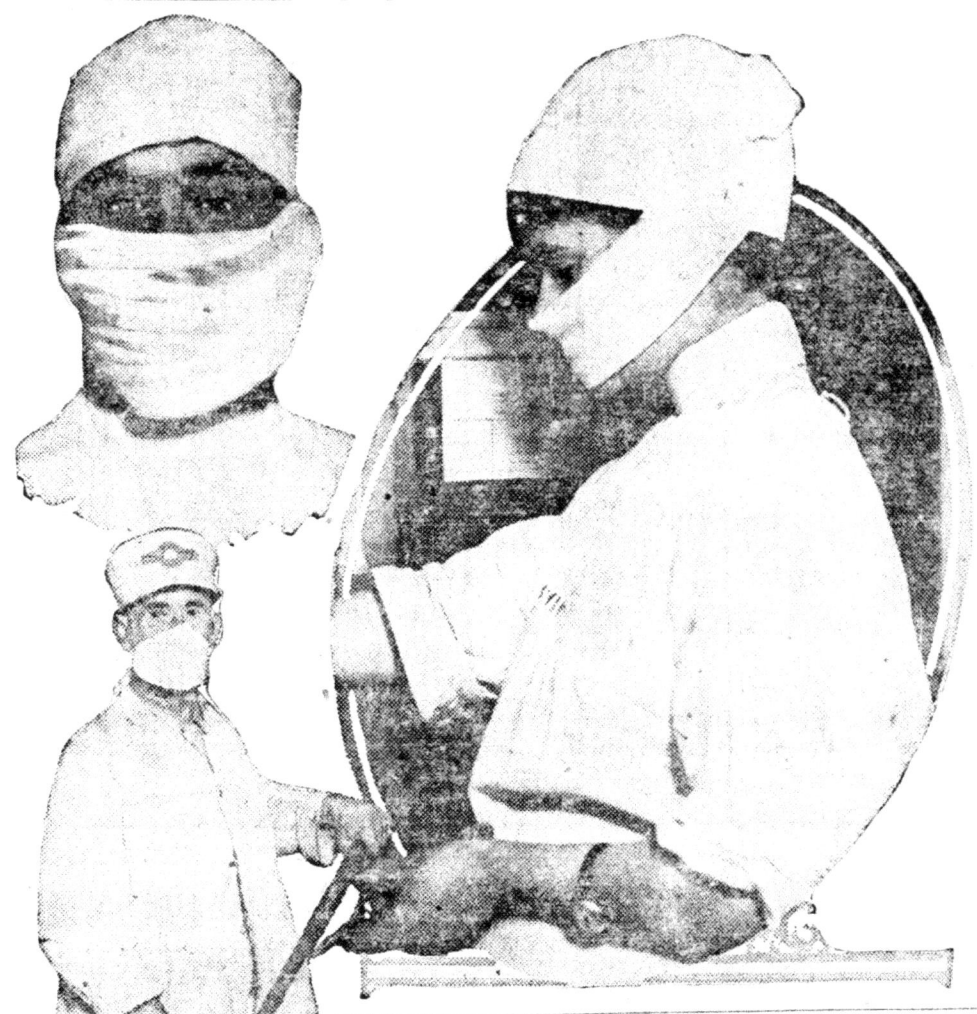

WEARING "GAS MASKS" IN CHICAGO

Street Sweeper Protecting Himself from Influenza Epidemic; County Hospital Nurse and Interne Adopting Precautionary Measures.

A Chicago composite photograph showing three people masked as they worked—part of a public relations campaign to move the populace over to the side of masking advocacy.

by the committee with much confidence as mitigants, while regular habits of living and education of the public as to the dangers of careless coughers, sneezers, and cheerers is thought of value. Discouragement of overcrowding in theaters, schools, churches, and other public gathering places is suggested, and the closing of saloons, theaters, and movie shows is believed a good idea. Necessary gatherings should be held to a minimum." Concerning masks, the committee of five concluded, "On the much discussed subject of masks the committee finds that the wearing of masks in a proper manner should be made compulsory in hospitals and for all who are directly exposed to infection and should be made compulsory for barbers, dentists, etc."[105]

Wisconsin

At a joint meeting, the Racine County Medical Association and members of the local health board in Racine tried to determine what steps to take to combat Spanish influenza on October 5. After debate, the group voted to close the Rupert Blue Protocol establishments and to require all stores except drug stores to close no later than 7 p.m. They also decided to request that the Milwaukee Electric Railway and Light Company not be permitted to allow its cars to be congested and that no passengers be carried beyond the seating capacity of each car. Saloon keepers were told not to permit crowds to assemble in their places of business. The order was to remain in force from the morning of October 7 until the evening of October 21. And the public was advised that it "should not become panic-stricken…. There is no reason for undue alarm, but of course, everyone must observe every health rule and keep away from afflicted ones."[106]

A change of heart quickly took place, and on October 7, John Sieb of the Racine Board of Health stated that the portion of the resolution calling for business closures no later than 7 p.m. would not become effective. He explained that business would not be interfered with at this time, "but there should be no crowding and every effort should be made to hold the number in the store at one time to 50 per cent of normal." Reportedly, there were many inquiries about whether the closure rule applied to bowling alleys and billiard halls. Sieb held that the ruling would not apply to such places because "they are usually well ventilated and there are few people in the places at any one time." However, Sieb did add that there could be a different ruling "at any time" and that there would be a "strict observance" of the public assembly ban. Public libraries would be closed for the two-week duration of the ban, although they had not been mentioned in the original order because "books carry contagion about as well as any other medium."[107]

On October 10, the Wisconsin Board of Health in Madison ordered all theaters, schools, churches, and other public gathering places to close. The order occurred after receiving an advisory order issued that morning by the state board directed to the local health boards throughout Wisconsin. The order from the state board was issued by the state health commissioner, A.A. Harper, as recommended by Surgeon General Rupert Blue of the United States Public Health Service.[108]

One week after that, the Racine Health Department held a meeting, deciding to extend the two-week closure order to be "indefinite." A notice was also sent to the street railway company ordering them to comply with the order not to allow crowding and to provide every passenger it carried with a seat. The local board also ordered all houses to be placarded when influenza patients were present. That was not a residential quarantine but a warning to people to keep out. The measure was done "at the request of the U.S. Public Health Service."[109]

Then, the local Racine Board received a communication from the Racine County Medical Association urging the board to close all business in the evenings, and the doctors declared, "It is the wish of a majority of the physicians of this city that the saloons, billiard halls and 10-cent stores be closed for an indefinite time to better the health conditions of our city."[110]

In response to that communication, the Racine Health Department held a meeting but decided it would not take any action on the medical society's request at that time. However, they did visit the saloons, pool halls, and ten-cent stores and warned them not to permit crowding in their establishments. At the same time, the Wisconsin Board of Health sent out an order that the statewide closing of the usual suspects would continue up to and including October 28.[111]

Then, acting on a communication from the state board, the local Racine Board announced that it would remove the restrictions imposed on the community through its closures and bans on public gatherings on Monday, November 4. Life would return to normal. The authorization for that move came in a letter from Dr. C.A. Harper of the state board. The letter authorized each local area to remove the ban when it saw fit.[112]

Other communities in Wisconsin closed on October 10 in compliance with the state board orders. Madison imposed closure, as did La Crosse. The latter city went a little further and ordered the pool and billiard halls to close.[113]

Green Bay went under a residential quarantine on December 3. City Hall established an ordinance to establish a quarantine over all the residences and buildings in which people ill with influenza resided. The closing ban that had closed theaters, cinemas, bowling alleys, pool rooms, churches, dance halls, and so forth was still in effect in Green Bay. It was to be lifted as soon as the residential quarantine took effect.[114]

With the hope of avoiding a second shutdown of the city, the Madison Board of Health, at the same time as the one in La Crosse, adopted a system of residential quarantine for influenza cases in the city. The quarantine was not to prohibit the wage earner in the family from continuing to work but would stop visits to the home in question and restrict the other household members from leaving the house. All houses containing an influenza patient were to be placarded. It was also strongly recommended that all dances be prohibited during the epidemic.[115]

The rush to impose residential quarantines continued when Stevens Point imposed one of its own a day after the others. Any ill person placed under quarantine had to remain in that category until released by a physician. Also, the local health board ruled that no more than ten people be permitted in any store, shop, saloon, or other business at any time (not counting staff). The rule also applied to banks. Police officers in the community were empowered to enter any store or business to check on compliance with the rule. No public gatherings, dances, meetings, or church activities were allowed except for regular services.[116]

The Wisconsin Medical Society held its annual convention in Milwaukee early in October. In a statement, it "demanded ... general and intelligent compliance with all lawful measures for the control" of the disease. It made several recommendations for the control of the disease, one of which was to recommend that influenza masks be used.[117]

A classic example of the state blaming the victim could be seen in the threat issued by the Racine Health Board in November. When the state imposed a measure on the populace and the situation improved, then the state took credit. When the state imposed a measure on the populace and the situation did not improve, the populace was blamed—the populace did not follow the measure, and so on. In reality, it was the state's fault for imposing a measure that had no chance of success. The Racine Board declared that unless the people were careful in avoiding the spread of the flu, the local board would order that everybody wear masks, whether in public places of assembly or on the streets. The people had to be careful and, most of all, compliant.[118]

In Stevens Point, the local officials declared that the cinemas must close or everyone in attendance would be compelled to wear a mask. This rule applied to the owners and employees of movie houses. The health authorities would close the venue if the mask rule were not complied with.[119]

When a few extra cases of influenza were reported in Kenosha, the local health officer sent a request to the town's people to take added precautions. He requested that members of all families where the disease had developed wear face masks. Commissioner Windsheim said, "These may be made very easily out of a piece of gauze and a small portion of absorbent cotton. A great deal of the danger of the spread of the disease may be eliminated if the people will take this simple precaution."[120]

A newspaper in Eau Claire, Wisconsin, announced that the anti-flu mask would appear there on October 14. On that date, all the workers in the Huebsch Laundry, totaling about 60, including a dozen men, and the 60 operatives in the Horn and Blum Factory would wear masks treated with a germicide when they arrived for work. The face coverings would be worn daily during working hours until the influenza danger passed. Laundry owner Huebsch declared the masks were made so that they caused minor wearer inconvenience, and he said, "if one individual is thus saved from the disease the effect will be well repaid."[121]

After wearing those masks for a day, a report stated that the first day of masking was a success, with no noticeable loss of efficiency and minor inconvenience resulting from the experiment. Most of the employees, the report said, were "entirely willing to wear the masks, but a few objected at first." At noon, when fresh gauze was put into the mask, the wearers were quite surprised to note the dust accumulations on the discarded gauze, and "objections to the 'flu-proof' policies of the establishments ceased." The staff of over 100 employees in the two plants was to continue wearing the masks, with a change every day at noon, until the epidemic was over. According to the story, "Masks of the same type are being worn in factories in many cities and also are worn by physicians and nurses attending the influenza patients."[122]

The health board in Eau Claire advised everyone ill with influenza, their attendants, "and all who meet the public to veil themselves below the eyes." The local chapter of the Red Cross assisted the board in making masks to be distributed free from drug stores. Each mask had to bear the following statement on its wrapper: "A face mask is used for the prevention of contagion in influenza cases." The board of health recommended that it be worn by bank clerks, ticket agents in railway stations, store clerks, and postal clerks. If the epidemic got worse, the board declared it would be wise for everyone to wear them on the streets or in railway trains. Detailed instructions on how to make a mask followed. This piece advised that the boiling period needed to sterilize the mask was ten minutes. While everybody everywhere recommended boiling to sterilize, the period needed to boil the mask varied from some 5 to 30 minutes.[123]

The Eau Claire Health Board continued to push for face coverings. One member of the board declared that "wearing a mask is just as sensible and necessary a precaution here and now as the wearing of gloves or a hat in cold weather or overshoes and umbrella in rain or slush. It is a protection the value of which has been proved in laboratories experimentally and in practical everyday use."[124]

All that gentle and not-so-gentle persuasion in Eau Claire seemed effective if the press could be believed, and, of course, it should not have been. A report in a local paper on November 19 claimed that "clerks in department and ten cent stores, in banks and in all the more popular of the local shops wore gauze masks yesterday and masks were frequently seen on the street."[125]

9

West North Central

Minnesota

In Minnesota, the state board of health met on October 8 with Minneapolis health commissioner, Dr. H.M. Guilford, to decide on the action to take in response to the influenza outbreak. A day later, no decision had been reached. Still, the restrictions had begun as communication was sent to the Minneapolis Street Railway Company, ordering them to keep at least three windows open in each streetcar. One day after that, Guilford banned all "unnecessary" public meetings.[1]

A resolution recommending closing the usual suspects was presented to the Hennepin County Medical Society. If adopted, the resolution—already said to be favored by a substantial majority—would be presented to the Minneapolis City Council, where it was expected to be quickly adopted.[2]

Finally, on October 11, the city health department ordered all schools, churches, theaters, cinemas, dance halls, pool rooms, and billiard halls in Minneapolis to close. All public assemblies were also prohibited. The order went into effect at midnight on October 12. The city health department acted with authority delegated to it by the state health board. The state board was acknowledged as having the real power in the decision, with the city council of Minneapolis just rubber stamping its recommendation.[3]

In this case, there was less than full harmony between the state and local boards. Dr. H.M. Bracken, executive officer of the state board, said he held unnecessary and inadvisable the Minneapolis order closing all public gatherings. Bracken explained by saying, "Consistency is a jewel. If you begin to close, where are you going to stop? When are you going to re-open, and what do you accomplish by opening?" He added, "You shut up your schools when you have trained teachers and nurses ready to keep watch on the children and detect symptoms of disease and take proper steps to prevent its spread." Continuing, Bracken declared, "But do you think that any program of shutting up a few things is going to stop this epidemic? I am not going to argue for the closing of St. Paul. If you ask me to close up Minneapolis, I'll do it, but you may as well be prepared to hibernate like a bear. If I begin, there will be no street cars running and no office elevators. You can close up the rest!" In support of his moves, Dr. Guilford showed a Surgeon General Rupert Blue telegram recommending the imposition of the Blue Protocols—the closing of the usual suspects.[4]

Strife continued to dominate the Minnesota situation. On October 19, the

Minneapolis Board of Education defied the city health board and voted to open the schools over the ban imposed by the city health commissioner, Dr. Guilford. The schools in Minneapolis opened for one-half day on Monday, October 21 but then closed again for the rest of the day and the following two weeks, at least. Then the board of education met again, reversed its action, and voted to keep the schools in the city shut. The school board members were aided in their decision to reverse when Guilford served an order on Lewis Harthill by the superintendent of the police. The order said, "Close the schools." Ultimately, a bitter school board capitulated but felt Guilford put the 60,000 kids within its system in danger and did not help the children. Guilford had never investigated conditions in the schools, for example, and just "blindly" followed the Blue Protocols.[5]

It all ended on Friday, November 15, at 11:30 a.m., after 36 days of quarantine, when the Minneapolis Board of Health removed all restrictions. All seven members of the city board agreed to remove the ban. But orders against public meetings and public funerals continued at least until the next state board of health meeting, due to occur on December 17. Bracken commented that local health officials could not remove a state ban. Other orders could be rescinded by those imposing them.[6]

In Winona, it was reported that flu masks had "invaded Minneapolis draft boards in the middle of October." Instructions sent out from the state draft headquarters required draft officials and their assistants to wear masks when conferring with registrants and for the registrants to be equipped when more than three congregated at one time.[7]

Around the same time, it was reported that barbers at a hotel were wearing masks. The direction for that came from the shop owner. It was thought that other barbers in Winona might follow suit. Nurses at Winona General Hospital were also wearing face coverings.[8]

Bracken made another pitch for masks when he said in a statement, "Wear a cheese cloth face mask over your mouth and nose.... The nurses and doctors wear them for their own protection." The article that featured his pronouncement also contained step-by-step instructions on how to make a face cover. He insisted that by wearing one, "every one can secure self-protection by the simple procedure of wearing the mask described above. It need not be worn at home if all members of the household are well, but it is suggested it be worn in the street cars, in passenger elevators, in the stores, and in workshops and factories."[9]

Minneapolis had not adopted the mask, but at the beginning of October, a paper featured a photo of a nurse from Boston wearing one while working. The caption with the photo was frivolous and lighthearted: "See the pretty nurse—if you can. Is she gagged? Well, hardly."[10]

By mid–October, Dr. Bracken of the Minnesota Board of Health urged that masks be worn "by every man, woman, and child in the state." Workers in the board of health office would continue to wear masks. Bracken noted that many people in Minneapolis, including barbers, nurses, and workers at draft board headquarters, were already wearing face coverings. The University of Minnesota medical authorities urged nursing mothers to wear masks when coming within eight feet of their babies.[11]

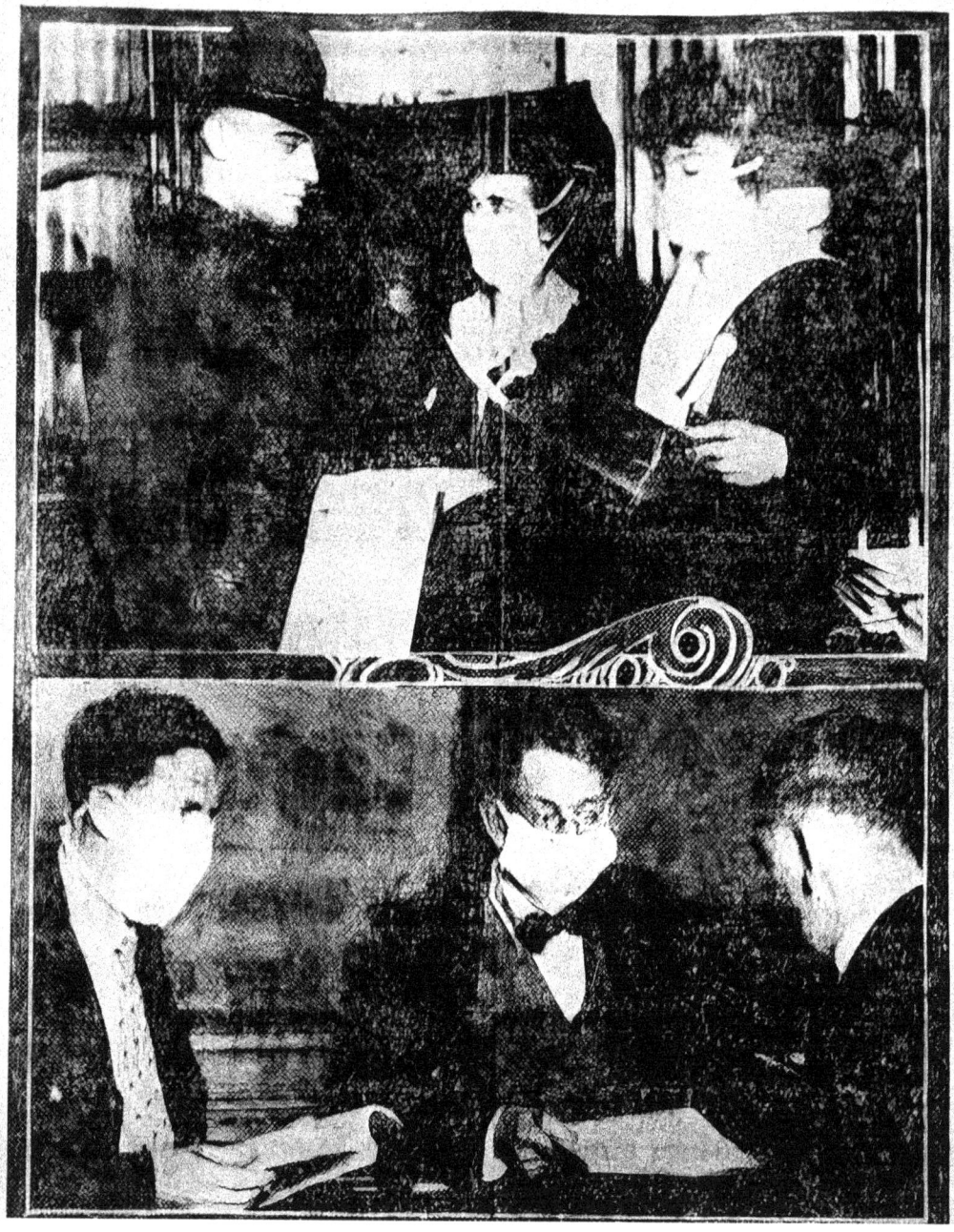

Minneapolis draft boards were "invaded" by flu masks. The military use of masks was pervasive in America, and it was one way the authorities tried to foster the spread of the use of face coverings.

Theaters and cinemas in Minneapolis could reopen on November 2 but declined to do so. The catch was that everyone involved, from actors to attendants to proprietors to patrons, had to wear gauze masks. Dr. Guilford explained that they might open whenever they pleased, provided all involved wore face coverings. I.H. Robie, speaking for the theater owners, said, "We might just as well hang smallpox signs in front of our theaters as to compel our patrons to wear masks. Not a single theater, to my knowledge, will open until the influenza ban is lifted." Restrictions in the churches remained in place, with every other row of seats having to be vacant, as well as every other seat in the occupied rows. Congregations had to be dismissed from the church in groups at staggered times.[12]

St. Paul, Minnesota, was put under strict closing orders as of November 4, with the usual suspects affected. Bracken once again urged masking. He said, oddly, "I would, however, advise the wearing of masks. I believe if all persons would wear masks they would be reasonably safe. I do not wear a mask myself because I personally prefer to take my chances."[13]

North Dakota

Dr. F.B. Strauss issued an order in Bismarck, North Dakota, on October 9, imposing the Blue Protocols on the city. A strict interpretation of Strauss's order closed all lodge, society, and club meetings, political rallies, and other events. Some communities across America used a looser interpretation and allowed certain events to continue, such as Liberty Loan drives and rallies, political events, and other "patriotic" things. Some used a stricter interpretation and banned all gatherings. A conference of Bismarck

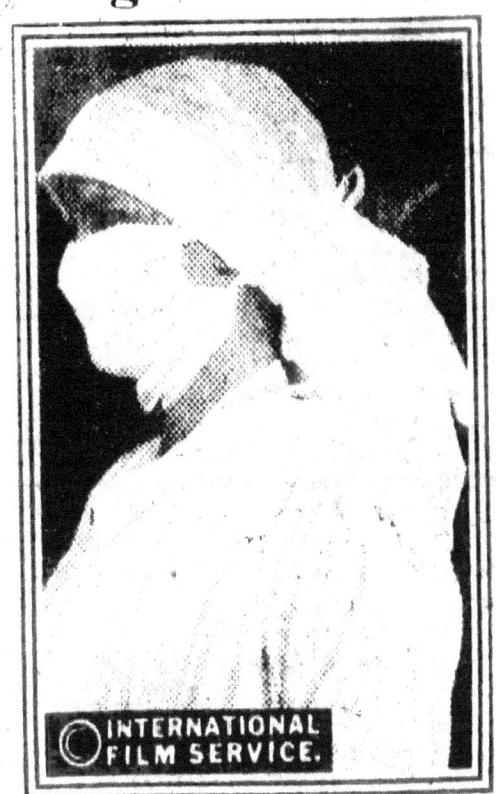

"See the pretty nurse—if you can. Is she gagged? Well, hardly." This facetious caption appeared in a Minneapolis newspaper on October 3 and served to introduce the mask to the public, which was unfamiliar with the item. Humor and sarcasm often attended such debuts.

physicians met on the morning that Strauss issued his order, with differing opinions on the wisdom of suspending public gatherings. While the meeting was in progress, Strauss received notice from Dr. C.J. McGurran, of the North Dakota Bureau of Health, requesting the imposition of restrictions. The notice was in accordance with the instructions Strauss had already received from Blue in Washington. Thus, Strauss overrode any objections from the local doctors and imposed closure.[14]

Fargo had already placed all "unnecessary" public meetings under its ban as of October 7 under an order issued by Dr. Paul Sorkness, Fargo health officer. However, no other measures were taken at that time against any other usual suspects. Using a word like "unnecessary" as applied to meetings meant that the authorities could exempt anything and everything from the ban they wished. The reprieve for the other suspects in Fargo was brief, as the Fargo City Commission ordered all the usual suspects to be closed with no exceptions. On October 9, enforcement was placed in the hands of the police department, which, that same day, notified theater owners and others. Other cities in North Dakota that shut down at the same time included Minot and Grand Forks.[15]

Then Strauss supplemented his orders with requests for the general use of masks by those who had any contact with flu patients. A journalist observed that dentists, barbers, doctors, and others whose work brought them into close contact with the public "are making use of masks in other cities, and it is probable that they will become common in Bismarck before the wave of influenza passes over. Everyone who had anything to do with influenza sufferers or who occupies the same house with a patient is urged to wear a mask."[16]

Strauss delivered harsher instructions to the Bismarck residents a few days later. People were told to stay at home, not to go downtown unless they had urgent business there, to keep off the streets, and not to congregate in stores or on the sidewalks. He said, "If you are coughing or sneezing, wear a mask," and "if you are compelled to be with others who are coughing or sneezing, wear a mask." Then there were the precautions Strauss ordered enforced to protect the general public. Taxicabs had to be kept clean, and the windows had to be open. All those engaged in handling food had to be masked. It was reiterated that citizens were not to assemble on the streets or elsewhere. Special police were detailed with instructions to keep the people moving: "These orders must be obeyed. Police have instructions to immediately arrest any citizen declining to comply." Strauss said, "Anyone with the interest of the community at heart will obey these simple regulations without question. Those who will not obey will be arrested and placed where they cannot endanger their own health and, that of their neighbors. Any business establishment which unnecessarily permits persons to congregate must be closed." Bismarck chief of police Martinson said, "By order of the national government as well as local authorities, people must not congregate on the streets. People can have no business on the streets in the evening when the stores are closed, and they must remain at home on their own premises. I have a corps of extra police on duty, with instructions to arrest, and imprison any persons found loitering or congregating." Servers in local hotels and cafés, employees at the customer windows at the post office, and others in other public places in Bismarck were wearing masks that day. A reporter speculated, "It is probable that the adoption of this precaution will become general."[17]

A reporter from Fargo, when discussing masks, first likened the face mask to a rabbit's foot used as a lucky charm. The surgical dressings department of the local chapter of the Red Cross had been swamped with applications from individuals looking for face coverings. The journalist remarked, "Hygiene and common sense all fall before the power of the face mask." He added, "It is an unnecessary precaution to wear a face mask in open, circulating air that is drenched with sunshine, the best disinfectant known."[18]

In mid–November, a report was received from Dr. C.J. McGurran, secretary of the state health board. The report was to the effect that influenza from the East was returning. Thus, McGurran said, "It is especially recommended that everyone supply themselves with a flu mask and wear it continually until the danger of the second epidemic has abated."[19]

South Dakota

Dr. F.W. Minty, health officer, received an order from Dr. Park B. Jenkins, superintendent of the South Dakota Board of Health, to stop all public gatherings in Rapid City, South Dakota. Schools were also closed. Minty hoped no residential quarantine would have to be placed on homes containing influenza patients. People were requested to stay at home "with the exception of those employed in needful occupation."[20]

Closures were announced a few days later for Aberdeen, Sioux Falls, and Minnehaha County. All the usual restrictions were imposed, except that the schools could remain open. It was believed that the children could be handled better in schools than if they were loose on the streets. People were requested to remain off the streets and in their houses as much as possible. Lodges were not specifically mentioned in the order but were "expected to comply."[21]

Two days later, the Sioux Falls Health Board decided to quarantine all residences with flu cases. Dr. W.E. Moore was the city health physician. Also that day, police were given strict orders to prevent groups of people from congregating either indoors or outdoors. Store managers were asked to perform the same function in their establishments. Dr. J.G. Parsons suggested "nose masks" as an effective public safety measure. At a meeting of medical people that included members of the Sioux Falls Medical Association, city commissioners, and others, with Parsons presiding, he argued that people who sneezed, sniffled, or coughed on the street should be compelled to wear the nose mask on public highways. Concerning limiting crowding or congregating, Parsons suggested that the standard should be one person for every square yard of store space. Dr. A.H. Tufts, county health physician, said people were becoming "far too alarmed." There was no occasion for fear, only for precautionary measures. Dr. D.L. Rundlett offered the opinion that the public was literally "scared to death."[22]

Keystone, South Dakota, imposed its restrictions later in October. Like most others, it banned all public gatherings. Unlike almost all other areas that took that step, Keystone defined the term rather than leaving the size of a gathering unstated or hopelessly vague. Keystone declared that a gathering was an assembly greater than two people. Schools were closed, and the kids there were to be kept under the supervision of parents and not allowed to mingle with other kids. Children could venture forth to do "errands" but not to "loiter" in business houses or other families' houses. No more than two people at a time could be in the post office. No visitors could enter Keystone unless authorized. Nobody from Keystone could visit other towns "without authorization by members of the School Board," who would arrange details of quarantine, if necessary, when that person returned to Keystone.[23]

On October 24, Mayor W.E. Robinson of Rapid City took steps to impose a strict residential quarantine. Someone under quarantine could only be released after receiving a doctor's certificate after five days without a fever. Homes under quarantine were placarded, and no gatherings were permitted. All pool halls, soft drink parlors, and soda fountains in the city were then closed, and serving soft drinks was stopped. No loitering on the streets was allowed. At the train station, only one person could go into the building and buy a ticket.[24]

Into this South Dakota contest to determine who could impose the quirkiest rules to live by came Custer (county and city). Among their restrictions were that no person could wait in the post office while mail was sorted, no person was allowed at the train depot except on necessary business, no chairs or stools were allowed in any place of business, no children were allowed on the streets, no public meetings of any kind could take place, and no person leaving Custer could return during the period of restrictions unless a permit from the health board was secured. Custer residents returning during the restriction period were to be isolated in their homes for one week. Nonresidents could not stop in Custer, and any suspected cases would be quarantined. Unnecessary visits within the town and county of Custer were to be discontinued.[25]

Then, in the first week of November, most restrictions were removed from most places. On November 4, all restrictions were lifted in Rapid City, except that the schools remained shut and the residential quarantine continued. Gregory, South Dakota, lifted its restrictions on November 6.[26]

Sioux Falls did not remove all restrictions until November 28, just in time for Thanksgiving. Dr. Moore announced the unanimous decision after a meeting with Mayor Burnside and a group of 15 other men (members of the city commissioners, the city attorney, the County Council of Defense, ministers, Commercial Club representatives, and the superintendent of schools). However, the residence quarantine remained in place. And people were still requested not to spend more time in the stores than was necessary and to avoid any unnecessary visits.[27]

As soon as the epidemic became apparent in other Black Hills towns, authorities in Hot Springs issued an order requiring all city residents to wear flu masks when on the street. The authorities declared that the order must be obeyed by "all, old and young."[28]

Beginning on December 19 in Aberdeen, South Dakota, no resident could appear on the street, in a theater, restaurant, church, business establishment, school, or other public place without wearing an influenza mask, by order of the Brown County Council of Defense and the Aberdeen Board of Health. Theaters, churches, and other public places were also required to see that the buildings were carefully fumigated and well ventilated and that any person who coughed or sneezed was "instantly remove[d]" from the place. All people were urged to be vaccinated, and school kids could get the shots for free. Schools would not be closed, but teachers and school nurses were to watch the pupils closely and send home any child who coughed, sneezed, or exhibited other signs of illness. All business houses, theaters, and churches were required to prevent overcrowding. A residential quarantine was put into place. These measures were all taken by Aberdeen as ways of dealing with the second wave of the disease as it traversed South Dakota.[29]

Within a week, the debate over masking heated up in Aberdeen. The discussion started when Dr. R.L. Murdy, described as a "leading" physician in the area, said in a newspaper interview that masking as a preventive of influenza was "all nonsense" and unclean, besides causing people wearing masks to rebreathe unclean air, a most unhealthful practice. At the same time, there was nothing to show that the masks prevented anyone from catching the disease. W.P. Butler, a "leading" socialist, endorsed Murdy's position, charging the physicians and the health board with selfish motives for requiring wearing masks. A.E. Joy, a leader of the Christian Science Church, wrote a newspaper article also contending the practice was wrong. On the other hand, the Aberdeen retail merchants' association, after a conference with the health board and physicians, issued resolutions announcing its adherence to the regulations and pledging its members to carry out the rules in every possible way. But the health board was buckling, as it announced it had abolished the requirement of wearing masks on the streets. It was also reported that some violators were arrested and fined, but the practice of donning masks was "generally being followed."[30]

By December 30, the Aberdeen Health Board had backtracked again. This time, it issued another order that rescinded what remained of the masking order. While masks were no longer mandatory anywhere, the Aberdeen Health Board "recommended" their continued use. And that meant the obvious would happen; as a journalist observed, "Following this action the 'flu mask' has practically disappeared from Aberdeen except in rare instances."[31]

Somewhat later, in mid–February 1919, an editor with a newspaper in Deadwood, South Dakota, republished an editorial that had first appeared in a Santa Barbara, California, newspaper. It spoke to the issue concerning masks that all too many scientists understood but which virtually nobody ever mentioned. "Queer, is it not, that germs that cannot be seen with the finest microscope and cannot be measured with the finest measurement are so disposed. They live in street cars or sidewalks. They thrive in barber shops and not in dentists' offices. They inhabit churches and theatres alike, but not restaurants nor cafeterias. Queer, is it not, that these little bugs, so very little they cannot be detected with the microscope, and that they can go thru cement and even glazed dishes, are yet so large that they can be held back by thin meshes of a handkerchief, or the thin stuff that goes into a mask?"[32]

Iowa

A general quarantine in Des Moines, Iowa, was established at 9 a.m. on Thursday, October 10, and involved the standard imposition outlined in the Rupert Blue

Protocols. In addition, the streetcars were limited to carrying the seating capacity of each car. A couple of days later, it was found necessary to modify the streetcar rules a little in order not to hamper the construction of the Fort Dodge military installation. Fort Dodge workers and coal miners could ride until 7:30 a.m. but could not exceed 25 percent of the car's seating capacity.[33]

Late on October 17, Dr. Guilford H. Sumner, secretary of the Iowa Board of Health, issued an order to impose the Blue Protocols statewide, closing the usual array of churches, schools, theaters, and all public gatherings. Muscatine had not yet ordered the closing of poolrooms, confectioneries, and the like. Because Blue had not specified establishments like those on his list of recommendations, some areas in America left them out. Some areas included them at the time of imposing the initial closing order, and some areas added them to the list of closures at a date after the original imposition of the protocols. The local health officers usually had discretion over whether to close those places. The statewide order also applied to Des Moines, which had already imposed a similar closure order a week earlier. Duplicating the order meant local officials in Des Moines could remove their closure order but not the state-imposed order, which remained in place until the state removed it. Sometimes, though, the state, after imposing statewide orders, would back away and leave the power to rescind to the local authorities.[34]

Giving an example of his authority, Sumner reiterated a few days later that he would not be lifting the quarantine on Des Moines until he did so for the whole state. Then, Sumner reversed himself just three days later and issued an order that permitted local health officials, such as those in Des Moines, to lift the ban. And in just a few more days, on October 29, Des Moines lifted all restrictions.[35]

When the second wave of influenza hit Iowa, the City of Muscatine imposed its restrictions for a second time. By order of the city health board, the usual suspects were closed, along with some additional measures. All business houses, except drugstores, had to be closed from 6 p.m. until 7 a.m. Before this second set of restrictions was imposed, there was vigorous debate over the quarantine and who had the authority to implement such things.[36]

When Davenport imposed its second quarantine on December 11, a reporter called it the most rigid one ever experienced in the city. Every business house, except factories, grocery stores, drugstores, meat markets, and milk depots, had to be closed. The city council recommended the action, and the local health board approved it. Every business was closed except for factories and those that sold food or drugs. Coal and wood dealers could also remain open. It was in effect for one week. Other cities followed suit in imposing second lockdowns. On December 21, Hampton and Keota imposed their second set of restrictions.[37]

Perhaps planning for future similar epidemics, Iowa issued a statewide set of rules in September 1919 for residential quarantines of flu patients. The attending physician had to certify recovery. If no doctor was attending to the patient, then recovery was defined as the patient's temperature being normal for three days in a row. In recovery, the convalescent had to have a complete change of clothing. The clothing worn during the illness had to be hung outdoors and thoroughly aired for at least eight hours, preferably in a place reached by the sun.[38]

A reporter writing in Davenport declared on October 18, "If you should happen to enter a Davenport barber shop and to see the barber approach with his face covered with a mask don't become frightened and think that there is any danger of a gas attack. The barbers are merely wearing the mask to prevent the spread of Spanish influenza." The Davenport Board of Health had not made it mandatory for barbers to wear face masks; it was "suggested" by the health officials, and as a result, most of the barbers in the city had adopted them. The Davenport chapter of the Red Cross supplied the barbers with disinfectant gauze for the masks. According to the report, if all of Davenport's barbers carried out the suggestion to wear masks, then the board would not issue a mandate. The board would not hesitate to issue such an order if some barbers refused.[39]

The idea of having more and more people wear masks was part of a plan underway by Davenport health officials. Barbers and street railway conductors were especially advised to wear them, as were people who rode daily to and from work on the streetcars and women shoppers. "This gauze mask is made of very light material and can be carried in the pocket, and a person riding on a street car could easily put it on before entering the car and remove it when they reached their point of destination." A journalist remarked, "The plan is a very good one and is one of the few that has produced any real results of the many that have been tried out."[40]

At the start of December, a reporter visited a Moline department store and was surprised to find a young clerk ducking her head under the counter. It turned out she was just bending over to adjust her flu mask. Most shop clerks wore them around their necks and adjusted them at a moment's notice. One clerk

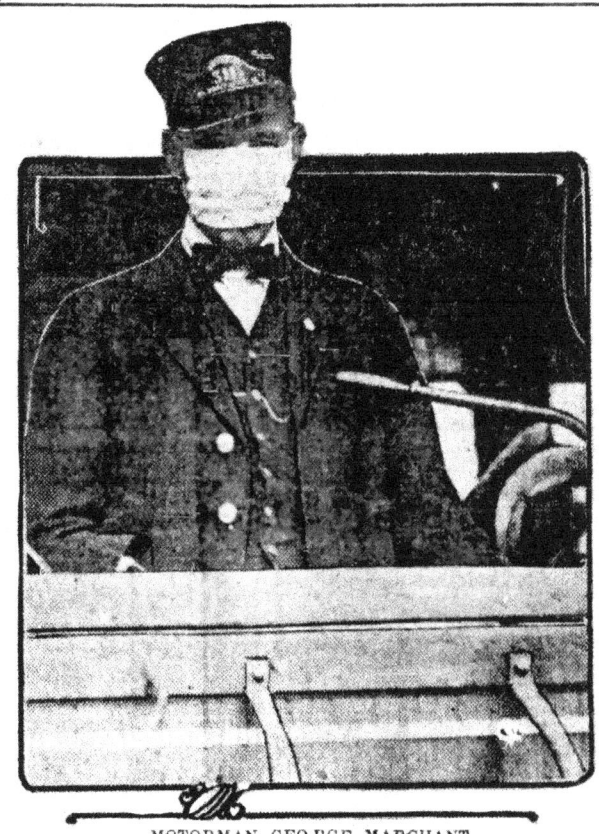

MOTORMAN GEORGE MARCHANT.

George Marchant, motorman, in Des Moines, Iowa, shown on October 10. While state and local health officials often lacked the nerve to impose mask mandates, they often successfully hectored private sector employers to do the work for them and force masks on their employees. Many did just that.

told him it was done just as the soldiers in the trenches donned gas masks before an impending gas attack. According to the reporter, the order of the board of health requesting all people entering and working in stores wear masks "has met with cheerful response."[41]

When the Davenport Board of Health met at the beginning of December, it adopted a series of lockdown moves. One was to order residential quarantines, with no one allowed to enter or leave the premises except medical personnel. Household members could not leave until the authorities removed the placard on the premises. People had to wear masks at public gatherings, including theaters, cinemas, and businesses.[42]

At the same time, masks were becoming more prevalent in Moline. Reportedly, the number of people observed on the streets who were masked up and in the stores and shops of the city was "increasing daily." Among the first to adopt masks for their employees were the local department stores. A reporter said, "So many people are realizing the seriousness of the second visit of the plague, that it is only a question of time when the person not wearing a face covering will be noticed, instead of it being just the opposite at present."[43]

In a meeting with Dr. Sumner, secretary of the state board of health, the Davenport Board of Health decided on December 4 to make wearing masks compulsory in all public places. It meant people had to wear face coverings in all theaters, dances, lodges, churches, and similar gatherings. It was noted that the compulsory wearing of masks was the only condition under which dance halls, theaters, and business houses could remain open. And it was reported, threateningly, "It is recommended that every business house enforce the order to prevent more drastic action on the part of the board of health." Manager Harry Blanchard of the Columbia Theater stated that he would order 10,000 masks at once for the use of his patrons, the masks to be furnished with every ticket, either free or at cost.[44]

In Sioux City, at Morningside College, the faculty ordered wearing masks as a precaution against the spread of influenza. Wearing gauze masks, the students reported to their classes "influenza proof," as the caption under a masked student would optimistically have it. The picture of part-time student and newspaper reporter Maurice Van Metze was under the headline "immune to influenza."[45]

Morningside College went even further a few days later when the institution announced a radical program to fight the flu. It included taking each student's temperature before classes each day and the "absolute compulsion" of wearing a mask during school hours. The action taken regarding wearing masks resulted from the discovery that the plan did not work out under the voluntary system. The student body had worn masks for only one day. Thereafter, everyone had to wear face coverings while in school—the faculty and the students.[46]

Even a rumor about forced masking in Keokuk, Iowa, caused some officials to get the jitters. At its regular board of education meeting, Superintendent of Education Aldrich explained, "We haven't required any wearing of masks." Board members suggested making that fact clear to all the children so they could tell their parents. Many children had erroneously reported at home that masks were required at school.[47]

In Muscatine, the local board of health issued an order requiring wearing masks by everyone in stores, factories, shops, and places where people congregated. The order had an immediate effect. The meeting of the board of health, which made the decision, was held after women representing the War Service League and other organizations had visited the mayor and other board members earlier that day and argued for adopting such a measure. Thus, wearing masks became compulsory everywhere except on the street. The local Red Cross chapter advised that they could not supply the necessary number of masks given the very short lead time, nor did they have enough material for the job. So, the article supplied detailed instructions so that readers could make their own.[48]

In Des Moines, the idea that people would have to mask up appeared in the press on November 27, when it was reported that a decision would be reached in a few days on the proposal that everyone in Des Moines would be compelled to wear a face mask.[49]

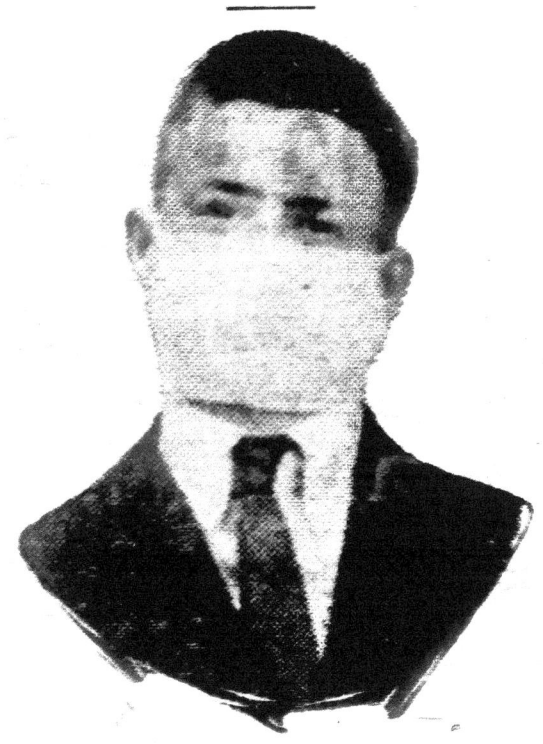

Maurice Van Metre, a student at Morningside College in Sioux City, Iowa, shown wearing a mask, which all students were forced to wear. According to the headline, Maurice received superpowers from that mask because it rendered him "immune to influenza."

Then what would become a disaster for the Des Moines authorities began. In order "to completely exterminate influenza," the special health board ordered, on the morning of November 29, the universal use of the flu mask. Those masks had to be donned immediately, although the order did not become legally mandatory until after November 30. Masks had to be worn on the street and in every type of public gathering. In short, when people were outside their homes, they had to wear it everywhere. The Des Moines City Council was to meet that afternoon to make noncompliance a misdemeanor and stipulate the punishment.[50]

A day later, the mask rule was modified when new rules were instituted. Under the new regulations to deal with the second wave, all schools were closed, additional streetcar regulations were imposed, and all public gatherings were banned beginning the following day unless the people in charge required all people who entered the gathering to wear a face mask—it was a rule that applied to all churches, theaters, and other public gatherings. If the rule was disregarded, it would result in the total closure of the event or gathering. The flu mask edict of a day earlier was modified to affect only theaters, churches, and public gatherings. Schools were ordered closed because it was considered "impractical" to attempt to enforce wearing masks during school recitations. It meant the mask had to be worn only at meetings and gatherings, not on the street.[51]

Speaking for the Des Moines churches, the Rev. C.S. Medbury advocated church closures because "people can't sing hymns through a mask very well and communion is out of the question." Representing the Christian Scientists, John L. Rendall called the mask an infringement of citizens' rights: "The mask has no validity, it is filthy, and does no good." He cited figures to show that death rates were lower in cities that did not employ the mask than in cities that imposed the face covering. Norman Wilchinsky, manager of Younker Brothers, speaking for the retail merchants, declared the flu mask regulation impractical and ineffective. "Business men are willing to cooperate in any measure necessary to save quarantine," he said, "but the situation has not been proven to be as serious as suggested." He, and others in opposition to the masking law, felt the residential quarantine should have been used earlier and wanted to see it in force now.[52]

Opposition continued to mount against the mask. A strict enforcement of the order to wear flu masks in all public places would make it impossible for the state-federal employment service to continue its work. At least, according to the statement of Mrs. Pauline Neufeld and Mrs. Marie V. West, in charge of the two main branches of the service in Des Moines, "We must be continually talking if we do our work properly. We sometimes have a difficult time making ourselves understood even without masks," explained Neufeld. "We are willing to do anything in reason to assist the board of health. Our rooms are well ventilated, besides we fumigate all the offices every night right after closing."[53]

The editor of a Des Moines newspaper expressed annoyance over the situation. "The *Evening Tribune* believes the scientific men ought to get together and issue some sort of definite program for the treatment of such epidemics as the flu. We have two wholly different sorts of quarantine ordered in Des Moines. First business was practically closed. Now everybody is to wear a mask." He concluded that unanimity was necessary and suggested that "a statement signed by twenty-five or thirty of the recognized scientific men of the city would go far to satisfy the public that the proper course is being pursued."[54]

After more stormy and controversial meetings, the mask order took effect at 6 p.m. on December 2. Masks had to be worn by the audience in all theaters, cinemas, and at all public gatherings. Masks did not have to be worn on the streets, in streetcars, offices, and stores. Colleges were open, but masks did not need to be worn. All public schools were closed. Public speakers and actors could appear on the rostrum or stage without masks.[55]

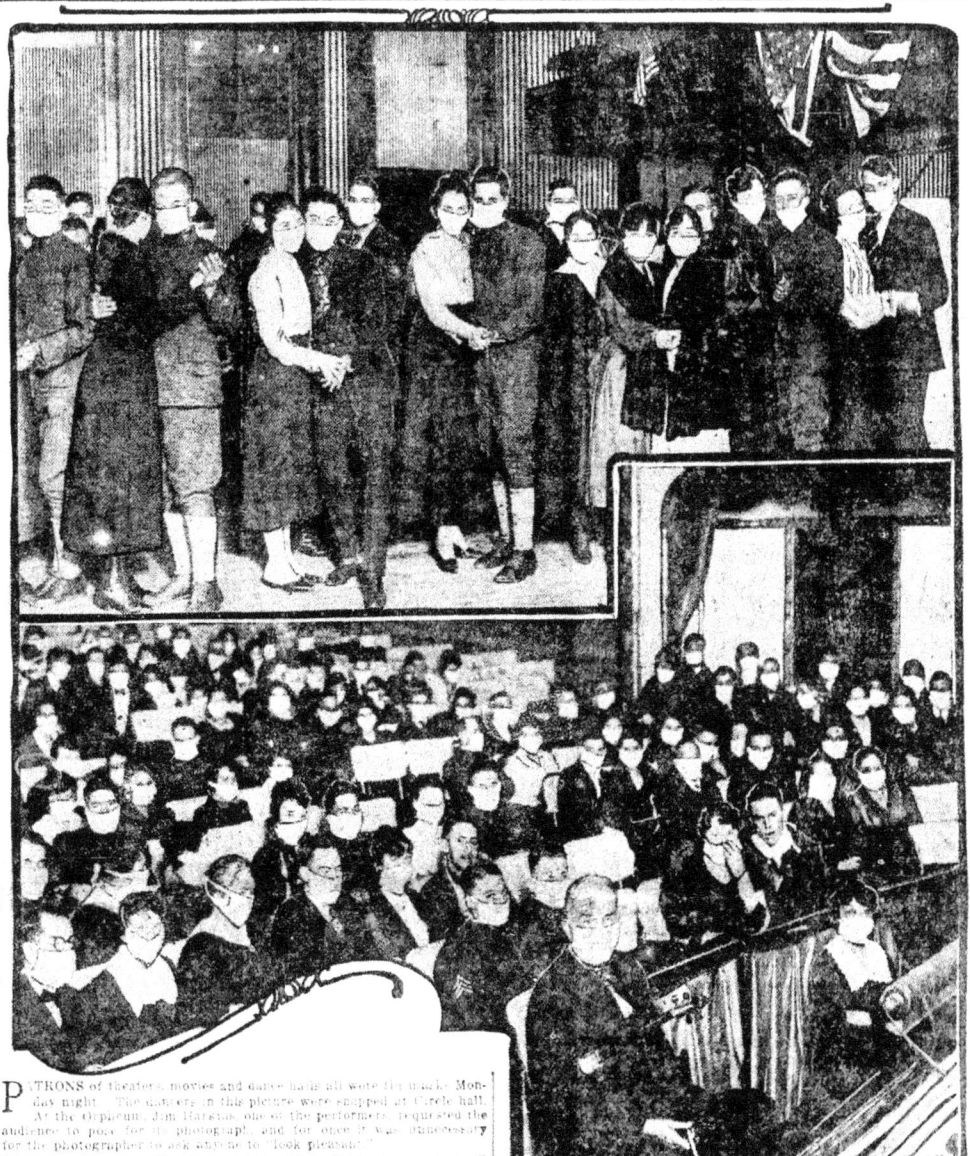

A theater crowd and a dance hall crowd in Des Moines were masked. See if you can spot the two in the theater crowd who are not masked. Rebels who do not understand the concept—question nothing, obey everything.

Just one day later, the masking mandate collapsed. The new order declared, "Wear a mask or not as you please at churches, theaters and public gatherings." Theater owners had argued that their venues were nearly empty. The influenza committee strongly recommended "the wearing of masks but leaves it up to the individual." Theater owners also noted that the few patrons who did show up were wearing masks, but most of them took them off during the performance.[56]

During their protests of the masking rule, at one point, the theater managers said they would not observe the masking requirement because the final form of the rule did not require mask wearing as they went about their usual daily business in stores, factories, offices, streetcars, and so on. The managers argued, "We feel that this resolution is unjust discrimination, and we will not ask our patrons to wear masks while attending our moving picture theaters and others, for we consider that if the mask is valuable and effective in one place, it certainly would be in another." Those theater owners threatened that they might have to take legal action.[57]

In a discussion of the rapid removal of the Des Moines mask law, Ralph Bolton, secretary of the Greater Des Moines Committee, said there was too much buck passing in the flu situation in his city. Dr. T.F. Duhigg, a member of the flu committee, denounced the regulations as an absolute failure. Bolton declared that the rules had been changed so frequently that no one took them seriously and that the mask edict "was laughed out of existence."[58]

A committee report from the American Public Health Association reached Des Moines and was published there on Christmas Day. It reached Iowa at the Iowa Bureau of Health office. It was the first report from that group on influenza, which arose from its convention in Chicago that month.

The report stated that there was no known laboratory test to determine when a person who had suffered from influenza ceases to transmit the disease to others. Also, there was no known test by which an attack of influenza could be differentiated from an ordinary cold, bronchitis, or other inflammation of the nose, pharynx, or throat mucous membranes. Wearing masks should be compulsory for barbers, dentists, hospitals, and all those directly exposed to infection. The committee's report did not suggest the general public wear masks, but members of the public could wear them if they so desired.[59]

Missouri

A proclamation directing the closing of schools, theaters, and other public gatherings was drawn up on October 7 in St. Louis for the signature of Mayor Henry Kiel. The action followed a conference among many city authorities, including medical officials, the army, and the Red Cross, among others, as well as the St. Louis Health Department office, which was headed by the health commissioner, Dr. Max D. Starkloff.[60]

The next day, under what was described as a "drastic order" from Starkloff and approved by Mayor Kiel, the usual shutdown was imposed on St. Louis, effective at noon that day. One exception was that ordinary church services could be held. Still, church events that involved gathering an "extraordinary number" of people were barred. Saloons were not affected, except loitering within them was prohibited. Library reading rooms were shut down, but issuing books was unaffected. A delegation of 15 cinema and theater owners visited Kiel that same day. It urged that the closing be extended to department stores, five- and ten-cent stores, and elevators. They did not ask for the part of the order that shuttered them to be rescinded.

Frank Tate, a spokesperson for the group, said it would cost theaters $150,000 a week to remain closed, and the government would lose revenue from them of $25,000 per month. Making a further point, the theater owners argued that if they could remain open, they could show propaganda concerning the flu on their screens. The theater men, through Tate, offered to pay for and post advertisements warning the public of the dangers of the flu. Meetings of clubs that held regular luncheons would not be stopped, but speaking at events that would "attract crowds" was forbidden.[61]

Dr. Starkloff then appealed to factories and large businesses, asking them to give full cooperation to his efforts to curb the flu. One way for them to do so was to institute medical supervision of their employees and refuse to let those showing symptoms of the disease work. Another was to ban customers with symptoms from their premises. He also made a special appeal to people to avoid gatherings, even congregations of five or six people. Starkloff met St. Louis Police Chief Young and all 14 police captains, who gave the officers their marching orders. Young directed the appointment of physicians to police stations so that all patrol officers might more easily report unattended influenza cases.[62]

On October 23, Dr. Starkloff said the limitation of store hours in downtown St. Louis (9:10 a.m. to 4:30 p.m.) would be rescinded immediately. The order had been designed to prevent crowding on streetcars. Still, it had caused much misunderstanding and confusion and had been a hardship for small dealers. At the same time, Starkloff called Melville L. Wilkinson, president of the Associated Retailers, and suggested the large department stores voluntarily continue with those limited hours. A week later, a committee conference that initially put the lockdown order in place adjourned its meeting without taking action. It meant the Blue Protocols would not be lifted for the present. Mayor Henry Kiel said he thought the ban on churches should be lifted, but he would abide by the opinion of the medical professionals. He explained that he had received many complaints against the order and that it was his duty to present them.[63]

One month after the original imposition of the quarantine in St. Louis, it was made even more drastic. Effective at 6 a.m. on November 9 (Saturday), the city was closed tight by order from the city health board. All department stores, general merchandise stores, saloons, candy and cigar stores, nonessential factories, and all other businesses not listed as essential were ordered closed. Offices had to be closed. A combined saloon and restaurant was allowed to stay open, but only to serve food. The closure order was extended for four days. And at midnight on November 12, it was lifted. The ban on theaters and churches, part of the first closure order, was also lifted.[64]

Toward the end of November, the regulations lifted two weeks earlier in St. Louis were partially reimposed due to a sudden increase in flu cases. Schools were closed, children were prohibited from Sunday schools, all "non-essential" gatherings were stopped, and strict rules for streetcar ventilation were adopted. Children under 16 were prohibited from places of amusement and larger retail stores. Starkloff lifted the ban on December 20, except for the parts involving children under 16.[65]

Kansas City, Missouri, passed an order from the health board forbidding the usual suspects, with a slight variation. Public gatherings were forbidden, but only if the size was more than 20. Also, meetings of "military necessity" were exempted. Mayor James Cowgill declared that an emergency existed. Streetcars were limited to carrying no more than 15 people standing in each car. Dr. W.P. Motley was the president of the Kansas City Health Board.[66]

When Dr. A.J. Gannon, head of infectious diseases in the health department, called P.J. Kealy, president of the Metropolitan (a streetcar company), and asked him to allow a maximum of 20 people standing in a car, Kealy refused to cooperate. Then Gannon went to police Chief Godley and asked the police to enforce the order. Still, other health department officials refused to back up Gannon. Dr. Bullock called off Gannon after an official with transit called Bullock and complained that Gannon was persecuting the company. Eventually, transit capitulated and agreed to limit standing to 20 to 25 people per car.[67]

Then, on October 14, the ban on public gatherings was lifted on the strength of an order from the city's health board. Permitted to reopen were the usual suspects, and the crowding of streetcars was also allowed again. Mayor Cowgill was the instigator of a meeting that ended the ban and the chief promoter of rescinding the closure order. Medical opinion was said to have been mixed, although the health board finally agreed.[68]

The order to rescind lasted precisely three days, at which point a more drastic lockdown order was imposed. Once again, streetcars were limited to no more than 20 standing in each car, and the windows had to be kept open. Music was stopped at hotels and cafés. All public gatherings of more than 20 people were stopped. Stores employing 25 or more people could not open before 9 a.m. and had to close no later than 4 p.m. Crowding in any store was forbidden. Health inspectors would be dispatched to exercise individual judgment in determining when the crowding was getting dangerous and to order the store closed until the crowd thinned. As to the rationale for the store hour limitations, it was said that "physicians asserted six hours' work in a store to be the greatest length of time a person should be exposed to the possibility of infection." Which, of course, didn't explain the seven-hour workday.[69]

Inspectors in Kansas City were quickly on the job. They found two business colleges were trying to get around the ban on holding classes with no more than 20 people in a classroom. Those colleges had more than 20, and they were both closed. Inspectors also found streetcars overcrowded and with their windows closed. Inspectors were sent to one of the five- and ten-cent stores and found it crowded. Since it was close to 4 p.m., the store was allowed to stay open as long as floorwalkers kept the crowd moving through the store.[70]

Mayor Cowgill ran into more differences of opinion when he tried again to rescind the order, and very little was accomplished, except that the lockdown order on the Kansas City, Kansas, side of the border was lifted at noon on November 9.[71]

In Maryville, a report observed, "When you call central [telephone exchange] today, and a muffled voice repeats your number don't imagine that she has not heard correctly and that you will get the wrong number. The muffled voice you will hear will be coming through a gauze mask." All the phone operators were wearing them. Manager H.C. Todd of the central phone exchange decided to ask the operators to use the gauze masks while at work. According to this piece, "the plan was readily agreed to."[72]

Dr. H. DeLamater, health officer in St. Joseph, Missouri, said at the start of December, "If the situation doesn't change for the better within the next twenty-four hours, the department will issue an order compelling all persons to wear influenza masks." The health officials also held out a possible second shutdown as a threat. The city's health department was receiving many protests from businesspeople against a second ban. And that type of lobbying was one reason for the authorities to move to masks in many parts of America. Another complaint from the businesspeople was their contention that some physicians called plain colds cases of influenza. From 1918 to 1920, there was no test of any kind that could determine if one had the flu or some other respiratory problem.[73]

In Columbia, it was observed that doctors and nurses wore masks while in the sick rooms to keep themselves from catching the flu, so why shouldn't everybody who came into contact with people wear one and prevent the spread of the present epidemic? Supposedly, that was the question that suggested itself to J.P. McBaine. He mentioned it to H.M. McPeters and Professor L.M. Defoe. They thought it was a good idea, and they started wearing masks. The idea was said to have spread quickly, and employees at the Columbia banks and workers at the Red Cross workrooms and the war activities office were wearing them. Then detailed instructions on how to make a mask at home were provided.[74]

When classes resumed in Columbia at the University of Missouri, all students were required to wear masks. Those masks were made by the local Red Cross and sold to the students for ten cents each. In case you didn't have a dime to spare, the reader of the article was given detailed instructions.[75]

A report from Kansas City on October 22 remarked that when a young woman got off a streetcar in the downtown area and strolled into a nearby store, "Hundreds of passersby turned to stare at her." She was claimed to be the first person seen on the streets of Kansas City wearing a gauze mask. According to the journalist, she was expected to have many copycats. One day earlier, Mayor James Cowgill agreed "that the only sure preventive against influenza appeared to be masks" and instructed Dr. Bullock to prepare the way for their general use. Bullock explained, "While we are requesting all persons serving the public and coming into contact with influenza patients to use them. Barbers, street car employees, waiters, elevator operators, nurses, doctors and, in fact, everybody should wear them." That same day, Bullock, Dr. A.J. Gannon (head of the contagious disease division), and W.P. Motley (president of the hospital and health board) visited all the retail stores and found them all to have complied with the health board's order to avoid crowding.[76]

Montgomery Ward and Company was the first big industrial concern to report having begun using gauze masks among its employees in Kansas City. The local Red Cross made 1,000 masks for the firm, with the company supplying the material. Superintendent of Merchandise Charles E. McCoy stated that "our employees found the masks were no great inconvenience and they had no difficulty speaking through them. We expect to supply all of the thirty-four hundred persons employed here with masks today." The Kansas City Railway Company (streetcars) asked the Red

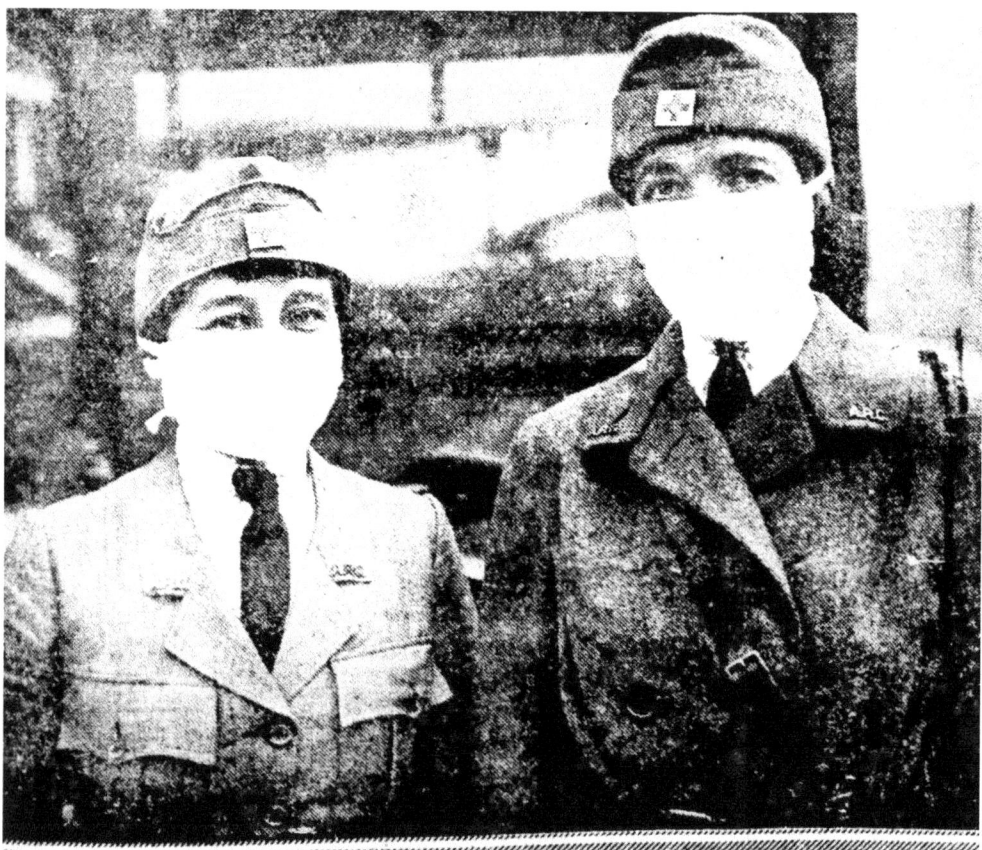

Miss Ida Britton (left) and Miss Grace Semple of the Red Cross Motor Ambulance Corps wearing influenza masks.

Two members of the masked Red Cross workers in St. Louis. Ida Britton (*left*) and Grace Semple were part of the ambulance corps that picked up flu-stricken residents of the city.

Cross for 3,500 masks for its employees. Several other firms had implied that they would soon adopt the mask for their workers. G.H. Clay, superintendent of Proctor and Gamble, said he was wearing a gauze mask at the plant and was prepared to adopt any emergency methods advised by the health authorities. Medicine was being provided to his employees at no cost for throat gargling. The American Radiator Company said that the 450 employees would be masked before the end of the week. However, a journalist noted that the recommendation of the health board that employees of business institutions serving the public should wear masks "has not yet been adopted by the downtown stores, cafes, hotel and other concerns of similar natures." It was a recommendation only, not an order. It was noted that city employees on the Kansas side of the border who came into contact with the public were wearing the gauze masks.[77]

The drive to get people in Kansas City to wear masks continued with a report that many more people on the streetcars wore masks, patrons as well as car employees. At the office of the Kansas City Railway Company, a sufficient number of masks had been ordered to supply three masks to each of the 2,000 streetcar conductors and motormen on the line. Those employees had already begun to wear face coverings while on duty. Several other Kansas City firms were reported as having their employees use masks or as thinking of doing so. However, it was admitted that in the retail sector, "some store managers are not as yet interested" in having their employees masked.[78]

In St. Louis, any drive to get people to mask up was doomed to failure. When Dr. George A. Jordan, assistant health commissioner in the city, returned from attending the American Public Health Association Chicago convention, he reported, "The opinion among the 1,000 physicians and surgeons who attended the meeting is that the flu masks worn in various parts of the country are absurd and inefficient." He added, "The health commissioner of San Francisco in an address, said he was strongly in favor of the masks—when the epidemic started in San Francisco. The masks were used. Now, the commissioner said, he knows they are of no value." As well, Jordan explained that all the medical providers at the convention agreed that the origins of the disease were still a mystery and that there was no specific treatment for the disease. No way of handling such epidemics was agreed upon.[79]

A couple of days later, F.H. Collier wrote an op-ed piece for a St. Louis paper on the topic of masking under the subhead "flu masks unmasked." Collier wrote, citing a resident of Seattle, "If Plato and Aristotle and some others among our ancient friends who lived over 2000 years ago should rise up to find themselves in enlightened America in the midst of a modern city of 400,000 inhabitants, most of whom were parading the streets in masks, I am sure they would feel that they had been cast on an island in some remote part of the world where the natives were still blindly worshiping an unknown god of decorating themselves with some symbol of fetishism."[80]

Back in Columbia, the University of Missouri at Columbia had difficulty giving up on masking everybody. When the university's basketball team hosted another from Ames, Iowa, for two games on January 10 and 11, it was stated that all people who attended those games were required to wear flu masks.[81]

Somewhat earlier, a newspaper in Columbia published an article on masks and science in more general terms. It captured the authoritarian view of so many health authorities and scientists. Boston physician Dr. Oliver P. Cranston stated, "If the threatened recurrence of influenza is to be checked, there should be a whole-hearted submission to the advice of the health authorities, and cranks should not be permitted to hamper the precautionary measures of the public officials." The article went on to cite a piece from the *Literary Digest*: "Large-meshed fish-net bears about the same sizal relation to a swarm of flies as the common gauze mask bears to the influenza germs it is supposed to stop; and for this reason doctors, and other persons who know something about germs, have been moved to comment either pitying or sarcastically on the common assumption that such masks afford protection." The openings in an influenza mask, as seen under a microscope, are enormous. In contrast, the influenza germ, even under high magnifying power, remains almost invisible. Another example of the authoritarian nature of the Boston physician came when he said that medical providers differed regarding the efficacy of masks, but there was hardly the slightest divergence of opinion regarding the necessity of preventing public gatherings. He said, "That is settled for all time, and the public should take it for granted without any fuss."[82]

Nebraska

Dr. Chapman, superintendent of the Lincoln Health Department in Nebraska, issued a statement on the morning of October 8, trying to ease public fears about the influenza outbreak causing panic all over America. He explained that he saw no necessity for closing schools, churches, and theaters. He believed they were all well ventilated, and people feeling ill were not likely to be going to places of amusement. The Lancaster County Medical Society recommended a residential quarantine, and the Lincoln City Council passed the recommendation. But it was a mild residential quarantine, as it only affected the patient, with all other household members able to come and go as usual. Chapman was asked why he and others in authority in Lincoln had not adopted the shutdown system imposed by many other jurisdictions across America and recommended in the Rupert Blue Protocols. He replied, "In my opinion this would only act as a makeshift and would accomplish nothing in the way of prevention." And there was no limit on closing once the process started, and it was simply extended.[83]

That resolve did not last very long because, as of noon on October 12, a closing order was in effect in Lincoln involving the usual suspects. All public assemblies were banned, and churches, schools, theaters, cinemas, pool halls, and all public and private dances were closed. The Lincoln City Council issued the order, and it went into effect as soon as it was passed. Children were to be kept "in or near" their homes, and streetcars were directed to keep all the cars well ventilated. However, the action was not taken on the recommendation of the city's doctors or even upon the suggestion of the superintendent of health. Commissioner Wright said it was on the initiative of the council, which believed public sentiment and the general conditions justified immediate action.[84]

A few weeks later, the restrictions were lifted in Lincoln, but then in late November, as the second wave moved through the state, the threat of closure loomed again in Lincoln. Other cities acted. At the Albion Board of Health meeting, measures were taken toward a more thorough and strict quarantine. People making store purchases were asked to stay no longer than necessary. News and cigar stands were ordered to be closed no later than 7 p.m., with no loitering there when they were open. Restaurants had to close no later than 8 p.m.[85]

Businesspeople in Beatrice, Nebraska, were angry over the end-of-November order issued by the local board of health, which banned all businesses except grocery and meat stores and restricted their activities to filling orders taken over the phone. A large protest meeting was held on the afternoon of November 30, attended by "practically all" the city's businesspeople. If the order were not modified, the city commission would be asked to modify it. The Beatrice business houses asserted that they were planning to reopen Monday as usual. The order for all to close went into effect at 6 p.m. on Saturday. Banks were among the businesses closed but could admit clients who might find it "imperative" to enter their doors after the closure order became effective. Beatrice chief of police Dillow said, "I have instructed the officers to see that there are no people on the downtown streets except those who can show good cause why they should leave their homes. Everybody will be expected to remain home." The order also shut down all factories and plants, throwing many people out of work.[86]

In an act of defiance, everything opened as usual on Monday. The authorities decided the matter needed to be rethought. It was pointed out that putting over 1,000 heads of families out of work was not helping the situation. Then one day later, on Tuesday, it was announced that the order was rescinded. All restrictions were lifted. As part of a face-saving measure, the local health board instituted a new regulation — each morning, the temperature of all factory workers and all schoolchildren would be taken.[87]

The initial closure order had been lifted in much of Nebraska on November 7. Still, removal came later for some communities. The local health board did not lift restrictions in Alliance until November 15. When that was announced, Alliance Mayor Rousey declared, in classic blame-the-victim style, "If the people will use a little judgment in their actions it will not be necessary to again put a halt to public meetings."[88]

The Norfolk Board of Health notified all its physicians in mid–December that arrests would follow failure to report influenza cases for quarantine, as they were legally required to do. All dances had been banned, but the local health officials had decided to fight influenza with a strict residential quarantine rather than reimposing the lockdown as they had during the first wave. A reporter observed, "A threat is made by the board to close the entire city if proper cooperation in the preventive schedule is not forthcoming."[89]

Around Christmas Day, the Nebraska Board of Health announced a statewide, strict residential quarantine for Spanish influenza following a recent conference with local health boards. Rules under the quarantine provided that no one could enter or leave the household in question except doctors, nurses, or clergy pursuing their duties. A person was not certified as recovered until four days after the fever had entirely subsided.[90]

Dr. W.J. McCrann of Omaha argued against many of the measures and said, "There is absolutely no benefit from quarantine or restrictions of public gatherings." He also decried making influenza a quarantinable disease. "You have nothing to accomplish by it, but you can only add more suffering to the already over-crowded and over-burdened wage-earners' homes ... where possibly from one to four, by their daily earnings are barely existing. By your quarantine there is absolutely no benefit to control the disease or spread of influenza which is an air-propagating disease."[91]

Most of the discussion was about flu regulations at a regular council meeting on November 12 in Broken Bow, Custer County, Nebraska. Dr. Sellon, the health officer, explained the rigid quarantine imposed a few days earlier. He said the rules governing the use of masks had been violated. Still, the investigation showed the ordinance did not cover the care of the mask, so Sellon requested the city attorney prepare a resolution covering wearing masks and embodying the other provisions of the regulations. When that was done, it was read to the audience. It said that beginning on

November 13 at 10 a.m., everyone should wear a mask, children under 16 should stay off the streets, those afflicted with the disease should be residentially quarantined, and not more than six people should congregate. The council could not agree on the full resolution, so it tackled it section by section. First to be considered was the section dealing with masks. Most of the council seemed opposed to compelling people to wear masks. The opinion was that it should not be done when the other towns in the county "were wide open, as it was antagonistic to the public." Some council members felt that if the county physician ordered the whole county to wear masks, then that problem would be solved. When the mask section was finally voted on, it lost by a vote of six to two. All other sections of the resolution were passed. Dr. Sellon then submitted his immediate resignation after 18 months as the health officer. He felt he had trouble getting the "proper backing" for his resolutions. A motion for him to reconsider was made, but he declined. He added that he resented people on the street making "slighting remarks about his orders and then disobeying them." The council then asked Sellon to stay in office until a replacement was found, but he declined.[92]

Health Commissioner Manning of Omaha advised employees in banks and other public places who came face-to-face with the public in business transactions throughout the day to wear flu masks. Ezra Millard of the Omaha National Bank replied, "It is our desire to co-operate with Mr. Manning in stopping the epidemic but we would be sorry to have to do it." He added, "We will do it readily just as soon as we get definite advice from Dr. Manning, although it would be an inconvenience to our employees and would have a depressing effect upon the public." The reporter working on the piece reported that at the United States National Bank, just one employee was wearing a mask.[93]

Fifty masks were provided for the Nebraska Power Company Omaha office employees. It was also reported that Jessie Briggs, a stenographer in the city health commissioner's office, had invented flu masks for the telephone. She provided the mouthpiece of her telephone with a mask of sterilized gauze furnished by the local Red Cross. Briggs explained it was not to block germs coming in over the wire but to prevent them from lurking on the mouthpiece in case someone who had the flu happened to use the telephone.[94]

A reporter toured some of the downtown businesses one day after Manning offered his advice. He found that very few bank clerks and others who had contact with the public wore masks. He asked Manning about that, and the commissioner replied that it was only a suggestion he had made for people's safety. He said, "I strongly advise it, but I do not propose further steps."[95]

The Nebraska Board of Health called together several hundred city and county officials in mid–December for a conference on methods of dealing with the flu epidemic. Its report concerning masks said, "Masks were argued for and against. The preponderance of evidence was to the effect that masks had, practically speaking, invariably proved inefficient, impracticable and unsanitary. The mask has its place in the sick room or operating room where sterile material can be used, where it can be changed often or worn but a few minutes. I am of the opinion that it is a filthy practice and should not be tolerated. Nurses and interns in hospitals who wore masks

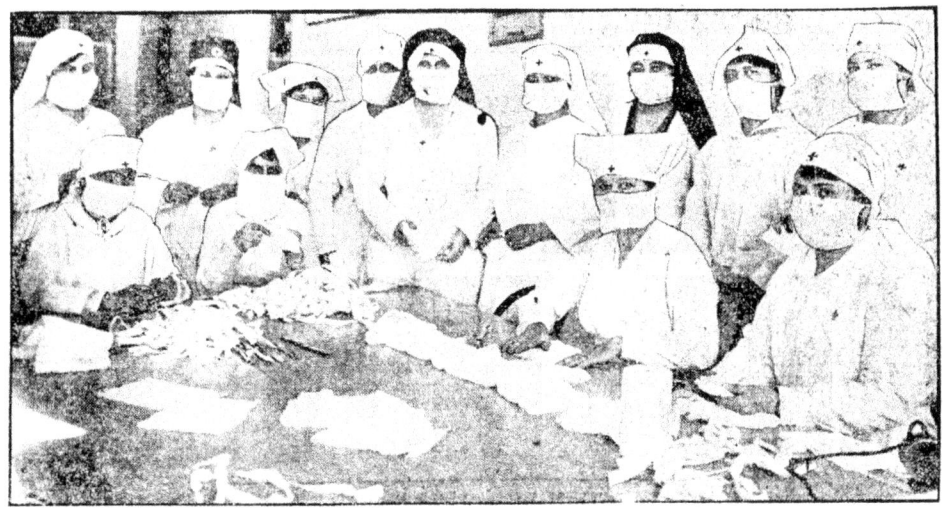

Thirteen Red Cross workers in Omaha, Nebraska, making masks for their area. It was a scene duplicated all over America, from the largest cities to the smallest towns.

continually contracted the disease as regularly as those who did not wear them. Some cities where the practice was in force claimed a noticeable subsidence after masks were installed. Other cities claimed there was an increase in the number of cases. No doubt both instances were true." The report argued the same for closure orders, with some places having a decrease in cases after closure orders were imposed and some places having an increase in cases after closure orders were imposed.[96]

At the conference, Dr. Manning told of tests about the distance the disease could be communicated. He claimed that in ordinary conversation, the germ would travel four feet, while in sneezing or coughing, the germs were communicable from 12 to 15 feet. Regarding taking steps in such emergencies as the flu epidemic, he said that health authorities such as himself should adopt the policy that "action should be taken at once, of any kind."[97]

A report from February 1919 indicated that the death rate in Lincoln from the flu was below the average of the larger cities in the United States. Statistics showed that the mask did "little or nothing" to curb the epidemic. San Francisco was the toughest on its citizens with masking mandates, yet only three other cities had higher death rates than San Francisco.[98]

Kansas

The city health officer, Dr. H.L. Clark of Topeka, Kansas, at noon on October 9, imposed the usual restrictions in the Blue Protocols on his city. All public gatherings were banned, but only those that involved more than 20 people. Exempted were any gatherings that involved "military necessities," such as Liberty Loan drives.[99]

Dr. S.J. Crumbine of the Kansas Board of Health imposed the usual lockdown statewide on Kansas, with the closure taking effect on October 12. Two weeks later, Crumbine announced that Kansas would stay under the restrictions until at least midnight on November 2. When the lifting date was only a couple of days away, it was announced that local health officials would receive a recommendation to place closure orders in effect in their communities if "marked improvement" in the influenza situation had not occurred in their areas. With the lifting of restrictions on November 2, the matter was in the hands of local officials. Still, the state authorities would continue to make recommendations. For example, in Kansas City, Kansas, the lockdown order remained in effect until the local officials removed it on November 15, leaving only a residential quarantine.[100]

When Wichita imposed new restrictions on its citizens as part of a second wave, the validity of those regulations was tested in Judge R.E. Bird's division of the local district court when an injunction was sought to prevent the Wichita authorities from interfering with the regular business affairs of the city. All the theaters (except one), business colleges, and churches were among the plaintiffs. Various Wichita officials and health authorities were the defendants. The quarantine that the city sought to impose was described in the suit as unnecessary and discriminatory.[101]

Dr. Thomas J. Carter was the city physician of Wichita. He had declared an emergency, and thus he declared he had the power to impose emergency restrictions on the city. All public gatherings were prohibited, not just some, but even those in banks, offices, and so forth. The only exceptions were when such gatherings were limited to one person per 100 square feet of floor area on the ground floor; for all other floors, the gathering was limited to one person per 300 square feet. The limit for business colleges, or colleges in general, was one person per 50 square feet. If the people were seated and grouped to prevent closer grouping, there was one person per 40 square feet. No room was to be used until it had been ventilated for at least five minutes. At least two windows were to be removed from all streetcars.[102]

Then, on the evening of November 30, this ban was lifted entirely in Wichita. The quarantine was declared illegal. Thus, it was business as usual. Judge Robert Bird declared that a quarantine affecting only certain classes of business without reference to the sanitary condition of such a business was discriminatory. A temporary restraining order was granted from the quarantine that had been issued on November 28. Bird suggested two remedies. One was to enforce a rigid quarantine on all unsanitary places. The second was to prohibit crowds of all kinds above a designated number.[103]

Salina, Kansas, imposed restrictions during the second wave simultaneously with Wichita. The usual suspects were closed, and a rigorous residential quarantine was implemented. Still, breadwinners in a household could come and go. Business establishments were allowed no more than 15 customers in their place of business at one time per 25 square feet of floor space. Children were kept at home as much as possible and not allowed to congregate "anywhere."[104]

Reportedly, influenza masks were used for the first time in Salina, Kansas, on

October 30 as part of a football game when St. John's military school in Salina met Wentworth Military Academy in Lexington, Missouri. Rather than cancel the game, the teams elected to play, but all were masked. Lexington won by a score of 78 to 3. Just a few days later, it was said that flu masks had appeared in Salina more generally. Clerks at the banks, the post office, and all the offices where people were served had donned face coverings.[105]

In Concordia, Dr. Beach, in conjunction with the community's mayor, issued an order in early December requiring all people to wear gauze masks while in a place of business and coming into contact with the public. The order was effective immediately and would remain in force until the danger of infection had passed. The masks were made of gauze of not less than four thicknesses and were to be worn in all stores, offices, et cetera. Wearing them on the streets was not compulsory, but it was recommended. According to the article, "The physicians agreed there is very little if any danger of the disease being communicated to a person wearing a mask or from one wearing a mask." They were to be changed every three to four hours and sterilized by boiling before reusing.[106]

Dr. A.W. Clark, Lawrence health officer, ordered all barbers to wear masks while serving clients. Barbers had to wear at least four thicknesses of gauze over their noses and mouths. Those who did not comply with the order would be ordered to close their barber shops.[107]

A few days after that, Dr. Ida Hyde of the University of Kansas at Lawrence law faculty issued a warning. She declared that masks were necessary but that a few thicknesses of gauze "commonly accepted as a mask are of really more danger than good" in the sense that wearers believed themselves protected when they were not. According to Hyde, experiments showed that the germ would be carried two feet from the mouth of the patient by ordinary conversation, four feet by loud speech, and from six to ten feet when the person was coughing.[108]

On October 22, it was reported that over 1,000 workers for one of Kansas City, Kansas's large mercantile establishments came to work that day wearing gauze masks. Many other large concerns in the city advocated the practice as a safeguard.[109]

By October 10, Wichita was locked down, along with the rest of the State of Kansas. A report appeared that all six physicians practicing medicine out of a particular suite of rooms were wearing flu masks—all six were named. Also, the receptionist at the desk was wearing one, and a journalist said, "It is probable that influenza masks, which cover the nose and lower part of the face, will become quite a common sight in Wichita until the influenza epidemic passes."[110]

Two weeks later, several hundred Wichita businesspeople met at the Crawford Theater to talk about the Liberty Loan campaign, each wearing a gauze mask. It was a spectacle to be matched in the following week, when several hundred livestock people were to attend a livestock sale at an arena. Several hundred flu masks had been purchased so each person could have one. A physician associated with the event said everyone, except the auctioneer, would have to wear a gauze mask.[111]

Dr. H.L. Clark and Commissioner W.L. Porter advised that people wear gauze masks in the streets of Topeka and places of business employing a considerable number of people. It was said that the citizens of Seattle were wearing masks with "marked good results." As a result, the health authorities in Topeka were considering the same action. The city health officials suggested that employers have their employees wear masks until the epidemic had abated.[112]

As the flu did not relinquish in Wichita, the threat of masking was brought out now and then. City health authorities considered asking store proprietors to have their clerks wear masks to benefit both the clerks and the public. People were advised that a mask should not be worn all day but should be changed after several hours. One person should never wear a mask worn by another before it had been soaked in some antiseptic solution. Dr. H.L. Clark recommended carbolic acid solutions, Lysol, or other similar products. Blanche Wier, an elevator operator at city hall, was wearing a mask at "the command" of Commissioner W.L. Porter. Only ten people at a time were let into one of the city hall rooms, and the elevator was limited to carrying no more than three passengers.[113]

On October 30, in anticipation of the shutdown being over, Dr. H.L. Clark said he hoped people could be induced to wear masks when attending shows, theaters, church, or political gatherings held indoors for the next several weeks. About ten days later, when the quarantine was lifted, on November 9, the public was urged to wear masks to theaters for at least one week.[114]

Later, near the end of November, when Wichita considered the possibility of a second lockdown, it looked at what Denver was doing. They thought it might be possible to allow schools, theaters, churches, and other public gathering places to operate, provided every person attending such places wore a mask. According to the news article, "It is said that the masks, if properly made and worn, are very effective in preventing the contraction of the disease."[115]

10

Mountain

Montana

Acting under the recommendations of Rupert Blue and his protocols, Dr. W.F. Cogswell, secretary of the Montana Board of Health, issued regulations for the control of Spanish influenza in Montana on October 7. Those regulations included closing schools and prohibiting all public gatherings in cities and towns. According to the order, when the flu appeared in any community, the health officer with jurisdiction was required to close the schools and prohibit all public gatherings.[1]

Bozeman, Montana, closed on October 16. Although there had not been a single case of influenza there, 14 cases originating among railroad workers and farm crews outside of the city had been brought to the nearest detention hospital outside Bozeman.[2] Helena closed one day later. A week after that, the local board of health ordered all the saloons in the city to close no later than 6 p.m. until further notice. When Bozeman closed, it was felt, at the time, that it would not be necessary to close the saloons entirely.[3]

Restrictions were lifted at different times and to various degrees in Montana. The health board in Butte lifted the ban on schools and theaters that had been closed for the previous month on November 9. Later that month, the quarantine in Missoula was partially lifted when poolrooms, churches, bowling alleys, and saloons could reopen. On November 27, the Butte Health Board lifted the advertising ban, which meant that department stores could advertise sales and special prices in the newspapers.[4]

During the first part of December, Washington sent a warning to Billings and every state in the union. Rupert Blue wrote that the pandemic was by no means over, as the reports received by the United States Public Health Service showed "a recrudescence of the disease practically from one end of the country to another." Blue advised closing the public schools at the first sign of a reappearance of the pandemic.[5] The warning from Blue caused no action to be taken in Billings, where the restrictions had been lifted for three weeks, and it was business as usual.[6]

At about the same time, at a meeting of the local health board in Helena, the city health board took no action to lift the quarantine that was in place, despite the views expressed by Dr. W.F. Cogswell, Montana health officer, at the meeting. After his return from Chicago and the American Public Health Association convention at which, as he told the meeting in Helena, the majority opinion "appeared to be that community quarantine measures have not been proven certain checks against the spread of the disease." Cogswell explained that he did not attempt to advise community health officers on lifting or not lifting restrictions but left it to the judgment of each health officer concerning conditions as they saw them in their localities.[7]

On December 22, the Helena Health Board lifted almost all restrictions except for dances, which would remain banned for "a while longer." Theaters could open that day but only for one performance each in the afternoon and one in the evening. Churches and public funerals received the order to resume. Dr. Max Barbour, city health officer, explained that schools could reopen but would not resume until after Christmas. The last of the restrictions in Helena was not lifted, after being in place for some three months, until January 9, 1919. At that time, public dances were allowed, and theaters could give more than one performance in each part of the day.[8]

The response on the part of the people of Missoula, Montana, that clerks, deliverymen, servers, and those coming "constantly" into contact with the public wear gauze masks at the request of the local health board was, a journalist wrote, "almost universal yesterday" on October 24. All the clerks in the stores, all the messengers, and all the newspaper agents were said to have complied with the request. The Montana Board of Health strongly favored everybody wearing masks and recommended that the practice become universal. In Victor, Montana, the council made masks mandatory for everybody. Visitors to the town had to wear one, or they could not stay there. According to a reporter, a huge sign on the town's main street proclaimed "in no uncertain words what the requirements are."[9]

In Great Falls, Montana, masks began to appear at the local office of the United States Employment Service. At the American Bank and Trust Company, the entire staff was wearing them, having obtained them from the local chapter of the Red Cross. The Great Falls Fire Department also obtained the firefighter's masks from the same source.[10]

Bearing in mind that there was too great a need for gauze for the proper care of soldiers at the battlefront and too little value in wearing the so-called gas masks on the street, Dr. J.H. Fairfield, one of the veteran physicians of Great Falls, said that he believed a mistake was being made by encouraging people to wear masks on the street. Fairfield believed they probably had value if one was traveling on the train and that they were okay when used by a nurse treating a flu patient. Still, he did not believe a wise course was being followed in using a large force of workers to turn them out for street use or the ordinary business office. He suggested substituting muslin for gauze for civilian use.[11]

In Lewistown, the health authorities amended the influenza regulations, allowing the churches and theaters to remain open but mandating that all who attended those places wear gauze masks. Once again, the local Red Cross undertook to supply all the needed face coverings.[12]

Starting late in November, all clerks in stores, banks, and railroad offices, bartenders, barbers, and everyone coming into contact with the public in doing business in Havre, Montana, were compelled to wear a flu mask. Although there was no change in the flu situation in the area, the city health officer, Dr. Hamilton, added the rule to the existing regulations. Chairs had been removed from the hotel lobbies, stores, barbershops, and poolrooms. An extra police officer was added to the force to see that people did not congregate or loiter on the streets.[13]

In a meeting, Mayor Tom McKenzie, police chief William McKinnon, and Dr. W.F. Hamilton decided that more rigid rules were needed to fight the flu. One day later, it was reported that nearly everyone in Havre was wearing a mask.[14]

When the situation did not improve in Havre, city authorities imposed even greater restrictions. It was decided to vaccinate people for free. However, "for clerks in store and others serving the public in any manner the order [to be vaccinated]" was "compulsory." People who had recovered from the flu and those who received the vaccine were given a health certificate. The authorities said, "When finally the right of public assemblage is again restored and the lid removed only those bearing health certificates will be admitted, for the time at least, to picture shows, churches and other public gatherings."[15]

In Butte, as the flu arrived in mid-October, an urgent call went out for more volunteer workers at the local Red Cross chapter to make face masks. The city's health board planned to distribute those masks to the public.[16]

On October 22, the Butte Health Board ordered all clerks and barbers to wear gauze masks and, among other measures, prohibited department stores from advertising in the newspapers. Within a few days, it was reported that numerous infractions of the board's rule regarding the wearing of antiseptic masks by clerks, servers, and others in places of business were reported to the county board of health. It was also noted that in many places where masks had been in use, they had subsequently been discarded. The board ordered an inspection and adopted a resolution whereby it would close any place of business subject to the mask rule if that establishment failed to comply with the order.[17]

When Butte ordered a new and sweeping set of restrictions on November 30 to be imposed on the citizenry, it included a section whereby all clerks, servers, and other workers serving the public had to wear masks while on duty, apparently ignoring the fact the order had already been imposed on the city over one month earlier.[18]

Dr. W.C. Matthews, Butte health officer, wrote to health officials all over America for information on what steps to take. One response was from San Francisco Health Officer William Hassler, who replied, "Wearing influenza masks considered 95 per cent protection." Matthews added, "I am a firm believer in the proper and universal using of the mask which, I believe, will permit the earlier opening of all places of business."[19]

A newspaper in Helena published a sizable public service ad from United States Surgeon General Rupert Blue giving the reader general advice on the flu pandemic. Many newspapers across America printed the advice from Blue, with the vast majority doing so in October. Blue did not mention face masks, except for people who attended to those ill with the flu. Even there, his advice was mild: "Nurses and attendants will do well to guard against breathing in dangerous disease germs by wearing a simple fold of gauze or mask while near the patient."[20]

Then, on October 24, Dr. W.F. Cogswell, secretary of the Montana Board of Health, asked the people of Montana to wear anti-influenza masks. The local health board and the Helena Chamber of Commerce added their appeal for the people of

Helena to comply with the request. The masks were to be obtained from the Red Cross or made at home.[21]

The masking mandate in Helena was part of a more extensive set of restrictions imposed on the city by Dr. Max Barbour, city health officer. The official order came from the Helena Health Board. Servers, cooks, and others engaged in preparing food had to wear masks, as did bartenders, barbers, hairdressers, clerks in retail stores and offices, and other classes of workers who came into close personal contact with people. Barbour said the face coverings should be sterilized no less than once a day by boiling in water for 15 to 20 minutes, then hung up to thoroughly dry. The executives and employees of two banks, Union Bank and Trust and American National Bank, began voluntarily wearing the "gas mask" in Helena even before the masking order. A newspaper article supplied detailed instructions for readers so they could make their own at home.[22]

Like many other places in America, the short lead time between issuing a masking mandate and when it became effective left Helena scrambling to find enough face coverings. A day after the order went into effect, it was noted that anti-flu masks were worn "to the extent that the supply was available by clerks, waiters and others." The volunteer workers making the coverings at the Red Cross building were working three shifts a day. As soon as enough were produced, they were donned by numerous others, such as streetcar conductors, who fell under the mandate.[23]

Any grace period concerning enforcement of the masking law in Helena ended within a couple of days. Reports reached the city health board that, in some cases, people affected by the order were not complying with the rule. The health board notified the police department with a request that it strictly enforce the law.[24]

Two more days passed, and the epidemic's scope was unabated in Helena. Yet, the city health board decided to modify the order regarding anti-flu masks, making wearing them optional instead of mandatory for certain classes of workers. However, the health board continued to recommend wearing masks. Rumor had it that if the mandate remained in effect, the board would have had to order numerous arrests for noncompliance, which they were reluctant to do. Thus, the board backed down and modified the order. Many people complained that constantly wearing masks subjected them to severe headaches and caused eyestrain, among other inconveniences. As county health officer, Dr. Barbour ordered a supply of gauze masks for the prisoners in the county jail. Wearing them in jail was optional.[25]

Upon his return from attending the three-day conference of the American Public Health Association in Chicago, Dr. Cogswell announced that, due to hearing the opinions of health experts from all over the United States and Canada, he had concluded that the closing-down plan for dealing with the situation could not be continued indefinitely and that the ban should be lifted gradually. He spoke of the great diversity of opinion at the convention, noting that everyone there had figures and observations, but he said, "no one knows what is the cause of influenza." Residential quarantines, he said, were of little value unless they were rigidly enforced because healthy people, "walking cases," were carriers of the disease. He asserted that "the flu mask is worthless." When he appraised Cogswell's report, Dr. Barbour, Helena's health officer, said a meeting would soon be held to consider the conclusions and the lifting of the restrictions.[26]

In an editorial on the flu epidemic, the editor of a Helena newspaper said, "Those who wear masks get air into their noses and mouths just as surely as those who do not wear masks. It is a tax upon credulity to assume that a flu germ cannot traverse the indirect route of the breathing current or cannot penetrate any gauze which admits enough air to sustain life."[27]

The same Helena paper printed some comments and thoughts from the American Public Health Association that were not printed elsewhere. Several physicians said that until a specific cure was found, it would be better for doctors to step aside and let nature work unhindered. Dr. Charles J. Hastings of Toronto, chair of the convention, said, "We are nature's skilled assistants. It requires a good deal of knowledge to know how little we know. A tremendous amount of damage is done by interfering with nature, when nature would have done better if she had been left alone." One of the attending physicians defined the art of medicine as "the art of entertaining patients while nature effects a cure."[28]

Idaho

In Idaho, on October 21, the state board of health ordered the closing of all public and private schools in the state. A few days later, it was reported that plans were being made by the Boise Health Board to have an ordinance passed that would require barbers and other people whose work placed them in close contact with their customers to wear gauze masks. At that time, there was no mandate in place. Still, some barbers had reportedly voluntarily adopted face coverings. And a reporter wrote, "Some three women were noticed Saturday on the streets of Boise who had courage enough to wear thick gauze veils over the lower portion of their faces in defiance of the attention which the curious crowds paid them."[29]

Near the end of October, all people in Franklin County, Idaho's offices and stores, were required to wear flu masks, and the entire county was under strict quarantine. One day after that, the announcement came from Washington, D.C., that all members of the SATC (student army training corps) had to wear masks. The SATC mask-wearing order was effective everywhere in America, and it took effect at the University of Idaho in Moscow. All members of the SATC were to be supplied with three masks, and a mask was to be worn at all times. Military authorities were very particular about the people who worked on the masks. No person with a cold or not in perfect physical condition could go near the material.[30]

A list of restrictions was imposed in Blackfoot, Bingham County, Idaho, on November 1. Under the regime, public gatherings were banned. People were told not to loiter in any store but to do their business quickly and leave. Stores had to close no later than 6 p.m., except for restaurants, which had to close no later than 9 p.m. Also required was that every person "upon the public highway or in public places, like stores, etc., shall wear a protective mask." On December 4, the community's mayor modified the rules to the extent of no longer requiring wearing the flu mask. As of December 16, all restrictions were ended, except for the residential quarantine, which remained on the books.[31]

Pocatello lifted the last of its flu restrictions on December 22. The Rathdrum Board of Education decided not to reopen its schools until after the Christmas break, on January 6, 1919. Moscow, Idaho, placed its residents under restrictions that involved the usual suspects and barred all public gatherings. It was to last for one week, starting on December 27.[32]

Just a few days into the new year of 1919, the Commercial Club in Boise, Idaho, held a meeting that lasted several hours and discussed the influenza situation. One of those present was the Rev. Willsie Martin, who declared wearing masks was commendable because it prevented people from spitting. He also believed that the psychological effect of mask wearing on the observer was argument enough for the use of masks. Dr. L.P. McCalla approved the suggestion and said that masks, if appropriately used, helped prevent the spread of the disease.[33]

Another example of a rule gone mad took place in Idaho, resulting in Sheriff W.K. Huntington of Custer County being ousted from office and Dr. C.L. Kirtley resigning from his position as county health officer after a controversy had waged for several weeks over quarantine restrictions. The sheriff arrested hunters for breaking a quarantine rule and held them in Challis, Custer County. They were held overnight notwithstanding a court order that the men be released. Huntington ignored that order. The judge who granted the release order was prevented from entering Challis by Huntington because of the quarantine rule. Upon more research it was found that no legal quarantine was in place because Kirtley had failed to take the necessary legal steps to establish a quarantine. Those two men both obeyed orders that did not legally exist (quarantine rule) and Huntington ignored a legal rule that did exist (judicial release order for the hunters). Both men lost their jobs.[34]

At the end of January, Burley finally lifted the restrictions, as the disease seemed to have run its course. A journalist observed, "Practically all known theories as to how the disease is spread have been exploded. Masks have been discarded as a means of avoiding the contagion, and public gatherings are no longer considered a source of danger. A strict quarantine of the premises where the disease exists, followed by thorough fumigation, seems to offer the best means of combating influenza at this time."[35]

Wyoming

On October 23, the town of Cody, Wyoming, passed regulations against people forming crowds, congregating, or loitering, but they did not close anything down. Under the rules, anyone with a "head cold" or who "commenced to sneeze" was mandated to go to a physician to examine their medical status. Nurses were "requested" to use face masks when dealing with patients ill with the flu.[36]

Dr. R.C. Montgomery of Riverton, recently appointed health commissioner for Fremont County, had a strenuous week late in October because he became overzealous in his attempts to control influenza. Early in the week, the stores and saloons were ordered closed in Riverton, with only employees allowed inside. Customers had to wait outside to be served. If they were lucky enough to have a telephone, they could call their order to the store and collect it at the door. If they did not have a phone, and two-thirds of households in America did not have a phone in 1920, then the customer had to shout his order out when he arrived outside the front door. A few days later, similar notices were sent to Mayor Hardin, who was directed to promulgate the same regulations in Lander. Hardin declined to do so and suggested that if Montgomery wanted to close Lander, he should go through his deputy in Lander, Dr. Replogie. The latter did not act, so Montgomery sent another deputy from Riverton. All the business houses in Lander were placarded. Citizens in Lander then held a mass meeting on the afternoon of October 23, at which it was decided to take down all those signs. The citizens at the meeting did precisely that on the same day. Mayor Hardin called Dr. C.Y. Beard, the Wyoming health officer, to discuss the matter and learned that Montgomery's actions were not authorized. Montgomery was informed of the conversation and agreed to remove the quarantine from Riverton.[37]

At the end of December in Kemmerer, Wyoming, the existing rigid quarantine was modified to the extent that public assemblies were allowed, but only if they did not exceed 20 people. That same month, Casper imposed a residential quarantine they expected to run for 15 to 20 days. Houses placed under quarantine had to remain that way until ten days after the patient's temperature had returned to normal. No one was allowed in or out of the quarantined house. In Lander, all restrictions were removed on December 10, except that school-age children (14 and under) were not to be admitted to certain areas. Kemmerer removed its restrictions and reimposed them in March 1919, closing the usual suspects of churches, schools, dances, and theaters.[38]

In November 1918, Dr. C.Y. Beard of the Wyoming Board of Health "emphatically condemned" masks to prevent the spread of the flu. He said a gauze mask with ten layers was worthless. In condemning the mask, Beard said the ordinary person did not thoroughly understand the sterilization process that would kill all germs. Hence, "the use of a mask, on again, off again, was more of a risk than a protection."[39]

A report published in a Cheyenne newspaper declared that doctors in Denver had finally concluded that masks were of little or no use against Spanish influenza, according to reports in the Denver papers. Dr. C.Y. Beard, secretary of the state health board, made that statement in November. Physicians from Denver did not unanimously agree, but the general opinion among the leading doctors was that they were of little or no use. However, a few did favor the mask. Doctors from Colorado Springs had joined the condemn masks camp, saying that the masks were nothing but "germ traps."[40]

Two chiropractors from Casper, Wyoming, took out a full-page ad in a local newspaper in late April 1919. They heavily criticized the conventional medical profession for mismanaging Spanish influenza, after it was over. They presented convincing statistics of the difference in death rates between cities that did no masking and no lockdowns against those that mandated masking and imposed rigid lockdowns. It was the latter group of cities that fared the worst.[41]

Colorado

The Denver Board of Health and city officials imposed the usual Blue Protocols on the city when it issued an order on October 5, taking effect on October 6 at 6 a.m.

Other communities took similar actions around the same time, including Pueblo, Colorado Springs, and Boulder. The entire state came under lockdown on October 8.[42]

One month later, the quarantine remained in place in Colorado. In Delta County, those ill with influenza were placed under a rigid residential quarantine until they fully recovered. Other household members could leave the residence only on such errands as were "absolutely necessary." In places of business, all people coming into contact with the public had to wear masks. Delivery men could not enter the quarantined house; they had to leave the parcels outside the door. Transients could pass through the county without stopping. People entering the county had to report to the health authorities and comply with all preventive restrictions. All public gatherings were prohibited. Violations of the regulations could lead to a fine of $50, 30 days in jail, or both.[43]

In mid-November, it was reported that Colorado school teachers would receive full pay during the entire period of public school closures. Attorney General Leslie E. Hubbard argued that the school districts had to pay full salaries. Heads of some school districts believed that the flu epidemic constituted an "act of God." Hence, they had no obligation to pay their teachers. Hubbard agreed that it was an "act of God," but teachers had to be paid as long as they were ready, willing, and able to carry out their end of the contract.[44]

Mayor Stover and health officials in Fort Collins put together recommendations for fighting the flu. The advisory board came out in strong support of a residential quarantine of the sick. The city's board of health was asked to implement those recommendations. The quarantine was applied to the individual who was sick, but not to the entire family. A special health officer was hired to see that the residential quarantine was obeyed. The Blue Protocols were implemented, including the closure of schools. Retail stores had to be measured by store managers, and only one patron was permitted entry per 30 square feet of space. The manager was held responsible for implementing and policing the measure. In admitting the problem of fighting influenza was a perplexing one, the advisory board remarked, "The majority of the men protest against one business being discriminated against but that the only effectual remedy is to quarantine and fight the disease wherever it is found. The flu mask goes into the discard but not so with other health provisions, which are to be promulgated at once."[45]

In Montrose, a petition was circulated near the end of January 1919 to secure the lifting or modification of the rigid restrictions that had been in effect for weeks. The Montrose merchants believed those regulations were driving away business from the city while accomplishing no good in stamping out the disease.[46]

By order of Mesa County physician Dr. Henderson, all polling places were well ventilated, and crowds could not congregate therein. Henderson declared, "The usual influenza mask is of course an absolute guarantee against contagion, authorities in Denver say that the ordinary chiffon veil worn by most women in motoring is a good protection, and to be on the safe side many women will wear these veils."[47]

As early as October 30 in Longmont, Colorado, because of the spread of the flu, the Longmont Commercial Association was giving out influenza masks to all residents of the area who applied for them.[48]

In Denver late in November, the first set of restrictions had been imposed and then lifted, as was the case in so many jurisdictions across America. And in so many of those places, the number of cases increased, usually in November, and left officials scrambling to do anything. In Denver, a renewed ban against public gatherings was imposed on November 22. A day later, city health authorities ruled that the churches, theaters, and schools could continue to operate, but with a requirement that masks had to be worn in stores, theaters, public offices, and on streetcars, but not on the street. Those revised rules by the health authorities were based on the presumption that wearing masks could prevent the spread of the disease. The regulation mandating masking was passed on November 22 and took effect at 6 a.m. the following day. As was often the case, the public was blamed for the situation. The official end of World War I led to huge celebrations across America on November 11 and 12, and many people mingled.[49]

Three days later, it was admitted that there was a general disregard for the masking law, which caused city officials to order drastic steps for its enforcement. Police officers were stationed on street corners in the downtown section of Denver that afternoon and ordered to prevent people who did not wear masks from boarding streetcars.[50]

An editorial that appeared in a newspaper shortly after the masking order was imposed explained what was behind the whole affair. It began by arguing that it was "outrageous that the theaters in Denver should be forced to remain closed with every other business open." The flu ban was imposed on Friday afternoon without warning and just as suddenly lifted on Saturday morning. Nobody was prepared when the city board of health announced on Friday that all the churches, schools, and theaters should be closed. Theater managers were all caught by surprise that closure was coming. Those theater managers had tolerated the first closure without complaint, but this time they did not. On Friday afternoon, they held an indignation meeting. On Saturday morning, they went in a body to city hall with a following of 150 people. As a result, the closure order was dropped, and they could remain open, but patrons had to be masked.[51]

A high-level conference was held at the Colorado State House, where the flu situation in Denver was discussed. Denver Mayor W.F. Mills announced that they had decided to enforce the recent orders regarding rigidly wearing flu masks in the city. The meeting involved Mills; E.E. Kennedy, secretary of the Colorado Board of Health; Dr. W.H. Sharpley; and Colorado Governor Julius Gunter.[52]

As of November 26, the public in Denver was not complying with the masking orders from the health authorities. A reporter thought it was due to the "considerable confusion in people's minds because of the orders and counter-orders." The latest change to the masking rule went from requiring that everyone on the streetcars wear them to the "mere recommendation" that masks be worn in the cars. Also, the previous order that masks had to be worn in department stores had been withdrawn entirely. Finally, the health officials backed down completely and removed the masking order entirely on December 1. No one had to wear a mask anywhere, with one exception: nurses, doctors, and others attending flu patients in hospitals or private homes had to wear them.[53]

Two weeks later, a story emerged that, the journalist said, showed how the streetcar conductors in Denver forced the mayor of the city and the board of health into a clear reversal, despite the efforts of those officials to keep the story quiet. First, the officials ordered everyone on streetcars to wear masks, including conductors. Then they permitted business to go on as usual, provided the patrons of theaters and stores wore face coverings. Sixty police officers were detailed to ensure streetcar riders complied with the order. The citizens, the story said, "took the order more as a joke and playfully fought with the police when the latter tried to enforce it. The mayor and the board of health reversed themselves again when they saw how strenuously the public objected" to wearing masks. The conductors had also been ordered to don masks or pay heavy fines. Those conductors met as a body and presented an ultimatum to the city that they would strike as a body if the order were enforced. It was not.[54]

New Mexico

All places were closed in Albuquerque, New Mexico, on the afternoon of October 5, per the recommendations from Surgeon General Rupert Blue. The board of health and the city commissioners of Albuquerque decided on the action at a joint meeting. To that point, there had been eight cases of flu in the city and two deaths. It was only on October 4 that the officials were informed the disease had been found in the city, and a meeting was held that night. At the meeting, a committee of three physicians was appointed to study the matter and report to the health board. The people of Albuquerque were advised to remain in their homes as much as possible, not to attend gatherings of people in houses or buildings, and to keep the windows in their houses open day and night. Open-air meetings were allowed.[55]

Rumors circulated in December that Albuquerque was getting ready to restore the influenza quarantine. The official word was that it would not happen "unless there is a sustained increase in the number of cases for a period of say a week or ten days. Even then it is only remotely possible that quarantine measures will be resorted to. If any action is taken, people probably will be required to wear masks in public or other regulative measures may be resorted to to check the spread of the disease." Even if the quarantine was effective (and doctors disagreed), a reporter commented that the flu would likely be around for months, "and we can't expect to keep movie shows, business houses, schools and churches closed for that length of time."[56]

Three weeks later, in Albuquerque, the city commissioners noted that the residential quarantines of people sick with influenza were regularly ignored, with "innumerable cases" in which members of families under quarantine went about their business normally, coming and going from the quarantined houses many times a day. Families had torn down the placard signs (that denoted the house as a quarantine dwelling) without permission from anybody. In the future, the commissioners scolded, such cases would not be ignored, but offenders would be taken to court. Also complained about was that laundry workers were picking up soiled laundry from quarantined homes, which was against the rules. In the future, offending laundry companies would find themselves closed. Under quarantine rules, laundries were not supposed to pick up from quarantined houses. The problem with quarantine rules here and in other cities was that it was not just the sick person who was confined to the house but all the other household members who needed to come and go for work, and so on.[57]

Albuquerque announced that the quarantine would be lifted on December 2. It had been established on October 5 at 4 p.m. Since that time in Albuquerque, 1,200 cases of influenza had been quarantined in their homes. As of November 23, there were an estimated 400 homes under quarantine, and according to a news story, "Spanish influenza [placard] cards still keep guard of as many houses." Of the 400, "quite a considerable proportion" were old cases of people who had recovered and who, for whatever reason, had neglected to inform the proper authorities to have the placard cards removed. "It has been suggested that a Spanish influenza card on a house is a very efficient and convenient way to keep out unwelcome visitors."[58]

As November ended, it was reported that Albuquerque would be "normal" again on Sunday, December 1. The city board of health voted to lift the quarantine that had been in effect since early October. Part of lifting the ban required churches to ventilate their premises at least three hours before services and for theaters to ventilate their places "thoroughly at all hours of the day and night when performances are being given." An editorial in a city newspaper on December 1 warned the public to be vigilant, and so on. The editor wrote, "The city board of commissioners has not required that everybody wear masks, nor has it required universal vaccination. Either one or both of these may have to be resorted to in cases of another outbreak."[59]

The Mountainair, New Mexico, community had a couple of single-sentence prescriptions in a local paper on November 7, something like mini-editorials to assist in adopting a mask-wearing order in that community. "Wearing a mask will not cure the flu, but it may prevent your taking it," and "An ounce of prevention is worth a pound of cure. Wear a mask." It was an oddly worded law. "Every person who is ill, all who have been ill, all who are in attendance upon the sick, all who appear on the streets, in public places or who interchange visits and intermingle with their neighbors, on business or otherwise, must wear gauze masks." And the order threatened, "Obey the law cheerfully or it will have to be invoked," signed by Dr. C.J. Amble, Torrance County health officer, and two acting assistant surgeons of the United States Public Health Service, Dr. C.E. Fisher and Dr. J.C. Tilt.[60]

A week later, it was reported that two people in Mountainair were arrested and taken before the local justice of the peace, charged with not wearing masks. Each was fined five dollars, and the sentence was suspended on the condition that the masks be worn covering the nose and mouth in the future, which both promised to do. According to the reporter, "The officers are meeting with very little opposition to their regulations, in their attempt to stamp out the epidemic, and are meeting with good success as the number of new cases is decreasing rapidly."[61]

A newspaper account that appeared in September 1919 explained that the State Department in New Mexico and the United States Public Health Service were preparing for the next flu epidemic. They had decided that the fumigation practiced in many jurisdictions was valueless. And they had about decided that wearing gauze masks, so much in vogue in San Francisco, San Diego, Denver, and other cities, was "utterly worthless." They said, "There will be few if any, of the white masked people walking around this winter, it is predicted." Dr. Royal Copeland, the health commissioner for New York City, stated, "Masks are no good, it has been demonstrated to the satisfaction of scientists. We are old fashioned here. We do not believe in closing schools or churches. We did everything unconventional here in 1918 and had the lowest death rate of all."[62]

Two days later, the New Mexico Health Department sent out a circular dealing with the best method of preventing the spread of flu during any epidemic that revisited the area. The communication stated, "Dependence should not be placed upon masks, sprays, drugs or vaccines for protection from influenza. That masks have any value in preventing infection is doubtful and it is believed that they may even favor it. The report found no use for sprays or disinfectants. This department also did not believe that restrictive measures such as closing of theaters and the prohibition of public gatherings have any effect upon the ultimate number of cases which occur in a community." It believed such lockdowns might be justified in small cities and towns to spread the outbreak over a more extended period.[63]

Utah

The Utah Board of Health ordered the closure of the usual suspects on October 10, 1918. All public gatherings ended with churches, schools, theaters, and other public amusements shuttered. The order applied to every town in Utah "where cases of the disease [had] been found."[64]

Logan, Utah, proudly touted the fact on October 22 that the lack of a large number of cases "which were expected in the beginning is no doubt due to the fact that the schools, picture houses, dances, churches and all other gathering places were closed promptly when the disease first appeared in the city." They remained closed, and all other public gatherings, such as funerals, conventions, and similar meetings, were held in the open air with as few people as necessary. All businesses were asked to delay any special sales that were planned. Roy Bullen, chair of the Logan Board of Health, advised people to spend as much time as possible on sleeping porches or in tents.[65]

On the afternoon of November 26, 1918, the mayor of Ogden, Utah, appointed a special health committee. The group met that same evening in the mayor's office and enacted rules and regulations that would "be rigidly enforced and to the obedience of which the entire population is requested to lend willing allegiance." Those new rules contained the following: Every house in which influenza existed was to be placarded, the sign to contain the word "influenza" and be posted on the house in a "conspicuous place." The quarantine was to last for at least ten days after the last day of fever for the last case in the house. No person was to enter or leave a quarantined house except a doctor or nurse without the special permission of the city's board of health. Any person who violated the rule and entered such a house had to remain there for the quarantine unless otherwise ordered by the health board.

People residing outside Ogden and where the quarantine rules were not of "equal strictness" with those of Ogden could not enter the city unless they could exhibit a certificate of good health. No special sale was to be held by any retailer, and no such sale was to be advertised. Streetcars were limited to carrying no more than their seating capacity, and no standing was allowed by passengers on those cars. All streetcars had to be fumigated before leaving the car barn. Streetcar operatives were "held personally responsible for violations of street car regulations." No public funerals were allowed, and funeral services would be no more than 30 minutes long. All people attending patients with influenza, including barbers, dentists, clerks, elevator operators, and others of similar occupations, and people coming into close contact with the public, had to wear masks. The rules further stated, "All masks shall be sterilized at least twice a day, by boiling for 15 minutes in water" or by placing the mask "in a newspaper in an oven and baking until the newspaper is brown." Parents were required to keep their children on their premises. All the rules were effective immediately.[66]

In Salt Lake City, Utah, on December 7, the state and city health boards voted unanimously to lift the ban against gatherings in churches and theaters, which had been closed for almost ten weeks. Churches were to open on the following day, while theaters were slated for two days hence. Lifting restrictions other than churches and theaters would occur as "conditions warranted."[67]

Due to the Salt Lake City decision to lift some of its restrictive measures, the health department and the city commissioners held a meeting in Ogden, presided over by Mayor T. Samuel Browning. The opinion in Ogden of the Salt Lake City decision was that, once again, commercialism had triumphed over everything in the capital city. The Salt Lake decision was seen as having caved to the pressure exerted by the business lobby. It was pointed out that Chicago, San Francisco, and Denver all had to reimpose restrictive measures on their cities after an initial lifting of a ban. John Spargo then made a motion that Ogden, by every means at its disposal, quarantine itself from Salt Lake by requiring all people entering Ogden by rail or by road from the outside to exhibit a clean bill of health from the health officer of the district from which they came, dated not more than 24 hours before arrival in Ogden. It was voted on, passed unanimously, and took immediate effect. Thus, Ogden was to become a city under guard. Every road leading into town and every rail station were policed for that clean bill of health. Refusal to comply with this new order was a misdemeanor.[68]

Two days later, offenses against the Ogden Board of Health regulations were the subject of charges against defendants whose names were called in Municipal Court that morning. None of the defendants except one were present in court, nor were any represented by lawyers. All were out on bail, and all forfeited that bail. Because of all the no-shows and lack of lawyers present, Judge Roberts huffed that he would not take the forfeiture of bail lightly: "It is contempt of court and I mean to treat it as such." Some had been charged with mask offenses and some for spitting on the sidewalk. Jim, described as a "chinaman," was arrested for not wearing a mask while serving customers in a restaurant. He pleaded guilty and was fined five dollars.[69]

Some restrictions in place in Ogden, Utah, were lifted on December 18, 1918, except for the strict quarantine on homes in the city. Streetcar regulations remained in place, and dancing and dance halls remained barred.[70]

Logan, Utah, passed an ordinance requiring all people to wear masks at all times except on their residential property. It went into effect at midnight on November 19. According to the article, "it is believed the step has been taken which will rid the city of the disease entirely before Thanksgiving [November 28 that year]." The report added, "With the universal protection [of masks] it is considered entirely safe for people to move freely about town to do necessary shopping or attend to any ordinary business. The Christmas season is approaching, and people have been advised to do their shopping early. The universal masking has removed the danger ... it is considered safe to go out in public wherever the mask ordinance is effective."[71]

On December 24, by order of the Logan Board of Health, wearing flu masks was no longer compulsory after that date. Beginning on Christmas Day, all people could go unmasked in all places. However, the board still recommended wearing masks where people congregated "for those who wish to assure their own safety." People were also advised to have their masks washed and sterilized for future use, should it prove to be necessary.[72]

In Brigham City, in mid-December, the regulations that made it mandatory for all people entering stores, offices, or other public places to wear gauze masks remained in effect. The board of health had also obtained a quantity of the Rosenow vaccine from the state board of health and planned to make an effort to have every person in Brigham City vaccinated.[73]

Vernal, Utah, and surrounding Uintah County had a mask mandate as late as January 17, 1919. Everyone entering stores or other public buildings had to wear a mask, but the employees did not. People on the street did not have to wear a mask unless two or more were congregating. All solicitors and collectors going door to door had to wear masks. Residents were advised not to admit them to their premises unless they were masked. And, under point four of the regulations, "Citizens, beware of people from outside points. Even your own relatives or friends may come to your home and expose you to influenza."[74]

On November 19, Provo, Utah, ordered the compulsory wearing of gauze face masks for every citizen in Provo engaged in public business. The city commission had enacted the order as a "final and desperate effort" to curb the further spread of the disease. At the same time, an urgent call for volunteers for the gauze room at the local Red Cross chapter was made after a huge demand was made for the masks. An official who was on hand and assisting in the effort to halt the disease, Captain J.N. Dolph of Washington, called attention to the fact that in several offices and factories where the masks were being worn, the wearers often reversed them when one side became soiled. Such a practice, he said, is almost sure to prove disastrous since germs would remain caught in the masks. He advocated boiling the masks for at least 30 minutes a day to sterilize them. Under the ordinance, every person in the city was compelled to wear a gauze face mask in public. The measure provided that clerks in all stores, servers, police officers, and all people on the streets provide themselves with a mask.[75]

The Utah Board of Health considered issuing an order making wearing masks compulsory, said Dr. T.B. Beatty, Utah health commissioner. At that time, an inadequate supply of material for manufacturing masks made the order impossible to adopt, even if the merits of the question had been undebatable and because such an order had not been adopted by any state in the Union. Late in November, Beatty received communication from W.H. Kellogg, secretary of the California Board of Health. Kellogg was responding to Beatty's request regarding the benefit derived from compulsory mask wearing. Kellogg wrote, "Comparison of the morbidity (number of cases) and mortality (number of deaths), curves (action of the disease) of the various cities shows little if any influence from the compulsory wearing of masks." He also said that "the United States public health service does not approve of the mask as a compulsory measure. The same regulations with regard to the wearing of masks adopted in Utah, are in use throughout the country, including the rules of the California state board of health which are its use in the sickroom and by every person coming in contact with an influenza patient."[76]

As of December 19, Provo had moderated its flu ordinance, and wearing masks on the street was not required after that time. The mask order was also lifted for store clerks, but customers in those stores still had to wear masks when entering public buildings.[77]

The influenza restrictions were lifted mainly in Provo and Utah County on December 27. On that day, theaters opened to the public after being closed for months. Schools reopened in the first week of January 1919. However, masks continued to be worn in public buildings after that date "for some time" as a precautionary measure. While customers in those buildings had to wear masks, the employees did not. People did not need to wear masks on the street, except those who had "recently recovered" from the illness.[78]

Some two dozen of the Chi Omega women from the University of Utah were working in Salt Lake City in mid–October, producing face masks for the local Red Cross chapter. According to the report, "These masks are becoming quite universal. Boy scouts and newsboys are now wearing them on the streets." The workforce at the Red Cross building was wearing them—not just the women working to make the masks but also the office staff. As in virtually every city where the Red Cross had a chapter, the Salt Lake City chapter sent out an urgent call for more women volunteers to come forward and help make face coverings.[79]

A couple of days later, it was reported that the Boy Scouts of Salt Lake City were busily engaged working the streets in selling war bonds, collecting tin foil, and gathering fruit pits (ground up and used as a filtering agent for World War I gas masks). The scouts also took the initiative in wearing the influenza masks, setting an example for the general public and being "objects of curiosity until the people became used to seeing them."[80]

On October 24, it was reported that every person in Salt Lake City would probably be compelled to wear a mask beginning the next day. Dr. T.B. Beatty, Utah health officer, said the order had been prepared and merely awaited his signature. "The situation has reached a stage where I feel the wearing of the mask is necessary. It will stamp the epidemic out in far quicker time than any other method. It will mean that all persons engaged in public business of any description must wear a mask. This order will be in effect in banks, stores, hotels, streetcars, railroad stations and in short in every place the public is accustomed to accumulate in numbers." According to Beatty, the mandatory masking order had been under consideration by the Utah Board of Health for several days.[81]

Beatty continued to favor masking. To that end, he consulted with federal health authorities and health personnel in other states and said he found "no instance where this order has been announced, but local health authorities express the opinion that the measure would aid in speedily checking the spread of the disease."[82]

On November 22, an open letter was published in a Salt Lake City newspaper and signed by 19 physicians from the area. Those doctors wanted other measures taken to stamp out the epidemic. They argued that residential quarantine regulations had been so feebly applied, if at all, that no appreciable results ensued. Quarantined houses had not even been placarded. "A feeble suggestion of the use of the mask was made, but no effort was put forth to enforce it." In mentioning their belief that masks were efficient, the example of San Francisco was cited. According to these doctors, "an order to make the wearing of masks universal would be easy to carry out because the very fact that any person is found outside of his own home without a mask on would make him an offender subject to punishment. But when you try to classify and limit the requirement to certain places or certain people, that is where you get lost. Of course, this thing would have to be done with vigor if it succeeded." Concluding their letter, the physicians declared, "We feel most emphatically that something of a more vigorous nature should be adopted if we are going to relieve ourselves of this menace to our health and life.... We urge therefore that the universal compulsory mask method be adopted forthwith."[83]

Various office workforces throughout Salt Lake City reportedly took to wearing masks over the following few days. At a Salt Lake County Medical Society meeting, the universal wearing of masks was vigorously favored by "almost all the doctors present." A resolution was adopted to advise the Salt Lake City health commissioner, Dr. Samuel G. Paul, that the organization was in favor of his recommending to the Salt Lake mayor the "immediate adoption of an ordinance compelling the universal wearing of masks in Salt Lake City."[84]

The issue of masking continued to be kicked around in Salt Lake City. On November 29, physicians, surgeons, theater operators, businesspeople, and the city board of health members gathered to discuss the flu. The consensus "was nearly unanimously against the adoption of mask wearing except, perhaps, in isolated instances." The meeting itself came about because of the resolution made by the medical society. Dr. J.F. Critchlow, leader of the doctors against masking, claimed that the medical society meeting was "packed" in favor of masking. W.H. Swanson, the owner of the American Theater, spoke for theater owners and opposed masking. It was pointed out again that research disclosed the fact that in no state or city in the country where the disease had been combated was the compulsory use of the mask adopted or approved, except in some cities in California.[85]

The letter signed by doctors favoring masking was countered on December 3, when an open letter signed by 22 area physicians was published against universal and compulsory masking. The letter read, "We the undersigned physicians of

Salt Lake City, having carefully considered the medical aspects of the wearing of the gauze mask for the prevention of influenza are of the opinion that under rigid restrictions as to cleaning, sterilizing, etc., such as can be secured in the sickroom, they are of value and their use for such purpose is to be recommended. We believe, however, that their adoption as a universal compulsory measure is not only impractical and ineffective, but may become a positive menace."[86]

On the same day, in another article in the same newspaper, a reporter declared, "The campaign for the adoption in Salt Lake of the influenza mask is practically dead." Salt Lake physicians had gone on record "following in the footsteps of leading health authorities of the United States in their condemnation of the use of the muzzle, characterizing the proposed adoption, as a universally compulsory measure, as not only impractical and ineffective, but likely to become a positive menace." Dr. Beatty had received a large number of telegrams from all over the United States showing there was "much skepticism regarding the efficacy of the gauze mask and that in many communities the compulsory use of the muzzle has had little, if any, influence in checking the disease." One of the most emphatic denunciations of the face coverings came in a telegram from Dr. J.N. Hurty, Indiana health commissioner, who said, "masks are useless, deleterious and unnecessary."[87]

While Salt Lake City never adopted compulsory masking, another community in Salt Lake County did so. On December 16, the town of Murray eased up on its flu restrictions. It removed the requirement for all people to wear masks in places of business and on streetcars. It marked the last day of wearing face masks anywhere in Salt Lake County.[88]

When the Ogden, Utah, health authorities published a sizable public service ad on October 14 in a local newspaper about how to deal with the flu, it did not mention masks, except for those working as attendants to sick influenza patients. The Utah Board of Health put together the ad, and it featured the standard advice given to people across America then.[89]

Just three days later, a report from Ogden indicated that masks were "the vogue from this day forward until further notice and it will make very little difference how much the appearance of any individual is improved or deteriorated by the wearing of them.... To look homely under the present circumstances is the demand of patriotism. The gauze mask is a friend indeed to every community infected with the flu." Instructions on making your own were provided since the local Red Cross chapter could not meet demand. After making a mask, this article advised the reader to pour eucalyptus or any good antiseptic on it. When washed, it should be boiled for 20 minutes and then given a new dose of antiseptic.[90]

In an editorial in an Ogden paper, the journalist wrote, "The *Standard* is firmly of the opinion that the general wearing of gauze masks would do more to check the epidemic now raging in Ogden than all the closing orders which may be issued against public place of assemblage." He complained that with schools, theaters, and churches shut, the people continued to mingle in the streets, and there was no attempt to quarantine the sick. "That being true, how is the spread of the disease to be checked unless we resort to the general wearing of the light gauze masks, which but little inconvenience the wearer? The great virtue in the masks, even though they are not kept highly medicated is the prevention of open sneezing which, when not obstructed, throws the germs into the air."[91]

Less than a week later, he returned with another editorial on influenza. He fretted because medical professionals could not provide information on the source of weaknesses that limited the possibility of curbing the epidemic. Perhaps, he mused, they could "devise a face mask which will as effectively exclude the germs as do gas masks keep out the deadly gas of war."[92]

Ogden newspapers followed the press pronouncements made by Dr. Beatty of the Utah Board of Health as he lobbied for compulsory, universal masking. While he lobbied endlessly to that end, he seemingly lacked the courage to attempt to impose the measure on his state. One Ogden account cited Beatty as having opined, "No person need fear influenza if the protective gauze mask is worn.... The mask need not be tied closely over the face, but is sufficient if it hangs over the nose and mouth."[93]

In mid-November, health inspector Shorten advised people in Ogden to take extra care by wearing the gauze mask. He exclaimed, "Even the barbers of Ogden have given up using it and they of all people ought to use it every day."[94]

An example of panic induced by public officials could be seen in the public service ad published by Ogden city and health officials on November 23. The ad outlined the new regulations, which included a mask mandate, but only for barbers while working. Children had to be kept at home. The ad was of the "we're all gonna die" immediately type with lots of words in capital letters.[95]

James Serras, a barber in the Marion Hotel in Ogden, was arrested on November 25 on a complaint from the special officers the city had hired to enforce its flu restriction for his persistent refusal to comply with the health department order that he must wear a mask while serving customers. Serras did not appear in court when called before Judge Barker in Municipal Court, and he forfeited his bail of ten dollars.[96]

Ogden finally implemented a masking rule at the end of November. The regulations stated, "All persons attending upon patients suffering from influenza, and all barbers, dentists, clerks, elevator operators, and others of similar occupations, and persons coming into close contact with the public, shall wear masks." Another part of the rules stated, "All masks shall be sterilized at least twice a day by boiling fifteen minutes or by placing in a newspaper in an oven and baking until the newspaper is brown." Even the number of people allowed to ride in an elevator was to be specified by the health board—no number was given in the printed regulations. Residential quarantine was imposed, with the patient having to remain quarantined for ten days after the last day of the fever.[97]

The Red Cross in Ogden did not have enough workers to increase its mask production, so it asked the various stores and corporations in Ogden to furnish themselves with gauze masks. Reportedly, some of the larger stores in the area had already equipped themselves with masks of their own making.[98]

Ogden officials were embarrassed to run another public service ad on November 29, detailing that, after making a canvas of the city, "only a dozen stores and markets have complied with the regulations as to the wearing of masks." Then came the threats in the ad. Readers were warned that another inspection would be made, and anyone violating the ordinance would be immediately prosecuted.[99]

WARNING!

HAVE YOU READ THE RULES ADOPTED BY THE BOARD OF HEALTH?

NOTICE After a complete canvass of this city only a dozen stores and markets have complied with the regulations as to the wearing of masks. Another inspection will be made and every person found violating this ordinance will be immediately prosecuted. Generally, the public is most willing to do all it possibly can to relieve the situation, others who make the work of the volunteers a greater hardship in putting the rules into effect by arguing and asking why other measures are not adopted.

No exceptions will be made after today.

THE BOARD OF HEALTH SAYS, WEAR THE MASKS, AND THE MASKS WILL BE WORN, OR ARRESTS WILL FOLLOW.

The masks should be worn properly.

By Order of CITY BOARD OF HEALTH

The rules in Ogden were not being followed by everybody. This infuriated officials, who furiously hectored the citizens in this ad that included "WEAR THE MASKS, AND THE MASKS WILL BE WORN, OR ARRESTS WILL FOLLOW."

On December 6, the Municipal Court in Ogden dealt with several people charged with failure to wear a mask. Judge Roberts explained at length that the court was not where the advisability or inadvisability of wearing the mask could be discussed. What the court intended to do throughout the epidemic, he stated, "is to back up by all means in its power the work of the health boards of the city and see that due penalty is exacted from those who willfully or in negligence disobey the rules as set forth." Rhoda Williams, a clerk in the W.H. Wright & Sons department store, pleaded guilty to not wearing a mask while serving customers. She explained that she could not wear the mask because she had asthma, and the mask was a misery for her. She had medical evidence, but Roberts found her guilty and fined her ten dollars. Mrs. Reynolds, an employee in the Hess Bakery, pleaded guilty and declared, "Rules are framed to hit those who have to work for their living the hardest." Roberts found her guilty but decided she did not refuse to don the mask willfully but carelessly, thus fining her five dollars. Henry Last of the firm of Last and Thomas answered a complaint that he allowed clerks in his store to wait on customers without wearing masks. Last said he had done his best to see that his employees wore masks, but it was not always possible to be aware of a clerk's momentary lapse. Roberts declared that the special officer who arrested Last had made a mistake and that he should have arrested the actual offenders. The case against Last was dismissed.[100]

The progressive national paper *Goodwin's Weekly*, published in Salt Lake City, Utah, editorialized on face coverings under the heading, "This mask bunk." The editor stated, "The wearing of masks consisting of three or four layers of gauze as a preventive for influenza is sheer nonsense, not to mention the fact that the practice is insanitary, if not absolutely dangerous." He added, "There are several reasons why masks should not be worn. Doesn't it stand to reason that the mask is bound to rapidly become a dirty thing with the filth from without, and the effluvia from within is spread over the face and the inner surface of the mask?" He concluded, "There can't be any question about the futility of the flu mask, according to the best authorities locally, and on the contrary, they are held to be a menace to those who affect them. From the common sense viewpoint, there should be a law compelling people to go without them rather than one making the wearing of them compulsory."[101]

Arizona

Louie Quong was the proprietor of the Peking Cafe in Phoenix. He was arrested on the night of October 26 for violating city ordinance number 236, commonly known as the influenza ordinance, for allowing a crowd to gather in his establishment. According to the police, only three of the roughly 30 people in the restaurant were eating; the rest were either dancing or looking on, with another large crowd outside looking in on the fun.[102]

Dr. O.H. Brown, the Arizona health officer, commented on the situation in Ray, Arizona, late in October. Ray had restrictions in and out of town, making it mandatory for travelers to show doctor's certificates before entering or leaving the district. Brown said he disapproved of such a quarantine as "it works too much of a hardship upon the people. The disease must run its course in this state as in other states. All we can do is to take such preventive measures as will keep it from spreading too rapidly. It is useless to attempt to stamp it out at once." On October 27, the Ray restrictions placed a strict quarantine over the area that included Ray, Ray Junction, and Ray Hercules. No one could leave or enter the district without a physician's certificate declaring the holder free from Spanish influenza. L.S. Cates, general manager of the Ray Consolidated Copper Company (Ray was a company town controlled by the mining interests and no longer exists—it is now a ghost town), stated, "The condition of the influenza epidemic in this section is excellent. We have no new cases and only about 30 who have not fully recovered. But we do not want any more of the disease brought in here, neither do we care to have people from here carry it to other communities. Hence the strict quarantine. Tickets will not be sold either way unless the purchaser has the necessary certificate. In this way we expect to entirely stamp out the influenza in a few days."[103]

As November began, an editor with a Bisbee, Arizona, newspaper remarked, "The Warren district [of Bisbee] is entering its fourth week of quarantine from the influenza, all meetings having been barred for the time. This quarantine is as irksome and as costly to many firms and individuals of the district as it is necessary." He added, "It should be raised as soon as possible with safety. It should be maintained to the last day needful with public health and the check of the disease and it should be lifted the first day the danger is passed."[104]

One week later, the same editor of the same Bisbee paper declared, "Boards of health in the west have generally been slow to lift the quarantine. In the east, where the disease was many times worse than in the west, quarantine was lifted promptly with the passing of the peak." Concerning the Bisbee quarantine, in its fifth week, he said, "Its usefulness has been served. Some announcement should surely be made soon as to the date of its suspension." He also noted the quarantine was "a most severe hardship" upon many businesses and people of the community and "when the sickness passes the epidemic stage, a quarantine is little short of a tyranny."[105]

With the passage of one more week, the quarantine situation remained the same in the Warren district of Bisbee. It was reported that Williams, Arizona, one of the first towns in Arizona to be placed in quarantine, was "up in arms against the continued enforcement of the quarantine." The town of Williams, through its town marshal Bobby Burns, had served notice on the state, which said that it "will regard a continued enforcement of the anti-influenza quarantine as an overt act against the village and forthwith will launch upon a war to the hilt against the Arizona State Board of Health." Brown countered that the restrictions imposed in Williams were identical to those put into effect throughout the entire state and involved the same measures advocated by Surgeon General Blue. Brown said, "While it may be true that there are only a few cases of influenza now in Williams, it is the belief of the state board of health that the situation there is yet too serious to allow the quarantine to be lifted." By stating it would launch a "war," the town of Williams meant it would launch legal action. Brown went on to state that even when the state board of health believed the danger had passed, lifting restrictions depended on all seven precautionary points being met, as laid down and agreed to by those at the recent meeting held in Phoenix. The seven points were as follows: (1) a thorough scrubbing with soap and water of theaters and all public buildings; (2) a rigorous neighborhood cleanup of streets, alleys, yards, and so forth; (3) the placarding of houses containing flu patients; (4) the competent inspection of food and drinking places to see health regulations were complied with; (6) a general survey of flies and fly-breeding places; (7) an "honest, serious, systematic effort to have all people vaccinated against the flu." Plus, they would have to look at similar communities that had permission to open and that had good results after their opening. Dr. Brown cited the example of

Flagstaff, Arizona, which opened without authority from the board of health, resulting in an "alarming increase" in the number of influenza cases.[106]

A reporter in Phoenix, Arizona, remarked on November 18 that whether the businesses in Phoenix, then closed for six weeks, were to be reopened or the entire city was to be placed under an "air-tight quarantine" could be decided that night at a meeting. Theater owners, the state health officer, Dr. Brown, at least one minister, two doctors, the city manager, the city attorney, and other "prominent" citizens attended the meeting. Two men had been appointed to a committee to secure the presence at the meeting of representatives from the Chamber of Commerce, Merchants' and Manufacturers' Association, Rotary and Kiwanis clubs, and "leading business men and citizens." The physicians were detailed to entice the medical fraternity to the meeting. The question of making it compulsory to wear masks when on the street would also be discussed.[107]

In Phoenix, at the close of the first 24 hours under the new health regulations, good results were noted by the citizens' committee in charge of enforcing

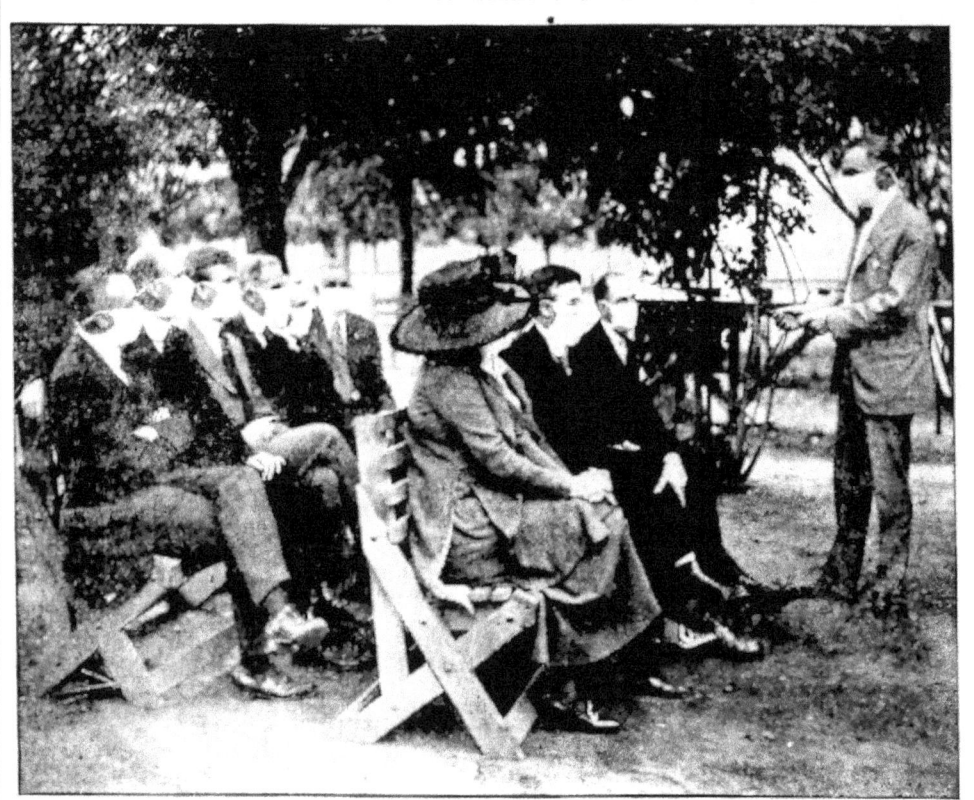

An open-air meeting was held in Phoenix. Despite moving their meeting to the outdoors, the participants still wore masks.

the regulations and by the committee of physicians with whom they were cooperating. Two surveys were started. One was the inspection of the downtown district to ascertain the number of people permitted in places of business at one time. Another survey reported, "More masks were worn yesterday than at any time since the appearance of the influenza in Phoenix."[108]

The new health regulations in Arizona prohibited people from being on the county highways without some "legitimate reason." One who objected was Frank Houston, who was stopped while returning to Phoenix from a hunting trip across the river. Somehow, he had gotten past the guards at the Center Street bridge when he was traveling out, but the guards stopped him at that point on his return. He was allowed to continue to his home in Phoenix, even though he was told he did not have a good reason for being on the highway. On arriving in Phoenix, he went to the police station to ask if the guards had a right to stop him the way they did. He was told they had the right. The county health officer, Dr. A.B. Nichols, stated that hunting was not a business and thus did not provide a sufficient excuse for a man to be traveling on county roads. He reiterated that he should stay home if he had no business duties that required him to be on the streets.[109]

On December 9, Mesa, Arizona, announced that it would remove its flu restrictions on December 13, and churches and theaters would reopen. Mayor Dan Kleinman signed the proclamation. However, removing the regulations in Mesa was contingent on whether Phoenix had any unexpected bad results from lifting their ban on December 8.[110]

On January 6, 1919, Phoenix announced that the schools would not reopen due to the recurrence of the Spanish influenza epidemic. An order closing all city schools for two weeks was issued that morning. The order had the unanimous sanction of the state, county, and city health officials and followed a meeting held the night before. In addition to school closures, the order prohibited all public and private dances and all social gatherings. Also, an "absolute" quarantine was placed on all houses with flu cases. It meant that no one was allowed in or out of a quarantined house without permission from the authorities, and the order allowed for the stationing of guards at those homes if it was deemed necessary. A placard giving the name of the disease had to be posted in a "conspicuous" place. Also prohibited was the "passing out of any material from the quarantined house." However, it did make "provision for conveying the necessities of life, under certain conditions, to those in quarantine." City police and county deputies were in charge of enforcement. Neighbors of quarantined houses were urged to report any infractions to the police. As a beginning, the new health measures were to be in effect for two weeks. "School children are not to be allowed to run about the city during the present closing of schools," John D. Loper, superintendent of schools, announced. "The police are to receive special instructions to be on the lookout for school children and to immediately arrest them if they are unaccompanied by their parents or are not on the street for some necessary purpose."[111]

At a meeting of the Bisbee, Arizona, city council on January 7, it was decided that a partial ban extending only to the dances within the city limits of Bisbee should be implemented immediately. The council took action at the request of Dr. D. Brown, city health officer. He argued for the ban because of the proximity of dancers and the large crowds that assembled in dance halls. Dr. N.C. Bledsoe, a council member, backed Brown's opinion.[112]

The influenza mask reportedly appeared in the Warren district of Bisbee, Arizona, on October 30. Following the example of people in numerous other cities, several residents of Bisbee went on the streets with masks on. "People turned to look and to remark, but the remark was that they would do the same. Later others were seen with a cloth mask that came down below the chin and was fastened behind the head…. The influenza mask wearers were pioneers yesterday but without a doubt, it will be a common sight by today."[113]

However, citizens in Bisbee were slow to take up the mask. An editorial in a Bisbee newspaper on November 19 discussed the situation. It declared that everyone in the city was frustrated with the existing restrictions and wanted relief. One thing the editor championed was the mask. He claimed that "there can be no harm in using a mask in any case. With this in view, why cannot the people of the Warren district be persuaded to use the mask? It must be conceded that it can do no harm and may be the cause of doing a great deal of good. The slight expense attached to the purchase of gauze masks will not be a deterrent against its use." He also noted that "the business people of the district are becoming vexed at the continuation of the quarantine." His solution was to "let the physician issue an order to the effect that every man, woman and child in the Warren district wear a mask. Bisbee can not go on all winter in its present condition. It is suicidal and must be alleviated in some manner. It is time for the authorities to act."[114]

Tucson, Arizona, imposed a mask ordinance on its residents, with the order taking effect on November 19. The order directed people to wear face coverings in places of business. Wearing them on the street was not required, but many did so. Regarding the first day with the order in effect, a reporter claimed it "was apparently accepted in good spirit." Supply of the masks was inadequate to meet demand, and they were not on sale until the afternoon of the first day.[115]

An editor with a Tucson newspaper discussed the subject of masks. He wrote, "Either the masks are a preventative against the flu or they are not. If they are a preventative, then there is no use keeping the theaters closed and preventing all public gatherings, provided that those who attend them wear masks. If the city health authorities believe that masks will stop the influenza germ, which is waiting around the corner to waylay you, then let us all wear them … we ought to be able to go about all of our pursuits undisturbed, provided that we wear them."[116]

When a reporter from another Tucson paper surveyed the situation on the first day that the masking mandate was in effect, he found all the leading politicians and health officials in his city scrupulously wearing them. The one exception was Mayor Parker, who claimed that he could not obtain one.[117]

Some ten days after the Tucson mask mandate was in force, the paper's editor returned with another screed about the situation. A member of the local health board let out that, in his opinion, masks were not an absolute preventive. That caused the editor to assert, "If they are not a hundred per cent effective they are no good at all. Either the so-called flu germ can enter through them or it cannot. If they are what they are claimed to be, then let us continue them and go about our business in the normal way. If they are no good, why burden the public with them?"[118]

On December 3, the regulations governing Tucson citizens were changed somewhat. The public was requested to wear masks in places of business and at all gatherings. Patrons would not be admitted to theaters unless they were masked. A plan was devised to open the schools but not burden the children with mask wearing. Half-day sessions were held so only half the pupils were in the schools at any time, and they would occupy every other desk. Three feet of distance would be maintained between the children at all possible times.[119]

The Tucson mask ordinance was enforced vigorously by the city's police officers. Nearly 50 people were arrested on December 16 as the result of a raid by the police on hotel lobbies. Thirteen appeared before City Recorder Cowan, with eight of them each paying a ten dollar fine and four having their cases dismissed because they were under the age limit. Cowan turned them over to their parents with a warning. One was fined but announced his intention to fight the ordinance. Tucson Police Chief Frank T. Bailey stated, "We are going to enforce this ordinance or close up the town entirely."[120]

A third editorial appeared in the Tucson paper on the subject, this one on December 20. Rumor had it that someone would appeal the ordinance's validity to a higher court. The editor felt it would not stand such a test. He added, "But whether or not the law requiring the wearing of masks is valid or invalid, the experience of Tucson has taught the people of this city that the whole business is a farce and incapable of enforcement. Not ten percent of the people engaged in business wear their masks all of the time, or attempt to comply with the ordinance. They simply will not do so and cannot be blamed for ignoring an order in the efficacy of which they have no confidence." The editor further wrote, "In view of the experiments and admissions by medical authorities, why stick to the little rag? The most enlightened authorities are now advising the people to use a little common sense, take care of themselves, eat and sleep regularly, keep clean and above all to refuse to be frightened."[121]

In Phoenix, it was mandated that visitors to hospitals and homes with cases of influenza be required to wear a gauze mask. Members of families with cases of influenza and all people suffering from colds in the head or acute coughs or showing other recognized symptoms of the malady should wear masks when mingling with other people.[122]

In Phoenix, on November 18, a meeting was held to discuss measures to control the flu. The city had been closed for six weeks after imposing the Blue Protocols. Different measures were discussed as the officials became more desperate. Among the new measures for discussion were closing every place people congregated, even in small numbers, and the residential quarantining of every residence containing a flu victim. Also under consideration was a compulsory masking order that would apply everywhere whenever a person left home.[123]

The next day, Phoenix announced that it was launching its fight against the flu in earnest. Everyone was ordered to stay at home, and people found on the streets of the communities in Maricopa County or on the country roads had to give an account of themselves, their destinations, their businesses, and the reasons for having left their residence. Special deputies roamed the area to enforce those rules. There was no loafing or congregating anywhere, and visiting was also banned. People were commanded to remain at least three feet away from the person with whom they were conversing. Also, people had to wear a gauze mask if they were in contact with cases of influenza or "in contact with many people on the streets."[124]

Then the next "logical" step took place in Phoenix. Beginning on Wednesday morning, November 27, everyone who appeared on the streets of Phoenix or anywhere outside their homes had to wear a flu mask. There were no exemptions to the order, which was made on Monday afternoon following a meeting of the citizens' committee with the committee of physicians appointed at a recent mass meeting. The committee explained that if wearing the flu mask was of benefit to any single individual in this epidemic, it was good for all. Masks could be purchased at drug stores for ten cents. As was often the case, instructions were provided in the article on how to make a mask. It was also suggested that a suitable mask was "a clean, close textured handkerchief."[125]

The headline of a story the next day claimed that 95 percent of the population obeyed the mask order in Phoenix. That number came from the citizens' committee, the same group that orchestrated the passage of the masking mandate. Supposedly, most of those used the "regulation" mask, with only a few using a handkerchief. A reporter said, "In ordinary times, the mask would have been laughed to scorn, but yesterday it was accepted as the usual part of a day's routine. The influenza mask had come into its own and claimed all Phoenix for its home." No arrests were made that day, as the first day was considered a grace period. Arrests were slated to begin the next day. There was at least one dissenter. The firm E.S. Wakelin Grocery Co. took out an ad in a local newspaper that warned those who favored the mask of its dangers of being dirty and unsanitary.[126]

The first person taken into custody the next day for failure to wear a mask was Edwin C. Moore, an E.S. Wakelin Grocery Company employee. It was thought Moore's arrest may have been deliberate, as his employer was against the masking order. Some others were also arrested. Despite the legality of the handkerchiefs, the police stopped some who were wearing them and "warned" them. The only explanation came from a reporter who stated, "The substitution of handkerchiefs for masks is not well looked upon by health officials, and the practice is being discouraged as much as possible."[127]

The flu mask order was abolished in Phoenix as of the morning of December 3, meaning no person needed to wear an influenza mask on the city streets. The order came after a meeting of the Maricopa County Medical Society, the physicians' advisory committee. The citizens' committee was told it no longer existed. Dr. O.H. Brown, Arizona health officer, was in charge of the campaign against the flu in Phoenix, replacing the citizens' committee. For people in sick rooms and those who came into contact with flu patients, mask wearing was still necessary.[128]

An editorial in a Phoenix newspaper on the flu epidemic pointed out the

Opposite: **An ad from a grocery store in Phoenix that took issue with the mask mandate then in force in Phoenix, Arizona.**

THANKSGIVING OFFER

To All Who Are In Favor of the Wearing of Masks

Please Take Notice

Cleanliness and the breathing of pure air have always been outraged by those who have the putrescent habit of sleeping with their heads under the bed-covering. Hiding behind a mask, like sleeping with the head under cover, is dirty, unsanitary, and psychologically in keeping with the ostrich's habit of getting away from danger by hiding its head and leaving its mammoth body exposed. Man is slow to learn that the more of his body he exposes to the air the better.

The great outside is filled with good, fresh air which is antiseptic. The sun purifies the atmosphere; the sun-light is indispensable as an air purifier; the earth and water needs it as much; it is the germicide par excellence. If it was not for pure air—if all the air could be made as impure as the blood is after sleeping one night with the head under cover, the human family would soon perish from off the face of the earth. The only mask that is antidotal to disease, is the mask of good cheer.

E. S. Wakelin Grocery Co.

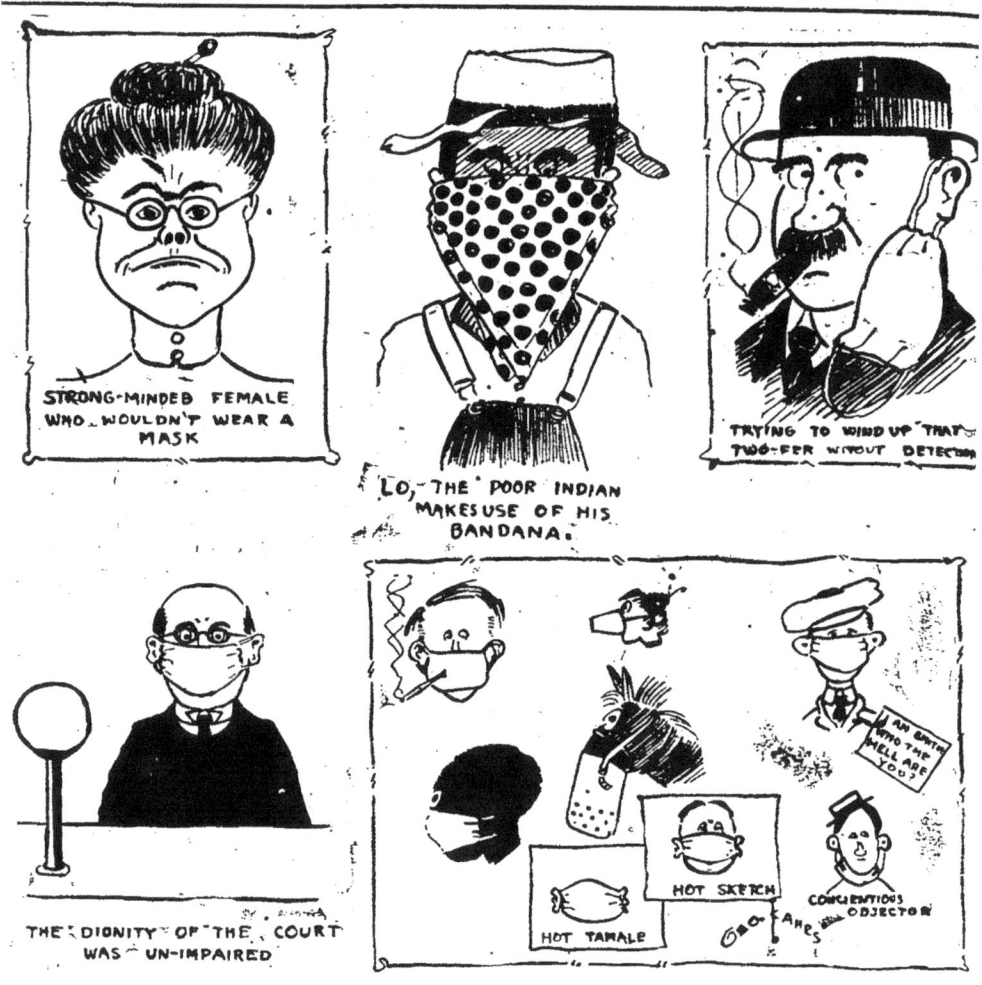

Editorial comment on the use of masks in Phoenix, Arizona.

inability of the authorities to agree on what to do and the overall inadequacy of their measures. "The schools, theaters, the latter at a great loss, have been closed longer than anywhere else in the country and yet we have no definite promise of relief," said the editor. And, he believed, the longer the situation went on, the less the people would willingly cooperate. "In the matter of the flu mask order there was a tendency to revolt and a disinclination to observe the spirit of the order though a show was made of complying with the letter of it. The result was that the mask was not given a fair chance. Worn merely over the left ear or on the chin it had no other effect than to keep those members warm. But they are not points of attack by influenza germs, so that the mask order fell short of its intended efficacy."[129]

A man named W.E. Copeland was fined ten dollars by Justice Wheeler for failure to obey the mask mandate. He was the only person convicted and sentenced. All the other arrests and cases were on hold because Moore was challenging the validity of the law. When the mask law was rescinded, all the other cases were dropped, and Moore's case was never resolved. Under the circumstances, Wheeler determined that Copeland should get his money back. Wheeler said, "If Copeland calls at my office I will return his check."[130]

When a Phoenix newspaper printed its summary of the American Public Health Association convention in Chicago in December, it showed its bias by choosing to highlight the remarks given there by Dr. Woods Hutchinson, who was a fanatic fan of masks, singing the praises of the use of the face coverings in San Francisco. Hutchinson was an outlier at the convention, with the majority of opinion against the masks and nobody as fanatically in favor as he was.[131]

The United States Public Health Service issued a report for the general public in September 1919 about what to expect and what to do if the flu should return in such an intense form. It did not urge the use of masks except, of course, in the sickroom. But concerning masking during the 1918–1919 period, it concluded that "the use of face masks has not been attended with the success predicted for them." In the fall of 1919, newspapers across America printed this story.[132]

Restrictions that had been in place in Douglas, Arizona, for several weeks were lifted in mid–December. Still, everyone appearing on the streets and in public was ordered to wear a flu mask. Beginning a day later, the police were stationed in the business district with orders to arrest anyone appearing in public without being masked. The order was enforced, with violators fined $2.50. Added to the order a week later was the mandate that every person entering hotel lobbies, including all guests, had to be masked. At the beginning of January 1919, the restrictions in Douglas were lifted, except that theater patrons were still required to wear masks while witnessing performances.[133]

Nevada

After discussing the danger of Spanish influenza for four days, the Reno Board of Health met on the evening of October 10 and decided that all theaters, churches, and high schools should be closed and all public gatherings should be banned. All these measures took effect at noon on October 12. While the public schools were allowed to remain open, restrictions were placed on them. Only half the school would attend simultaneously; those in attendance would be placed in alternate seats; and the children would not be allowed to mingle on the playground.[134]

Restrictions were increased over the following days: all schools were closed, cabarets had to discontinue music, and saloons were ordered to remove the chairs from the card rooms. Then, after 34 days of restrictions, they were all dropped as of November 15. The most significant effect of those restrictions was said to have been the ban on political meetings during the height of the election season.[135]

An article in a newspaper in Goldfield, Nevada, in December observed that just as other places had suffered when protective measures against the flu had been relaxed, Goldfield was suffering due to carelessness over the previous few days. So, after a meeting of the Board of County Commissioners and Dr. J.L. McCarthy about the situation, they decided that schools could not reopen until, at the earliest, the new year. They also decided to enforce the mask-wearing ordinance again strictly, and the officers promised to enforce it rigidly and arrest the unmasked. And "it was decided that the masks must not only be worn but must be worn properly." The journalist added, "It would be well for some people to wash their masks at least occasionally and replace them with new ones when they become so ragged that they are nothing short of a disgrace."[136]

The health board met in Tonopah, Nevada, on January 7, 1919, lifting all the flu regulations. All social and lodge gatherings could resume, theaters could operate, and masks were no longer compulsory. The entire flu legislation of the previous three months was erased from the books. One board member noted there was no sense in retaining the masks "since there is no enforcement of the ordinance."[137]

In October, it was decided that all trains entering Nevada would be inspected and disinfected. All suspected cases of influenza would be quarantined as soon as the proper medical officers could be appointed and arrangements made with the railroad authorities. Reno Mayor Frank Byington contacted Nevada Governor Emmet Boyle. He asked that the state restrict trains and travelers entering Nevada. Boyle approved the plan and said, "The state board of health has authority to appoint any doctor or other qualified person who may be selected to inspect passengers at the state line points. They will be made members of the state police."[138]

The city council of Elko, Nevada, adopted an ordinance at the end of October, making it compulsory for all citizens to wear influenza masks while on the streets of Elko and in all public places. Another Nevada community with a masking ordinance was Ely. Four men were fined five dollars each in that town for appearing in public without wearing a mask.[139]

Early in November, the Las Vegas city commissioners passed an order that required everyone to wear a flu mask. The order was, according to a reporter, "being very faithfully obeyed by the people." The story added that it was essential to wear masks. Still, the precaution was worse than useless unless the masks were sterilized frequently and kept clean.[140]

In Reno, Nevada, it was reported on October 22 that the local Red Cross chapter was busy making masks. They were being supplied free to different concerns in Reno for their employees' use. People were also urged to make them at home, and the usual instructions for making one were part of the article.[141]

One day later, a brief editorial appeared in a Reno newspaper. It stated, "If by wearing gauze masks or any other kind of masks, the people of Reno can stop the spread of influenza and perhaps save lives, there ought to be no hesitancy in wearing them. Any precaution that needs to be taken ought to be taken. It is not only one's self that is protected, but one is also protecting the community."[142]

When the Reno Board of Health met on the evening of December 2, it came close to ordering city residents to wear flu masks. After the motion to do so was introduced at the meeting and duly seconded, it was decided to obtain some official information from San Francisco on the effects of masks there. If the information received was satisfactory, then Reno would be masked. The reply received in a telegram from San Francisco stated, "No data available to show whether masks were effective in stamping out epidemic or not. Best authorities are divided as to effect of use of masks and each community must work out its own problems."[143]

Later in December, Dr. J.A. Ascher, Washoe County (Reno) health officer, said, "Knowing that my views on the following suggestion will meet with opposition I am nevertheless of the opinion, based on the results proven by available statistics that the gauze mask is of great benefit as a preventive measure." He added, "I would unhesitatingly recommend the general compulsory use of masks until such time as those desiring were immunized through the use of the vaccine, or the pandemic abated." And, like bureaucrats all over, he concluded by declaring, "The responsibility in the final analysis rests with the public."[144]

11

Pacific

Alaska

Judge James Wickersham, in Juneau, Alaska, deliberately violated the influenza quarantine regulations on the night of October 31, 1918, by attempting to hold a political meeting and speaking at a public hall. The police dispersed the meeting, although the door had been locked against them and the lights had been turned out by a guard at the door to try to fool the authorities. Also present at the meeting was Senator Dan Sutherland of Juneau. Police Chief Dargan, in Juneau, said to Wickersham, "I ought to arrest you, but don't let it happen again." The order to prohibit all public meetings went into effect on October 26. At the meeting that was broken up, an estimated 20 to 25 people were in attendance.[1]

Increasing cases of influenza made it necessary to reestablish a quarantine in Juneau, Alaska, reported Dr. L.O. Sloane, city health officer. After 6 p.m. on December 18, by order of Mayor Valentine, "it will be necessary to wear gauze masks." Also, all theaters and places of public gatherings were ordered shut.[2]

Starting around November 11, in Douglas, Alaska, health officials, with the sanction of the Territorial Board of Health, made it compulsory for everyone in Douglas to wear a mask while away from their homes. Those officials also swore in J.D. Bagley as a special officer to see that the law was obeyed. There were a few arrests during the first days of the imposition. The maximum penalty of $25 was assessed against those disobeying the orders. Due to that, a reporter wrote, "the wearing of masks has now become general."[3]

At noon on December 5, the health board of Douglas Island decided that the flu situation had improved enough that the masks could be discarded. All the other restrictions that governed the area were also removed over the following week or so.[4]

With other parts of the quarantine lifted on December 9, there was a sudden reversal by the health officials in Douglas when the restrictions were all reimposed on December 17. Schools and churches were all closed, along with all places of amusement. Also, residents were once again ordered to wear flu masks whenever they were outside their homes.[5]

Instructions for making masks for influenza prevention from the San Francisco Board of Health's circular were received in the mail in Juneau, Alaska, on November 1. They were made of four layers of fine gauze and were five by seven inches. According to the circular, the masks should not be medicated in any way and should be cleaned by boiling for 15 minutes. Dr. L.O. Sloane was the Juneau health officer, and his office approved the instructions.[6]

Four days later, a news story declared the masks had appeared in many public places in Juneau, with the post office and the Gastineau Hotel and Cafe being the first to have their employees don the "germ destroyers." All the employees at the post office were wearing them. At the Gastineau Cafe, masks were first worn by the servers, while at the Gastineau Hotel, the cleaning staff were wearing them that morning. Besides being the city health officer, Dr. Sloane was also the territorial quarantine officer. Acting under the authority of Alaska Governor Thomas Riggs, Jr., and Juneau Mayor Emery Valentine, he signed a request that all residents of Juneau and all others while in the city wear flu masks. The report added, "The wearing of influenza masks is compulsory in many states, including California and Washington."[7]

The Juneau Common Council introduced a resolution on November 13 making wearing a flu mask mandatory in the city and providing a $25 fine for those not wearing one. The final passage of the ordinance was still a few days away then. In hyping the idea to the public, the council declared, "This is a duty you owe not only to yourself but to your fellow citizens, for is not the saving of one human life recompense enough for the few days of discomfort that the wearing of the masks may cause? Show that Juneau spirit, wear your mask for a few days so that we may again open our schools and our commercial activity may become normal once more."[8]

The ordinance passed on November 15 and required people in Juneau to wear masks everywhere when not in their residences. In Juneau at the time, all the usual suspects were closed as the Rupert Blue Protocols were followed. When this ordinance was passed, the Juneau council also voted to hire three special officers to assist the local police force in enforcing the ordinance.[9]

Juneau Mayor Valentine raised all the restrictions in Juneau on November 27 at midnight. The churches, schools, theaters, and places of public gatherings were all allowed to reopen. However, he emphasized that the mask ordinance remained in force. He held out the hope that he might raise that one in a few days. While churches could conduct services again, the Presbyterian Church in Juneau announced that it would not hold its usual Thanksgiving service (November 28 that year), "owing to the fact that people are compelled to wear masks." The mask ordinance in Juneau was lifted at midnight on November 30.[10]

Normality did not last long in Juneau because, as of 6 p.m. on December 18, the restrictions were reimposed on the city, including the masking order. Douglas and Douglas Island were both included this time. The following section from the ordinance said, "All places wherein people congregate shall be closed. This shall include all schools of whatsoever nature, all churches, all poolhalls, hotel lobbies, the post office and all other public places, and not more than four people shall be allowed to congregate on the street or other public place, at one time and all such persons shall wear masks of not less than six layers of cheese cloth or similar goods."[11]

In Douglas, the Island Board of Health lifted the restriction that masks had to be worn on the street on December 28. All other restrictions remained in place, including the mandate to wear masks everywhere except in one's home and on the street.[12]

Then all the restrictions were lifted again, starting after 6 p.m. on December 30. Masks did not need to be worn anywhere. The only restriction left was the residential quarantine imposed on anyone diagnosed with the disease. That continued until the last of those cases was pronounced cured.[13]

Washington

In Kennewick, Washington, the influenza restrictions that were to be lifted after October 20 were clamped on tighter than ever on October 21, when Health Officer Morrison received instructions that a statewide quarantine had been implemented. Schoolchildren who had been ready to return to school were banished back to their homes. In addition to the ban on schools, churches, and cinemas, the closing order was extended to pool halls and card rooms.[14]

In Seattle, Washington, police Chief Warren detailed the mounted police on Saturday morning, October 26, to patrol all car lines in the city's central section and stop all streetcars that did not have at least one-third of their windows open before they could proceed. A shortage of masks meant it was not then possible to issue orders for certain classes of employees to wear them, said Commissioner McBride. McBride emphasized that people should stay at home and keep their homes well ventilated. Crowds were to be avoided, and people were warned not to sneeze or expectorate "promiscuously." If people were well, they should stay in the open air; if sick, they should stay home and breathe fresh air. McBride said, "Seattle people would do more than all the doctors toward stopping the spread of influenza if they would stay at home for two days." Police were instructed to prevent anything resembling congestion in department stores and sales establishments downtown and to arrest proprietors who did not cooperate.[15]

Dr. J.S. McBride, Seattle health commissioner, when asked to comment on the mask wearing underway in San Francisco, said he thought the average individual didn't have to wear a gauze mask but recommended, however, that all clerks, particularly those who sold or served food, be required to wear gauze masks.[16]

A retail outlet placed an advertisement announcing the end of the influenza restrictions in Seattle, as far as retail outlets were concerned. The store, in the ad, congratulated itself for how it came through the crisis. Also noted in the ad was the fact that regulations concerning wearing influenza masks in all places of public assembly would remain effective until further notice.[17]

Pullman, Washington, Health Officer J.L. Gilleland placed an ad on page one of the local newspaper on November 15, 1918, that outlined the lifting of restrictions for his city and listed the slightly staggered days when various places could reopen.[18]

Spokane, Washington, announced the extension of the influenza quarantine to mass meetings, community singing groups, and crowding in theater lobbies on December 4. Theaters and churches would remain open.[19]

Seattle launched its fear and panic campaign when a local paper published a lengthy article. It was headlined, "Spanish flu has Boston in tragic grip." The subhead was about the "strange new malady that takes huge death toll." There was no

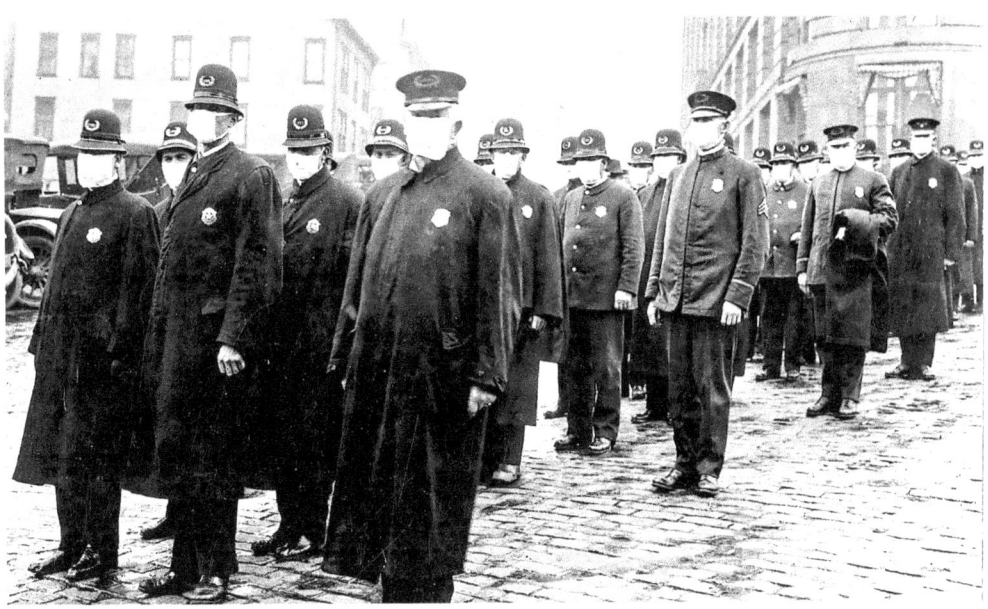

Seattle police wearing masks while on duty.

treatment for the disease, and the suggested measures were limited to the isolation of the sick. However, the article admitted there "was no practical quarantine and disinfection can only be general. Attending nurses may wear a gauze mask." And nothing else was mentioned about masks other than general and mild recommendations. Also mentioned was that all kinds of cures and prophylactics were being advertised. Patent medicine quacks were all jumping on the bandwagon after suddenly discovering that the cure for baldness or arthritic knees was just as effective for the Spanish flu—but no mention of masks.[20]

A warning about the rising number of flu cases in Seattle appeared on October 25, issued by Dr. J.S. McBride, Seattle health commissioner. He classically blamed the victim. He said the caseload was rising due to "the negligence of a large part of the populace regarding the health regulations." Agreeing with McBride was Dr. T.D. Tuttle, then the Washington state health commissioner. "Seattle will not be placed in the position of San Francisco whose citizens are compelled to wear masks on the streets, if the people here will adhere to the prescribed health rules laid down by the health department," he whined. "I wish to emphasize the fact that the disease is spread mainly by the people coming downtown unnecessarily, and frequenting the stores and soft drink establishments, etc. People should stay at home, unless compelled to go downtown by absolute necessity."[21]

Despite the difficulty of obtaining masks in Seattle, the authorities ordered residents to don gauze masks "wherever people congregate" on Monday, October 28. That meant indoors and outdoors, and it left residents confused about whether the outdoor area they were in was crowded or not. Red Cross masks were available by then to some degree, and block-long lineups were reported outside some of the drug stores where they were available. McBride issued the new orders on Sunday after consultation with Seattle Mayor Ole Hanson. Seattle residents could get the masks for free at the drug stores, and that irritated Hanson, who helped deliver Red Cross masks from the organization's workrooms to the city drug stores. He said, "The one trouble with the distribution is the fact that people don't have to pay for the masks, and getting them for nothing means that they are careless with them." According to McBride and Hanson, it was the attitude of negligence on the part of the public that had to be overcome, as in the following report: "Monday morning, crowds of workers, coming downtown, unaware of the new edict, congested the street cars without masks. Few street cars had the required number of windows open." Could it all have been the fault of the so-called health authorities? People had less than 24 hours' notice of the need for masks, and much of that time was on a Sunday. Masks were not readily available. How could a worker find the time on a Monday morning to get in line to obtain a mask and still get to work on time? One of the bizarre rules implemented by the authorities, supposedly to avoid crowding and make people stay home, was the instruction to streetcar crews to "pass up" shoppers as nearly as they could distinguish them and bring only workers to the city.[22]

The gauze masks had their distribution taken over by the City of Seattle the following day. A charge of five cents was levied, with the proceeds used to combat influenza. Residents continued to get their masks at drug stores. As some passengers on streetcars persisted in closing windows that were ordered open all the time, the officials were considering nailing the windows open. McBride stressed that it was not compulsory to wear the masks on the streets in the open air but that it must be in readiness to slip over the nostrils and mouth when an individual enters a building. "It is foolish to wear the masks in the open air," said McBride. "The regulation makes no mention of it." The city took over mask distribution and implemented a charge for them, mainly due to "apparent negligence" on the part of at least some of the public. According to McBride, masks had been used and thrown aside "by thoughtless or careless individuals, who apparently have no appreciation" for them. It was also announced that people would not be allowed to board streetcars or enter department stores if they could not obtain a mask. "If the supply is short and people cannot get masks at their drug store they must make them at home," declared Hanson. "As a last resort they can use a handkerchief." According to a survey by a reporter, about 25 percent of all streetcar passengers on Tuesday morning were not wearing face coverings. The Bon Marché continued to display subservience to the authorities, pointing out their compliance and even going so far in one of their ads to advise parents to keep their children at home. It had even set up its own "Red Cross auxiliary" and had its employees make masks and sell them to the public, who came unprepared, for the same five cents each.[23]

An editorial in a Seattle newspaper on October 30 was, dramatically, printed on the front page above the masthead and perhaps hinted at resistance and non-compliance. "Put on that gauze mask and smile" was how the headline began. "As to other preventive regulations the thing to do is to conscientiously observe them. Don't lose any sleep trying to figure out why it is that gauze masks have proven effective in preventing the spread of the disease…. The thing to do is to wear a mask and be thankful you can benefit by it," asserted the editor. "It is easy to be cynical and skeptical, to deride gauze masks and serums, the closing of theaters and schools

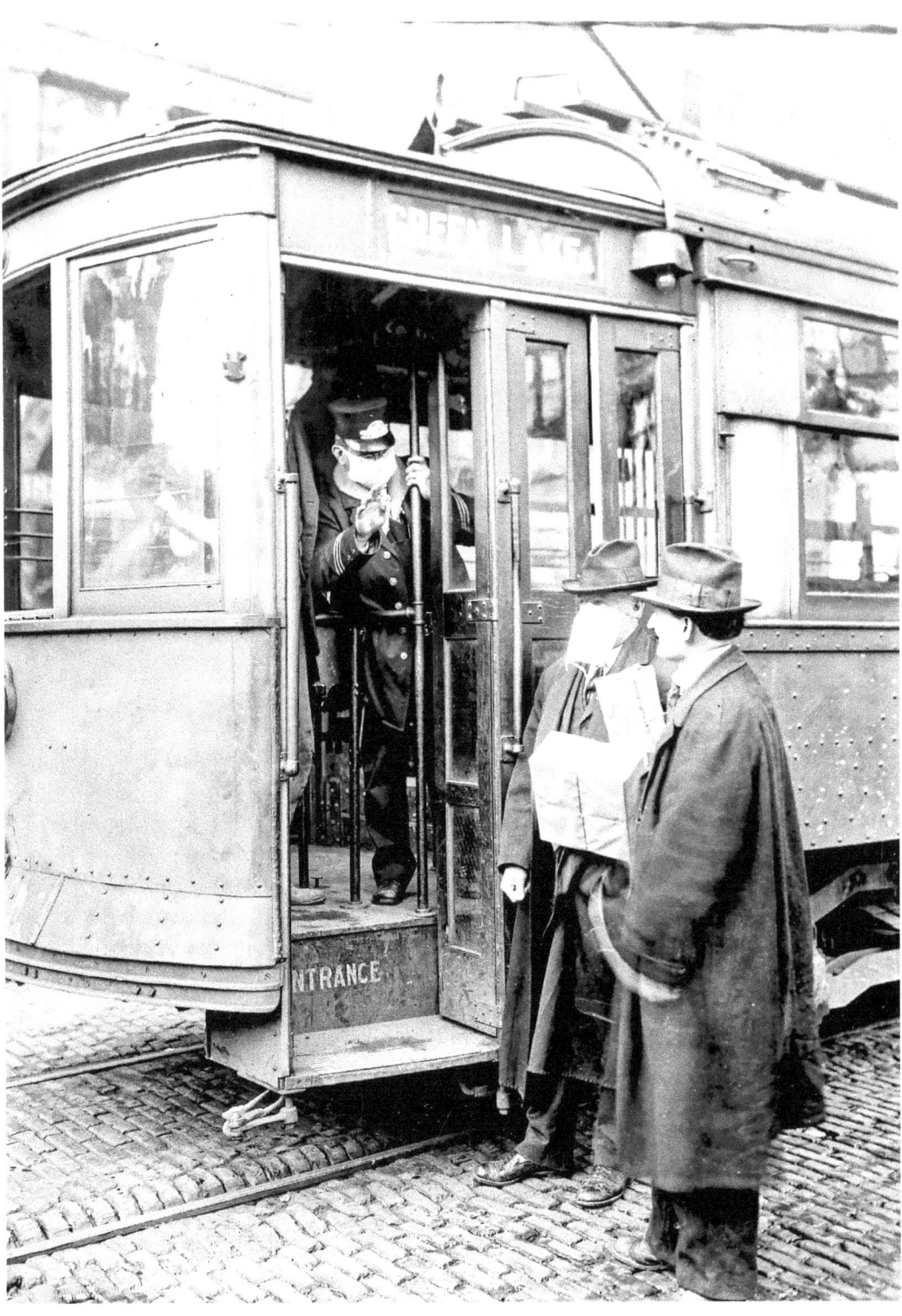

An unmasked man tries unsuccessfully to board a Seattle streetcar when the mask mandate was in effect.

and churches.... Our health authorities are giving scientific study to the influenza problem. What they have to say is plainly more reliable than the sneering, disputing, purely argumentative objections of a few smart Alecks."[24]

Seattle police made seven arrests on the morning of October 29, all for failure to wear a mask. One officer, G.W. Wilson, made six of the arrests. All were processed and released on bail for five or ten dollars. When a journalist described the scene, he wrote, "In open defiance of regulations, people rode to work in the street cars Wednesday morning without masks or excuses, conductors jammed and congested their cars, and in many of the cars, but two or three windows were open. A far larger percentage wore masks Wednesday than Tuesday, however, the bare-faced individual being conspicuous by his openness of countenance, which generally was defiant or contrite." Police were instructed to board the cars as they entered the business section and arrest those who were unmasked or compel them to wear masks. Guards were stationed at department store entrances with instructions to allow no one to enter who was not masked. In at least one case, a passenger took on a vigilante role. When an unmasked passenger tried to board an East Union line car early Wednesday, a firefighter on board as a passenger knocked him off the boarding step.[25]

On Thursday, October 31, it got crazier as Mayor Hanson imposed even more drastic rules. All stores, offices, and wholesale houses in the city had to close that day at 3 p.m. On the next day, Friday, they could open at 10 a.m., close no later than 3 p.m., and remain closed Saturday and Sunday. Exceptions to the rule were drug and food stores and doctors' and dentists' offices. More rigorous enforcement of mask mandates was promised. Reportedly, by Thursday, almost everyone seen on a streetcar was masked.[26]

McBride spent an increasing amount of time hectoring the public. He whined almost daily about how the masks, though being worn by most people most of the time, were not clean enough. He badgered people to be sure to sterilize their masks at least once a day by boiling them for five minutes. After a few days, an additional whine was that people were getting careless about how the masks were worn. He admonished that the mask had to cover the nostrils and mouth thoroughly.[27]

As of 8 a.m. Tuesday, November 12, all the restrictions in place in Seattle were lifted, except that face masks still had to be worn by the citizens. The ban on churches and theaters was lifted, and all stores could resume their regular hours.[28]

As the panic subsided in Seattle in mid–December, a brief article presented the commissioner's rules for people to follow. His first rule was to be vaccinated. If one wanted to be "certain not to contract influenza or be a carrier," then one should follow these nine rules, as laid down by McBride: (1) do not overeat or eat indigestible foods; (2) sleep only in well-ventilated rooms; (3) keep the intestines clean; (4) wear warm clothes; (5) keep in the open air; (6) avoid crowds as much as possible; (7) sleep at least eight hours out of 24; (8) exercise physically every day; (9) bathe often.[29]

On October 10, in Tacoma, Washington, C.H. Woolsey of the United States Public Health Service recommended gauze masks for city residents who were forced to ride to and from their homes during the hours of the day when the streetcars were jammed. Seeing a streetcar filled with people wearing gauze masks "would be ludicrous he admits," but he thought it was better to be safe. It was also reported that

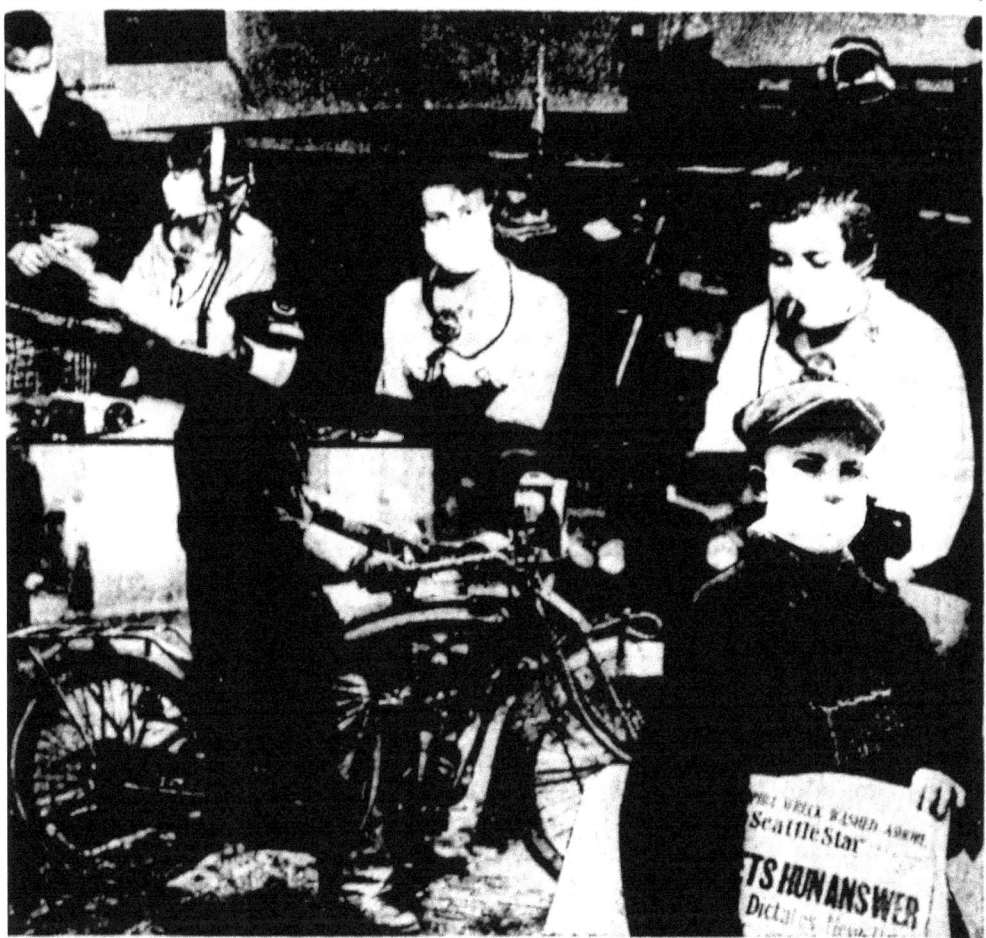

SEATTLEITES WAR ON FLU GERMS

Nearly everybody downtown was masked Monday in accordance with health department orders in an ort to check the spread of Spanish influenza.
Above are Western Union telegraph girls at the Fourth ave. and Union st. station, masked to protect mselves from germs that might be carried into their quarters by patrons who come and go all day long
Below is Motorcycle Policeman George Reynolds, who was kept busy breaking up groups on the street d checking on street cars that failed to keep windows open.
To the right is a downtown Star newsie, who deals with hundreds of pedestrians daily.

A composite photograph showing people in different occupations going about their work while wearing flu masks.

streetcar employees found it impossible to keep the car windows open as passengers continued to close them.[30]

Two weeks later, in Tacoma, Dr. Woolsey expanded his recommendations somewhat. At that time, he advocated wearing gauze masks by clerks in stores and others "whose occupations require them to meet the public in considerable numbers." Dr. Robert D. Wilson, Tacoma health officer, came up with a bizarre recommendation. He advised people with influenza in their families to dip the sick person's clothing and bed linen, et cetera, into a formaldehyde solution before sending them to a laundry.[31]

A few days later, Dr. Wilson joined the chorus hyping the mask when he declared that barbers, servers, clerks, and streetcar employees were among those who would do well to follow the practice adopted in many other cities and wear gauze masks. He added, "The appearance of solicitors on the streets making their pleas for money for the soldiers' and sailors' tobacco fund through gauze masks was helpful yesterday in showing the public what it might do in the way of self-protection."[32]

On October 28, Tacoma Mayor C.M. Riddell ordered that all people coming into contact with the public through business relations wear masks. The order specified that the following people wear flu masks: all store clerks, barbers, servers, elevator operators, all people handling foodstuffs, city hall employees, and courthouse employees. Health officers also made an urgent plea to everyone to stay home, going out only if necessary.[33]

On October 30, it was reported from Tacoma that "the opposition of the public is so strong in some quarters, however, that a sweeping order is considered of debatable wisdom. Barbers, clerks and others were reported yesterday as in some instances quitting their jobs rather than abide by the order to wear masks." Tacoma Police Chief Harry Smith reported to Mayor Riddell that a few merchants declared they would not "muzzle" their employees. Riddell instructed him to give the merchants an ultimatum to mask their employees or be shut down. "The ultimatum was sufficient to bring compliance," according to the story.[34]

Dr. C.H. Woolsey of the United States Public Health Service offered his opinions in Tacoma and Seattle. In Tacoma, on November 3, he said the people of Tacoma were not sufficiently impressed with the seriousness of the situation. "I can go about the city at any hour of the day and see persons who are not wearing gauze masks that should be. In barber shops, on the street cars, in department stores, everywhere people are careless about wearing these masks. It should be remembered that we are not out of the woods as yet, and that we should take advantage of the experience of other cities where such practices have resulted in a serious relapse in the epidemic."[35]

In Spokane, one of the local newspapers published, on October 22, a full-page ad that gave the standard advice and information about influenza. It was the advice that appeared all over the United States, mainly during October. No mention was made of masks, except for attendants in the sick room. Most of those ads credited the source as the United States Public Health Service. However, this ad, being in a much larger format, gave credit to some companies, all listed, who had previously paid the publishing costs.[36]

Masks began to appear in Spokane on October 26, when instructions were received from the war department for all soldiers who were on duty in the city to wear masks. Western Union messengers and many barber shop employees followed suit and were wearing the "white face." There was an order for telephone operators to don the coverings, and they were expected to do so shortly. Dr. J.B. Anderson, Spokane health officer, said, "I have no personal objection to anyone wearing the influenza masks. I think it is a very good plan here; people have to meet the public to a great extent."[37]

One minor rebellion was reported from a Spokane bank. On Saturday, October 26, clerks who came into contact with the public at the Exchange National Bank

BANK TELLERS WARD OFF FLU BUG

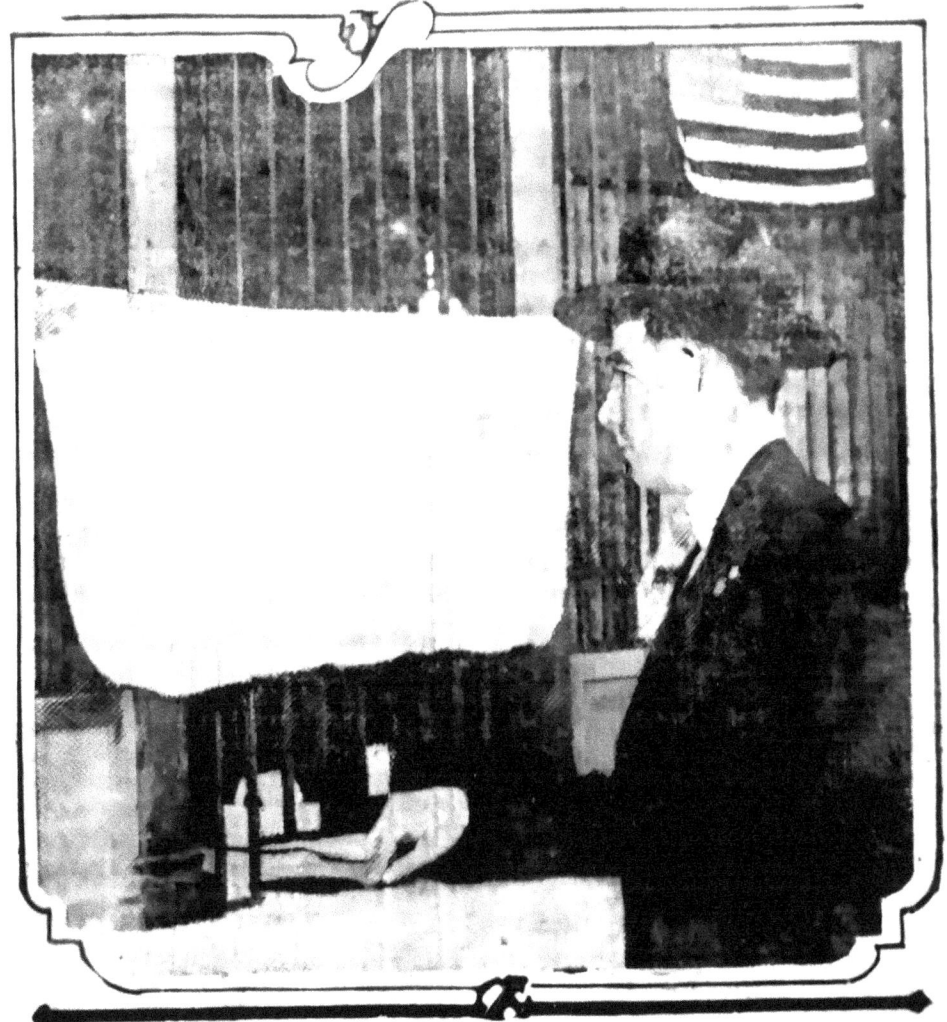

Banks are among the first institutions to see the necessity of guarding against influenza germs. The photograph above shows a teller's cage in a Cincinnati bank, where gauze screens are used as shields. Spokane tellers may soon all be wearing flu masks.

A Spokane bank teller has hung a rag in front of his teller's cage as he deals with a customer. The customer and teller are now, thanks to the rag, fully protected.

wore them. Then on Monday morning, several of those clerks did not don the coverings, and by that afternoon, none of the employees were wearing them.[38]

Then, the Washington State Board of Health stepped in and, on November 3, ordered wearing masks throughout the state. The mask was to be made of gauze of fineness not less than 20 to 24 mesh, five by six inches, composed of not less than six layers sewed and bound together and entirely covering the mouth and nose. The masks were to be worn on streetcars, trains, cabs, jitney buses, hotel buses, elevators, and all public conveyances. They were to be worn in corridors, lobbies, hallways, and all public places in buildings, hotels, and lodging houses. In all stores where merchandise was bought and sold, in all offices, and in other places where people dealt with or transacted business with the public. They were to be worn in all restaurants, cafés, and other places serving food, except that customers need not wear masks while eating. They were to be worn in all places where food was prepared or offered for sale, whether such places were within buildings or not. They were to be worn in all barbershops, laundries, washhouses, and dry-cleaning establishments. They were to be worn until the state authorities decreed that the danger was over.[39]

The Washington State Board of Health rescinded the regulations enforcing wearing masks. The masks came off in Spokane on the evening of November 11. The state board also rescinded the ban on public gatherings imposed on November 3. However, the City of Spokane's ban on public gatherings, imposed on October 9, remained in place.[40]

After the state board imposed the statewide masking order, it was reported that the people of Walla Walla were against accepting the order. Some firms had reportedly already arranged with attorneys to defend cases of violation by their clerks. Other stores threatened to close their doors before they would wear their masks. The health officer, Dr. J.E. Vanderpool, gave verbal orders to the chief of police, John Haven to enforce the health orders. Haven countered with a written statement to the health officer demanding more explicit orders and stating, "At the outset I am confronted with resistance." He added that he had nothing to do with the execution of state laws; his authority was limited to and by city ordinances, which he said did not cover wearing masks.[41]

Two days later, it was reported that the masking order was generally ignored in Walla Walla. It would be tested in court for validity, as two attorneys, E.L. Casey and C.M. Rader, had both been charged with failing to wear a mask in a public place. Meanwhile, in Yakima, Washington, 18 people appeared in court before Judge R.B. Milroy on charges of not wearing masks. Five paid fines of one dollar each, one forfeited his five-dollar bail (as a no-show in court), and the remainder had their cases dismissed. Though those cases were looked upon as tests of the validity of the local and state health boards, the court held that there was ample authority behind the regulations.[42]

On November 9, in Walla Walla, a jury acquitted Casey and Radar of violating the mask-wearing order imposed by the state board of health. Much amusement was said to have been created in court when the defendants caused the county health officer to remove his mask while testifying on the grounds that the constitution required that a man be brought face-to-face with his accuser. None of the jury members wore a mask except for a barber, who wore a towel with two holes for his eyes over his head. The prosecuting attorney and his assistants wore masks. One of those assistants, after adjusting his mask several times, stated, "Confound the things, I hate them myself."[43]

When the Washington State Board of Health masking order was rescinded on November 11, just eight days after being imposed, rumors spread that little cooperation had been shown to the state by the counties in enforcing the ban. Dr. Thomas D. Tuttle, Washington state health commissioner, denied any problems such as that to a reporter. The journalist stated, "Dr. Tuttle informs me that he did not say that the county prosecuting attorneys had refused to co-operate with him in enforcing the mask order. He says that he had had the best of assistance from this office and that only three counties in the whole state have neglected to enforce the influenza restrictions."[44]

Oregon

In Oregon, on October 8, the Oregon Board of Health ordered all schools, churches, and public amusement places throughout the state to be closed immediately upon the appearance of an outbreak of Spanish influenza in the community. They were following the Rupert Blue Protocols from Washington, D.C., by imposing those recommendations but leaving the actual triggering of the imposition to the discretion of the local health authorities. Portland issued its closure orders two days later.[45]

Klamath Falls, Oregon, went a step further than most places when, on December 13, it published in the local newspaper a list with the names and addresses of the influenza patients then isolated in the city. Also listed were the other family members, if any, who were also isolated.[46]

Judge James A. Fee drafted a proposed new ordinance for flu regulations in Pendleton, Oregon, at the very beginning of 1919. It would not close the stores or cinemas but would permit their being open under regulations based on air space in the room. As recommended, cinemas would open with patrons occupying every other seat in every other row (25 percent maximum capacity). Churches and stores would probably be regulated the same way.[47]

When the ordinance was presented to the Pendleton City Council, other

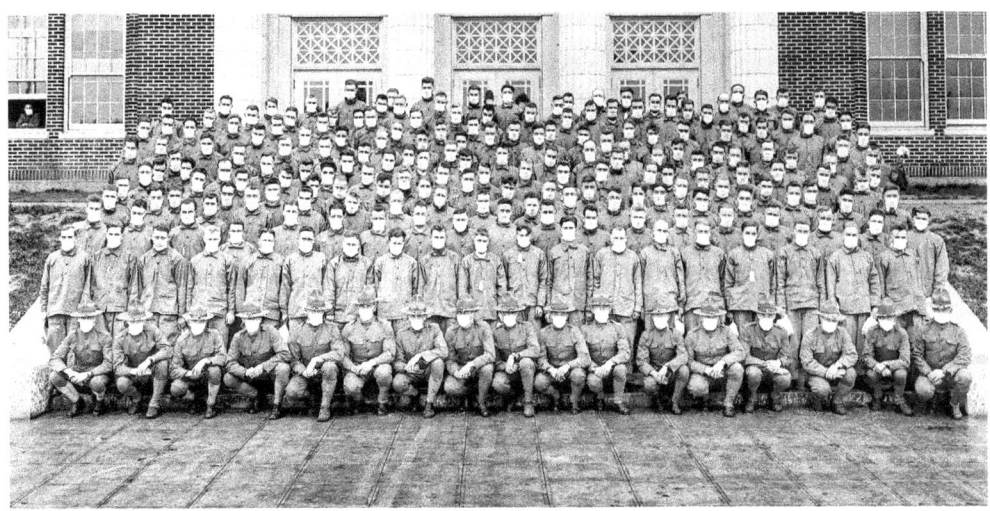

A Benson Polytechnic College in Portland class in the student army training corps.

measures included one that did not permit crowds to gather at transit depots and stated that people were not to go to transit depots unless they had special business. Meeting a friend arriving or saying goodbye to a departing person was "not allowed." In transacting business, people could not get closer than four feet to each other. Cinemas could open, but every other row had to be vacant. In rows with seating allowed, every other seat had to be vacant. Pool rooms could open, but only two patrons were allowed per table, with no spectators permitted. Bowling alleys limited players to two per alley.[48]

All barbers, dentists, shoe shiners, tailors, doctors and nurses while attending to patients, and servers while delivering meals were the only people allowed to get closer than four feet to the people with whom they were transacting business in Pendleton. The city ordinance required that all "shall wear proper flu masks over the mouth and nose while engaged in said occupation." While the regulation was in effect, citizens could not get closer than four feet to each other as they conversed on the street, passed each other, or transacted their business in the stores. A special city council meeting was held to enforce the new influenza rules and the stricter quarantine and to regulate the number of people allowed in stores, cinemas, and other public places in Pendleton. The ordinances were all passed, with one of them allowing for the appointment of special officers to look after the enforcement of the regulations.[49]

A day later, a reporter observed that flu masks were "much in evidence today in Pendleton, and those wearing the masks are making the best of the situation and doing it good naturedly as a rule." Barbers were said to be "generally" observing the rules, and those not wearing masks would be reported. Some restaurants had equipped their servers with masks, and some had not. Thirteen special flu officers could be seen on the street. They wore a blue ribbon on which were printed the words "Flu Officer." They were stationed at the entrance of the leading stores, where they kept count of the number of people entering, and when the limit was reached, they stopped others from entering. Guy C. Matlock, manager of the Pastime Theater, had voluntarily closed his venue because he said he found it impossible to stay open with the limit of every other seat occupied and every other row left vacant. Listed in this article were the names of the business houses where guards were placed and the number of people allowed in the building simultaneously. For example, American National Bank (25), J.C. Penney (35), Sayres (35, if the back door was used), and French Restaurant (20). All 13 of the special flu officers were listed by name, four women and nine men.[50]

Louis Pinson, the proprietor of the Office Lunch restaurant on Main Street in Pendleton, was arrested on January 9 for serving meals while not wearing an influenza mask.[51]

Then there was a sudden change of direction in Pendleton. On January 10, 1919, just days after enacting flu rules, a special city council meeting was called to repeal the part of the ordinance that required certain occupations to wear flu masks. Enforcement of the ordinance, the council said, threatened to close a number of the restaurants and dining rooms through servers' refusals to wear the mask and their threats to quit their jobs rather than do so. "The doctors of the city did not uphold the ordinance, in fact, themselves refusing to wear masks, and the restaurant workers and others required to wear them used this as leverage, taking the ground that it was not a proper requirement," explained a journalist. Louis Pinson's arrest a day earlier precipitated the trouble. With the repeal of the mask ordinance, the case against Pinson was dropped. The city council voted six to nil to repeal the mask law, with two council members absent. Other parts of the law remained in effect. The number of people allowed in stores was still limited to one person per 100 square feet of floor space. The four-foot rule stayed in effect. Churches could open, provided those attending were limited to one person per 100 square feet. The 13 flu officers remained on duty. Nothing else changed except the dropping of the mask law.[52]

As late as January 29, 1920, in Pendleton, Oregon, nine new families were placed under influenza quarantine, while eight were released from quarantine. At that time, there were about 140 homes under quarantine in Pendleton, representing 300 to 400 people. A reporter commented that Pendleton seemed to have more influenza than any town in the west, but the worst was thought to be over. The reporter said that the "voluntary quarantine" of people with colds and other symptoms had been "highly successful it is believed." Until conditions returned to normal in Pendleton, no lodges or other societies would hold any meetings.[53]

As of December 9, restrictions in Medford, Oregon, were imposed, closing schools, theaters, churches, poolrooms, and billiard halls for the second time. Once again, the city officials imposed the Blue Protocols. This time, though, they ordered wearing influenza masks. Medford Mayor C.E. Gates and Dr. E.E. Pickle, city health officer, signed the orders. The mask ordinance stated, "It shall be the duty of every person employed in stores, hotels and all places of business within the city of Medford to wear a mask as a preventative against Spanish influenza until this ban is lifted by order of the board of health of the city of Medford." The following section said, "It shall also be the duty of every person who rides or walks on the streets, sidewalks or thoroughfares of the city of Medford to wear a mask as a preventative against Spanish influenza until this ban is lifted by order of the board of health of the city of Medford." Punishment for each violation was a fine of not less than five dollars nor more than ten dollars.[54]

Five Medford citizens were arrested two days later for violating the flu mask ordinance. They were all fined five dollars, and they paid their fines. One of them was J.A. Westerland, who was arrested for wearing his mask on his chin while smoking after a second warning. Westerland gave notice that he would hire a lawyer and fight the charge in court. That irritated Mayor Gates, who complained, "This is no time for our leading citizens to oppose a measure designed for the protection of the people of this city. The only possible objection to the flu ordinance is based on technical grounds. I don't care about the strictly legal phase of the matter, and no other loyal citizen should call up such a question now." City Health Officer Pickle remarked, "There is apparently some objection to the flu mask ordinance…. With flu masks the individual can shop down town without danger; without them there would be danger on every side…. It is an absolute protection to the individual and a check to the spread of the disease."[55]

On the evening of December 17, opponents of the flu mask ordinance, "including a small representation of business men and a goodly representation of Christian Scientists" invaded the city council meeting in its chambers in a vain effort to get the mask law repealed. When the council finished its debate on the issue, it did what politicians always do, if possible. They passed the buck and voted to leave any question of repealing the order to the discretion of the city's health department.[56] The Medford Board of Health ordered on December 23 that flu masks no longer had to be worn on the city streets, effective immediately. However, the order to wear the masks inside stores, churches, theaters, places of business, and all other public gatherings "must be strictly carried out."[57]

Ten days after Portland, Oregon, imposed the lockdown order, issued two days earlier by the Oregon Health Board to be implemented by each local area as the disease struck, it was reported that efforts to have the closing order canceled had been made by representatives of certain churches and educators, but the state board had refused to respond. There was no talk of masks in Portland, although a photo accompanying the October 20 article features a barber wearing one and giving what was described as a "hygienic haircut."[58]

The Portland chapter of the American Red Cross warned mask wearers on October 27: "Gauze masks are worse than useless if they are used with alternate sides to the face. They must always be worn with the same side out. They will accomplish no good unless sterilized daily. Gauze masks to be sterilized and must first be washed thoroughly with soap and water. After rinsing well, boil for 15 minutes. This is the only method of insuring perfect sterilization. While disinfectants are useful in some instances, they cannot positively be guaranteed to kill the germs that may have lodged on the mask."[59] Over a few days in Portland, the local Red Cross had made 40,000 masks, with 20,000 of them sold at the cost of the material only to large plants in the area for their employees. Other plants could obtain the items from the organization upon request. Masks would go on sale for individuals the next day at all department stores and large drug stores.[60]

The next day, it was noted that the United States Army had sent word that physicians and nurses had to wear masks while attending to flu patients. But as far as the general public was concerned, the health authorities said, "The public may use its own discretion in the matter of wearing masks." According to a journalist, "the local and state health officials had put the mask problem up to the federal authorities because of the agitation in favor of the safeguard which had been made in Portland." However, attempting to pass the buck in that fashion could not work because the United States Public Health Service in Washington never recommended using masks anywhere or anytime except for attendants in the sick room.[61]

In the opinion of Dr. George Parrish, Portland health officer, wearing gauze masks by people with colds using streetcars to go to and from doctors' offices might become necessary. He declared on November 1 that it might be necessary to pass an ordinance compelling such people to wear masks when out in public to protect others.[62]

Things continued to deteriorate in Portland, Oregon, and on January 11, 1919, new regulations were imposed. Dr. E.A. Sommer of the health board declared that cooperation was the keynote of his "new" approach. "We wish to coerce no one but on the contrary ask the cooperation of all Portland citizens. If the results are not

DANCING
NOT STOPPED
DANCING TONIGHT

Under the regulations of the Health Board as outlined by Dr. Sommers, limiting the capacity of the halls to 40 square feet for each couple, with 5 minute dances and 4 minute intermission.

(Signed)

COTILLION HALL MOOSE HALL
CHRISTENSEN'S TEMPLE APOLLO
HALL MURLARK HALL

Public dances were not stopped in Portland if each couple had 40 square feet of the dance floor to themselves, if the dance lasted no longer than five minutes, and if a minimum four-minute mandatory rest period was inserted between each dance.

satisfactory, of course, compulsory methods must be instituted, but we will first attempt to eradicate this disease by cooperation." The plan to put a ban on dancing was abandoned, and regulation by the "consolidated health bureau," as the new organization was known, took its place. Thus, public dancing was allowed to continue as long as only one person was present per 20 square feet of floor space; each dance lasted no longer than five minutes, followed by an intermission of at least four minutes. The masking situation was to be handled in the same way. "All persons are asked to have masks available at all times, although it is not compulsory. When the person is exposed by a cough or sneezing, the mask should be immediately donned."[63]

A day later, the new regulations in Portland were formally announced, supposedly done under the guise of cooperation, but in reality, it was a de facto set of mandated orders. There were two medical experts, two physicians, and two clerks in the "consolidated health bureau," the newly established organization in charge of fighting the flu. A strict residential quarantine was part of the new regulations, with the quarantine to continue for ten days after the fever had gone. The number of people on streetcars was limited, and the regulation would be carried out with the aid of police officers—so much for the idea of cooperation only and no coercion. Restaurants were to place a vertical screen at least two feet high on each table to "protect" guests at the same table from each other or seat all the guests at a table on the same side. Part of its resolution stated, "The most fundamental procedure in the control of the spread of the disease is the judicious wearing of masks. It is recommended that masks be worn by all persons attending the sick, by all people who enter where people congregate, as public meetings, theaters, churches, hospitals, department stores, etc., and that sterile masks in envelopes to be furnished by the consolidated health board, shall be put on upon entering such places and deposited on leaving."[64]

A day later, a resolution adopted at a meeting of the citizens' advisory committee, selected to aid in the fight against influenza, advised the compulsory wearing of flu masks at all public gatherings and on the streetcars. The resolution called upon city and county officials to take the necessary steps to establish such an ordinance. Dr. Sommer explained, "Everyone in close contact with other individuals should wear a mask and it should be sterilized several times a day. Doctors should also wear them. Only 5 percent of the physicians wear them now." An intensive public relations campaign was also mounted, with four-minute speakers detailed to theaters and other venues to hector the audiences. The consolidated health bureau requested that all gatherings and meetings that could be delayed be postponed and that if meetings were held, "all participants should be masked."[65]

The idea of cooperation quickly disappeared in Portland. On Monday, January 13, the city council drafted a resolution making it unlawful for someone to enter a store, shop, hotel, poolroom, theater, office building, taxi, or streetcar without wearing a mask. The mask had to have four layers of gauze the thickness of butter cloth. The penalty for violation of the ordinance was set at a maximum fine of $500 or 60 days imprisonment.[66]

Surprisingly, two days later, when the city council brought the mask proposal up for a vote, it was defeated by one vote. Had it passed unanimously, it could have taken immediate effect as an emergency measure. However, Commissioner John H. Mann refused to vote for the measure. That stripped the proposal of its emergency status, and if it passed, it would require 27 days for the measure to be put into effect, seven days before the third reading, and 20 more days to become effective. Mann explained, "Since this ordinance has been under consideration I have talked to no less than 100 medical authorities, and the consensus of opinion is that the disease can be stopped without compulsory wearing of the mask, through strict enforcement of the quarantine. Those who wish to wear the mask may do so; it is optional. I will cast my vote against this ordinance."[67]

In the wake of that defeat, an editor with a Portland newspaper mused, "Why not wear the flu mask?" He went on to add, after citing the false figures from San Francisco, "it is difficult to see why there should be reasonable objection to masks

Wear a Mask

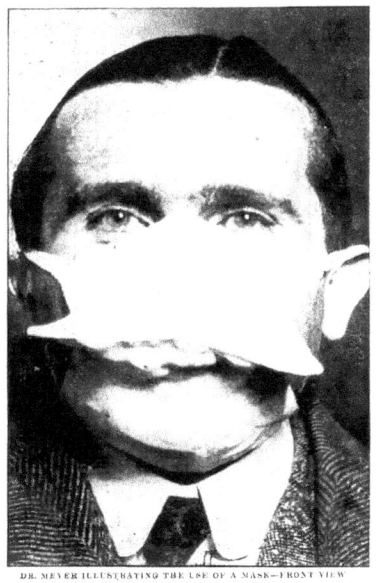
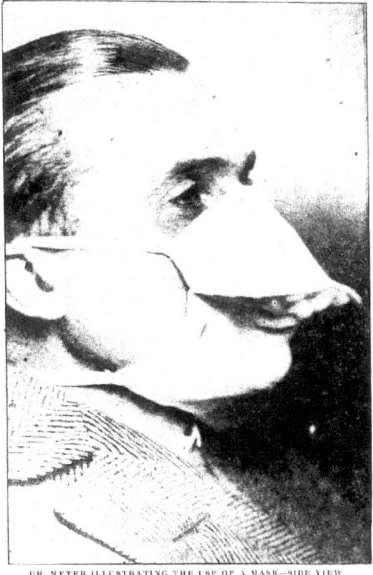

DR. MEYER ILLUSTRATING THE USE OF A MASK—FRONT VIEW   DR. MEYER ILLUSTRATING THE USE OF A MASK—SIDE VIEW

We appeal to your civic patriotism to co-operate with us in our effort to

STAMP OUT THE
Spanish Influenza
or "Flu" Plague in Portland
By Wearing a Mask

You should willingly co-operate in doing this and not necessitate the passing of an ordinance which will make the wearing of a mask compulsory.

OBSERVE THE FOLLOWING RULES

Mask should be worn when you enter crowds, streetcars, stores, theatres, moving picture houses, churches, schools, and even at home.

After you have worn the mask sterilize it by boiling at least five minutes before you wear it again. Never wear a mask the second time, after having removed it to go from one place to another.

Realize that the outside of the mask is contaminated after use—you can very readily infect your fingers, and in this manner transmit the infection.

The mask should consist of four layers of butter cloth. Pattern of it will be shown in the big stores.

Never visit people who suffer from a cold without wearing a mask, because they may have influenza, if only in a mild form.

SIGNED:
K. F. MEYER
Associate Professor of Tropical Medicine, George Williams Hooper Foundation for Medical Research, University of California Medical School, San Francisco, California.

SIGNED:
THE CONSOLIDATED HEALTH BUREAUS
By E. A. SOMMER
Director-General

Dr. K. F. Meyer of the University of California, San Francisco, demonstrates the proper way to wear a proper mask in a typical mug shot pose for the enlightenment of the residents of Portland, Oregon.

since to wear one is so easy and simple a matter with no possible chance of harm. It isn't proposed to wear masks for a lifetime. It is for a few weeks only."[68]

Portland Health Officer John G. Abele proclaimed on February 8 that masks would not be worn in Portland, although, of course, there was no mandatory masking order in effect in Portland. The consolidated health bureau closed its doors on the same day, and city or county health officials would treat any new cases that developed. Dr. Sommer believed the epidemic to be over.[69]

When case numbers in Salem, Oregon, increased in January 1919, it was announced that physicians and members of the board of health were divided as to the advisability of compelling the public to wear masks, but it was thought that definite action one way or the other would be taken within the coming few days.[70]

A week later, nothing had been decided about masks, but health officials began to talk about cooperation first, and then the coercion of restrictions would be lifted, probably copying that buzzword from Portland. Residents were encouraged to call the police or personally visit any of their neighbors they suspected of being sick. Tipster anonymity was promised. It was proposed that when the theaters were reopened, if anyone coughed, the ushers would bring them a mask, and if they refused to wear the mask, they would be ordered out of the venue. Theater managers had reportedly agreed to keep a supply of sterilized masks on hand at their venues to meet the needs of their patrons. Mayor C.E. Albin explained, "If we get the proper cooperation we can open the city very soon. That time cannot be decided until we learn to what degree our recommendations will be carried out if necessary, a large health police squad will be put on to enforce our orders."[71]

As of January 27, all restrictions were lifted in Salem, Oregon, and the city got back to business as usual, more or less. Loitering anywhere was not permitted. People in churches, schools, theaters and other public assemblies had either to leave the premises or provide themselves with "an appropriate and approved mask." Children were hit the hardest in the newly "free" Salem. Children from homes where the quarantine placard was still up were not admitted to school. No child was required to wear a mask, but the teachers were to "observe" any children who coughed or sneezed. Each morning at 9 a.m., every teacher was mandated to inspect the pupils in their room. Each school principal was to "determine" the condition of the teachers' health regarding colds. The teacher was mandated to conduct a "health quiz" in her school room each morning, receiving a report from her pupils "in regard to sickness in their own immediate family or in the vicinity." Children who had contracted the flu had to remain out of school for two weeks after the ten-day quarantine period (that is, the residential quarantine ended ten days after the disappearance of fever), and then admittance was only allowed after receiving written permission from either Dr. Pemberton, the city health physician, or from Dr. Cashatt, the school physician.[72]

California

The situation developed rapidly in California, moving into hysteria before the end of October. A report that appeared in print on October 6 noted that the

California Board of Health had sent a communication to Dr. J.L. Pomeroy, Los Angeles County health officer—and to all the other counties in California—to inform them that influenza had been made a reportable disease and cases had to be isolated in California. This meant that all reported cases would be quarantined to prevent the spread of the pandemic that had swept over the East. Pomeroy admitted that the spread of the disease to the West Coast appeared inevitable and that they hoped to check the disease in Los Angeles city and county by promptly quarantining all cases that came to the attention of the authorities.[73]

Less than a week later, a Long Beach paper published the lengthy article from U.S. Surgeon General Rupert Blue and his agency, the United States Public Health Service. The article gave the reader an explanation of the malady and how best to deal with it. The piece was published in papers all over America, mainly in October. In it, Blue made no mention of masks, except that attendants should use them in the sickroom when caring for flu patients.[74]

Despite those words from Blue, Sacramento, California, officials spoke very differently just five days later. On October 21, the California Board of Health instructed all local and county health officers throughout the state about wearing masks during Spanish influenza. The board cited the authority under which it acted as Section 2979A of the Political Code. The state board declared that not only were doctors, nurses, attendants, and visitors to hospitals or homes where patients were being treated required to use a gauze mask, but all members of families having the disease in their homes and every person suffering from a cold in the head or acute cough, or having any of the recognized symptoms of influenza, would be compelled to wear the mask. Dr. W.H. Kellogg, secretary and executive officer of the state board, issued the orders. The part about people suffering from a head cold, acute cough, or other recognized flu symptoms stated that they "shall wear a mask of approved type while outside their living arrangements." An acceptable type of mask was made of two to four layers of fine mesh gauze or six to eight layers of coarser gauze or three layers of butter cloth, five inches by eight inches, and held firmly over the face using tapes attached to the corners. Another acceptable type was folding cornerwise a clean, closely woven handkerchief. When trying to justify their use of the mask, many jurisdictions would point to the "success" achieved with the mask in California, mainly San Francisco. At a time when nobody in America was under any masking mandates, this article stated, "The properly made gauze mask has proven to be the most valuable single measure which can be adopted for the prevention of influenza and health officers are urged to encourage its use beyond the above mentioned requirements." California cited no authority for the supposed efficiency of the mask since, of course, none existed. Nobody, anywhere, had ever used it before for influenza prevention. In his mandate order, Kellogg enthused further: "In many instances department store managers can be prevailed upon to require their clerks to wear them, and it will be of the utmost value if barbers, dentists and particularly druggists would also wear them." The greatest publicity should be given to the mask as a preventive measure, and the public should be encouraged to wear them generally both inside and outside. And so the groundwork was laid for the enthusiastic and widespread use of the mask and the imposition of masking orders all over California. And it was so. And the madness began.[75]

Cities across California imposed the usual Blue Protocols, mainly in October, and then removed them, mostly in November. In many cases, they reimposed those bans, often in November. During the second imposition, conditions were often harsher. Escondido lifted its quarantine on November 16 for churches, schools, public gatherings, et cetera. The ban was off for only two weeks before the reimposition. Effective at midnight on November 30, the usual suspects were again shut down. This time there was a ban on outdoor meetings, which had not existed during the first closure. As well, the request was made that people telephone their orders for goods to the stores and stay at home as much as possible.[76]

Pasadena again banned public gatherings on November 26 after lifting the first set of restrictions ten days earlier. In enacting the second closure by resolution, the city council avoided the necessity of passing an ordinance. A unanimous vote was required for ordinances. In Riverside, the health board again closed schools, churches, theaters, and poolrooms on November 27. This time, Riverside decreed that masks would be worn in public places, including on the streets.[77]

The ban against public gatherings that had been in force in Los Angeles for more than seven weeks was lifted on December 3 by repealing an emergency ordinance. Motion picture production was resumed, although regulations against more than a dozen people congregating anywhere barred all but small scenes.[78]

A week later, on December 10, the authorities imposed a new ban in Los Angeles, imposing a residential quarantine on the cases themselves instead of closing down outside activities. The idea was that the rest of the city would go about its business as usual. The city council also appropriated extra money to pay for a group of inspectors using placards to monitor and enforce the residential quarantines. Officials also threatened to take unspecified action against the "walking"

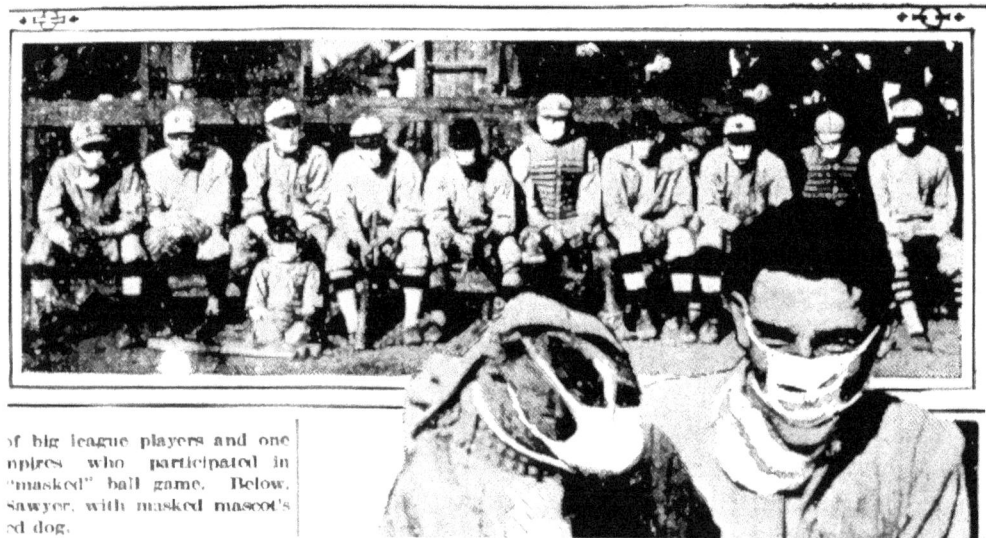

Players from a baseball game in Pasadena. The players and the spectators were all masked. It was reported that the players wore their masks for the entire game.

cases—those not fully recovered from the flu but well enough to go out and mingle with people.[79]

The first complaint charging violation of the quarantine law in Los Angeles was issued on December 20 at the request of Dr. J.L. Pomeroy, Los Angeles County health officer. The warrant was for the arrest of Mrs. W.T. Haile of Lancaster. According to the complaint, she left her home while suffering from influenza, and her husband was confined to his bed. Pomeroy said, "Every case of violation of the quarantine law that is called to my attention will result in vigorous prosecution." The maximum penalty involved was a fine of $200, 30 days in jail, or both.[80]

Three days later, three more arrest warrants for violating the quarantine rules were issued, all at Pomeroy's request. Mrs. Chris Machada of Culver City allegedly left her home while her family members were quarantined with influenza. Dr. C.J. Hinman of Belvedere and Dr. L.B. Nelson of Los Angeles were each charged with failing to report influenza cases to the authorities.[81]

In San Diego, the health department warned city residents on October 16, blaming the victim by pointing out that the disease appeared only in those who had neglected "the simple precautions provided as preventives. The avoidance of crowds and the use, after each meal of the quinine bisulphate spray will preclude much danger from the malady." In addition to the warning, the health board prepared a notice that was mailed to all employers. Along with the notice, the employers were told the health board would enforce the measures to the letter. The notice declared, "Spray the nose and throat of all employees, with bisulphate of quinine solution, twice daily, once upon reporting for work, and again upon leaving in the evening." Employers were also told to immediately send home all suspicious cases and report "promptly" the names and addresses of all employees sent home under suspicion. Point six of the notice to employees stated, "It is the urgent request of the board of health that all employees, during business hours, make use of gauze masks, same to be of sufficient size to cover both the nose and mouth." Point seven required that all gauze masks be boiled daily to sterilize them. The Red Cross was to provide nurses to take charge of all spraying. However, firms could use their employees for that purpose upon satisfactory arrangements with the health department. As was true all over America, the Red Cross urgently appealed for volunteer workers to come to the organization's building to help make masks. Helene Richards, director of the Red Cross Bureau of Production, said, "We ask high school girls, wives and daughters of officers, and young women who are not employed to come to the bureau of production. They should bring their thimbles, scissors, and aprons, and report this morning if possible." According to the account, whenever anyone visited the Red Cross Bureau of Production, the question asked of every visitor was, "Have you been sprayed?"[82]

A couple of days later, it was reported in San Diego that "throughout the city yesterday, was manifested a disposition to obey the regulations laid down by the board of health. In many places of business the employees wore gauze masks, and the practice is expected to be generally adopted today. Those who wear the masks declare that one quickly becomes accustomed to them and little, if any, discomfort is noticed. Their use is regarded as a certain preventative of contagion."[83]

Those optimistic words about the public rushing to embrace the mask were all false. According to a more accurate version of events, a reporter remarked on October 24: "Consequent upon the failure of many San Diegans, especially those who are engaged in occupations which bring them into direct contact with the general public, to comply with the suggestions and requests of the health department, that body has taken steps to make the wearing of gauze masks compulsory by all who are in public business." To that end, John G. Buerkele, a member of the health board, appeared before the city council and asked for the adoption of an ordinance making the rulings of the health department mandatory. One reason for asking for a mandate was the knowledge that the Red Cross produced more masks as volunteers responded to the group's pleadings for help. San Diego would have pushed earlier for a mask mandate but realized that earlier, the Red Cross was in no position to supply the number needed, so the city waited a bit. Other cities in America in the same position ignored the supply shortages and enacted mask mandates anyway, leaving an impossible situation in the hands of the public, who were thus also forced to make masks themselves at home.[84]

Since later mask advocates often cited California, especially San Francisco, as the "proof" masks worked, who did Californians cite? Mostly nobody. An exception was in San Diego, where Dr. E.P. Chartres-Martin, city health officer, was a believer. He cited Dr. Woods Hutchinson, "a recognized national health authority," and said that the San Diego Health Board endorsed his views on the face mask. Woods said, "If one-half or even one-third of the population would wear masks, the number of attacks and deaths due to Spanish influenza would be cut from one-half to two-thirds. A mask is the only single thing with the exception of vaccine, that I have any confidence in. The vaccine is almost unprocurable.... You are 99 percent safe if you wear your mask faithfully." And, of course, Woods Hutchinson cited no support for his numbers. He was a nationally syndicated columnist, which was not the same as being a national health authority.[85]

Then, on October 24, the San Diego Health Board passed an order asking the city council to pass an ordinance making wearing the mask compulsory everywhere. Wearing a mask or staying at home was the result. But the city board of health did not wait for the council to act. After midnight on October 25, any unmasked people appearing on the street or inside in any public space where they came into contact with people were violating the new order of the health board. The board asked the San Diego Police Department to cooperate in enforcing the rule. At first, members of the board of health advocated the arrest of anybody appearing without a mask but later changed it to ask that any such person found by the police be "sent home." Dr. Chartres-Martin explained, "We realize that it will be difficult for the population to equip itself with masks by midnight tomorrow but it must be done. The Red Cross will supply all who apply with patterns for making the masks."[86]

At the end of October, the health authorities could still not get the civic authorities to act on the request for the council to pass a universal masking mandate. People largely ignored the order issued by the board of health. So the medical people threatened to establish a quarantine of the entire City of San Diego, meaning nobody in and nobody out of the city, or that the universal wearing of masks be made compulsory. This prompted the Merchants Association of San Diego to come out and vow to fight to prevent the imposition of a city quarantine. The president of the association, John A. Gillons, stated that his group would not seriously protest wearing masks if it were made a universal requirement but that the proposed city quarantine would be opposed as a detriment to business.[87]

Then the caseload eased, and the flu passed through the down cycle of one of its waves, and everything about masks and a city quarantine was put aside for a time. On November 16, San Diego lifted the Blue Protocols that had been imposed earlier. School reopened a week later, and all seemed to be returning to normal.[88]

And then the caseload grew worse. On December 5, the battle between forces resumed in San Diego. The city attorney's office prepared an ordinance described as "drastic," as it intended to close every business house or other place where the public assembled, except for those deemed "extremely necessary." The definition of what was necessary was to be left to the discretion of the city council when it dealt with the ordinance. A large delegation of businesspeople was present. Their spokesperson, A.J. Morganstern, addressed the council, argued against closing business houses, and urged legislation that would require a universal masking mandate.[89]

At midnight on December 5, San Diego imposed a most drastic closure order. The order ended after four days, at midnight on December 9, unless the city council decided to extend it. During those four days, every place of business in the city except those dispensing the "absolute necessities of life" were closed. Masks had to be worn in business places—that is, the very few that were open. Businesses that could remain open were those selling food, drugs, doctor's supplies, stock supplies, and fuel. Newspapers were considered essential and allowed to remain open. Banks, public utilities, laundries, gas stations, and hotels could remain open under certain restrictions. Hotel lobbies had to be cleared of chairs and tables. Any restaurant with a liquor license could stay open, but it could not sell liquor. The Druggists' Association published a list of articles available in their stores that could not be sold during the shutdown. Those products included perfume, shaving supplies, toothpaste, stationery, or any article "not used as a remedy or preventive or in a sick room."[90]

A day later, a dozen miscreants appeared before Police Judge Schuermeyer's court, charged with not wearing a flu mask. All were found guilty and were fined five dollars each. The excuses included, "It just slipped down," "I couldn't breathe," "The baby tore it up," "My wife lost it," and "I couldn't buy one." The judge accepted no excuses.[91]

On the afternoon of December 9, the San Diego City Council met, as previously planned, to consider whether to extend the draconian shutdown. By a unanimous vote, except for one councilman, the council adopted an ordinance that compelled all people to wear the gauze face mask to cover their mouth and nose at all times, with certain exceptions. Those exceptions were, in their own homes, when eating, drinking, smoking, or being shaved in a barber shop. The ordinance went into effect at midnight on December 9 and was to run until midnight on December 19, unless extended. It replaced the drastic lockdown. Punishment for violation of the masking law was a fine of not less than five dollars and not more than $100, 30 days in jail, or both. If a fine was assessed and left unpaid, the violator had to serve jail time at the rate of one day in jail for every two dollars of the fine imposed.[92]

Then the caseload decreased as the disease passed through another downward part of a wave. As a result, the compulsory wearing of flu masks ended in San Diego at midnight on December 24.[93]

In Grass Valley, California, on October 24, the city board of health and the city health officer issued new orders requiring everyone appearing in public to wear masks and a committee to meet people arriving from out of town requiring them to don masks. Those refusing to do so would be subject to quarantine. Grass Valley Mayor Micheil was empowered to name a committee responsible for meeting all arriving trains. Part of the resolution read as follows: "Whereas, many people are in the habit of visiting Marysville, Sacramento, Roseville, Auburn, and other places on Sundays where the epidemic is very prevalent, be it, therefore, Resolved: That all persons be requested during the period of the epidemic to refrain from visiting these places of pleasure and as far as possible arrange their business affairs so it will not be necessary to go out of the city until after the epidemic has subsided, be it further Resolved: That where people do go out of the city by automobile, that they be required on their return to Grass Valley to wear a mask, and any such person found not wearing a mask be subject to quarantine."[94]

On October 19, it was reported from Fresno that the flu mask had "made its way from New York to Fresno. Women with chiffon veils and even with cheesecloth masks were observed near the Federal building yesterday." And "people laughed to themselves after passing a girl with a ... harem veil or whatever it was she wore to keep the germs at a respectful distance from her nose. Some are said to be perfumed."[95]

Five days later, every man, woman, and child who walked the streets in Fresno had to wear a gauze flu mask. No exceptions were allowed. The police had been ordered to stop anyone who appeared in public without a mask. Those regulations came into effect on October 24 following a conference the night before between Mayor Toomey and city Health Officer Mathewson because so many people had ignored the order from a day earlier. The earlier order had imposed masking on those involved in serving the public and in other specific circumstances. So many had ignored the order that they decided to make the order general and universal. Mayor William Toomey thundered, "The public is given two alternatives one of these alternatives is to obey the order. The other is to force the city officials to close up the city completely until the epidemic has passed." The latter masking order required everyone to wear a mask everywhere once they had left their residence. Adding further to the threat, Toomey warned that if the city were shut tight, the grocery stores would be allowed to remain open for only two hours each morning, just long enough for people to buy necessities. Continuing his tirade, Toomey whined, "It will not be just for the indifferent or the selfish to put these hardships upon the general business public simply because they feel that their personal appearance is not enhanced by wearing the masks. For this reason and in justice to those who obey the rules of the board of health every effort will be made to enforce the order before we take the extreme step of closing up the city. All police officers have been ordered to stop every man and woman and child appearing on the streets and in the belief that we have power, under the health laws of the state, to protect the public health by the use of the city's police powers, those who fail to comply with this order will be placed under arrest." Masks were available for ten cents from the Red Cross and sold for 15 to 25 cents at drug stores.[96]

On October 31, ten violators of the masking law made their appearances before Judge Smith. They were each fined $25 in court. The penalty for violating the mask ordinance was a cash fine of $25 or 25 days in jail.[97]

Fresno removed the masking law in November, only to reimpose it again around the end of November. Then, as of February 3, 1919, masks were no longer required. That coincided with the reopening of schools at that time. And it was argued that wearing masks was incompatible with work in the classroom. Nevertheless, Dr. Carleton Matheson, city physician, advised all those attending theaters, churches, and other public gatherings to continue wearing masks. He also recommended that those serving customers in stores and other places of similar nature continue to wear masks.[98]

In Sacramento, in compliance with the "urgent demands" of both city and state health officials, gauze masks were beginning to be "quite generally worn here," according to a report. While the clerks in various stores in Sacramento were the first to wear the masks, many were seen on the streets. In office buildings and the state capitol, the elevator operators mostly donned face coverings. That was also true of many of the state employees. Dr. G.C. Simmons declared, "The use of gauze masks prevents 95 per cent of cases of influenza among those who use them." Simmons was described as "the best authority," although no evidence was cited to back up such a claim. Simmons continued by noting, "The mask ought to be changed every two hours, and the same side always worn on the outside. The outside should be designated by a small mark of some kind. Every two hours the mask should be boiled and dried out."[99]

Speaking from Sacramento at the same time, on October 23, California Governor William Stephens urged every state resident to cooperate with state, county, and city officials in combating the spread of the Spanish flu, especially by wearing a mask. He said, "As an aid in winning the war it is a patriotic duty for every American citizen to assist in preserving the health of himself and his fellow citizens. Strict observance of the rules prescribed by our health authorities is essential to the speedy eradication of the influenza. Our health authorities advise it is imperative that all persons wear a mask over the nose and mouth, thus preventing the spread of this disease. Compliance with this temporary edict means but little discomfort and means a service rendered to our fellow men and to our country.… I therefore earnestly request that this precaution and protection be followed immediately."[100]

Commissioner G.C. Simmons introduced an emergency ordinance at a meeting of the Sacramento city commissioners on the morning of October 24, requiring every person in the city to wear a flu mask in all places where they might contact the public. Commissioner Haynes declared himself against the proposal, as he found it too extreme. He opposed mask wearing, and he did not believe in forcing people to do something he did not care to do himself. Commissioner Carmichael expressed himself against the ordinance, as he did not think it was workable. The proposal was then altered to eliminate the clause compelling people to wear masks on the streets.

When the vote was held, it was two for and two against, and thus it was defeated. Because they could not pass an ordinance compelling mask wearing, they passed one that "requested" people to wear a mask. The language used in their "request" was as follows: "Be it resolved by the City Commission of the city of Sacramento, that every person in the city of Sacramento be urgently requested, as a measure of public health and safety and for their own good and benefit in order to prevent the spread of influenza to wear a mask."[101]

Sacramento Commissioner Edward Haynes blocked a compulsory mask-wearing ordinance again, for the third time, on October 28. Haynes was pressured and lobbied, but he would not change his vote. An angry state controller thundered that "the people should and must know where to lay the blame for this criminal negligence."[102]

The ordinance finally passed on October 29, when the city commissioners held a second meeting and vote. A previously absent commissioner was present, and his vote enabled the measure to achieve a majority. It was the original masking ordinance that applied to everybody in the city. All had to wear a mask everywhere, at all times, when they were out of their own homes. The penalty was a fine ranging from $5 to $100, up to 30 days in jail, or both.[103]

The California Board of Health reported in mid–November that mortality resulting from the influenza epidemic in California had "not been reduced by the wearing of masks or even the closing of schools and theaters." The board's data showed that death rates in Los Angeles, with no masking ordinance, were lower than in San Francisco and Sacramento, both with such ordinances.[104]

Police proved overzealous in Sacramento on November 16 when plainclothes police raided hotels in Sacramento and arrested more than 40 hotel guests in hotel lobbies for not wearing their flu masks. The hotel owners complained to G.C. Simmons, commissioner of public health and safety. They received a promise that such raids would not happen in the future. In return, the hotel managers promised to see that the ordinance was enforced and uniformed police would visit the hotels to warn new guests of the ordinance before any arrests were made.[105]

On November 26, the people of Sacramento could discard their masks when the city revoked the masking ordinance. The reason was said to be a decrease in the number of cases.[106]

As in many other places all over America, the disease went into an increasing cycle again. Sacramento tried to reimpose the masking mandate on its citizens. The city health authorities recommended the reimposition, but on December 17, the city commissioners refused to agree and vetoed the recommendation.[107]

Late in January 1919, Dr. G.C. Simmons, commissioner of public health and safety in Sacramento, asked California Board of Health members to show themselves "as leaders and men of action." He continued, "We are closing the second phase of the influenza epidemic in the State of California, and the experience gathered proves again that where masks were worn, those communities brought the number of cases to the minimum in the shortest time and reduced the death rate more rapidly than where the 'let alone' policy was followed." That was, of course, a lie. Simmons argued that three weeks of applying the gauze mask in all California cities would wipe out the state's influenza. Simmons was still stinging from his city's rebuke when he argued to reimpose the mask law. He was trying then to get the state to act where he had failed.[108]

When the mask law was imposed in Stockton, California, barbers were reportedly one of the hardest-hit occupations. A barber reported that three days earlier, before November 1, he had worked on nine men in his shop; the next day, on five men; and even fewer since the mask law was mandated.[109]

In Stockton, at the request of the city health officer, Dr. Goodman, Commissioner C.O. Smith appointed 25 special officers to enforce the mask ordinance. They dressed in civilian clothing with instructions to arrest all offenders. They were on the job on November 16, patrolling the streets and shops of the city.[110]

Stockton repealed its masking law at noon on November 28. It was left in place for the major Thanksgiving celebration in Stockton in the morning, as the city did not want "to take any chances." But when the fire whistle blew at noon, it was a signal to unmask.[111]

As early as October 24 in Los Angeles, Dr. L.M. Powers, city health commissioner, stated he was making a special investigation into the results obtained from the use of gauze masks. He explained, "During the past two days I have received numerous requests from doctors and others asking an order be issued advising the general wearing of gauze masks." Powers added, "I do not feel this action would make much difference among people whose business does not bring them in close contact with the general public." Powers, however, planned to study the issue, and his committee, he reasoned, "may see fit to recommend the wearing of gauze masks. If this is done, it would be merely a recommendation and not an order. The choice of wearing a mask would be optional with each citizen."[112]

Later that day, it was announced that the City of Los Angeles could issue an order for masking at any time. Mayor Frederic T. Woodman had been conferring with the Medical Advisory Board, and Woodman said the plan was favorably considered. The local Red Cross had sent the mayor a couple of masks, and for part of the day, he wore one.[113]

A day later, it was announced that the general use of masks would not be made mandatory in Los Angeles, at least for the present. However, the board of health requested that, beginning on November 25, all dentists, barbers, vendors of food, servers, doctors and nurses, and others brought into intimate contact with the public wear masks. Even that was only a request.[114]

On November 9, the Theater Owners' Association of Los Angeles asked Dr. Powers and the City of Los Angeles to order the closing of all places of business except drug stores, grocery stores, and meat markets for an indefinite period. The authorities were also asked to order the general public to wear masks when appearing in any public place. The discrimination that the theater owners saw in the current shutdown angered them because the Blue Protocols closed theaters, churches, and schools but permitted crowds to gather in other institutions.[115]

On November 7, Dr. Woods Hutchinson appeared before a special conference committee in the Los Angeles Council chamber, where the "self-constituted regulator of the city's health measures, and single-handed exponent of compulsory mask-wearing for the prevention of flu, had rather a bad time." Instead of swatting the flu, the special committee swatted Dr. Hutchinson. At the end of the two-hour meeting, President Farmer of the council remarked, "All this talk about making the wearing of masks compulsory sounds to me like bunk." Hutchinson made a lengthy opening address, declaring that nothing but the mask could stop the flu. "In regard to serum, he said that one shot in the arm would prevent death from the flu, two shots would prevent it from turning into pneumonia, and three would keep you from getting the disease at all. What four would do he did not state." An exception was taken to the fact that Hutchinson removed his mask while talking. He explained that he did so because he had been made immune and could not scatter germs. When asked why he wore one, he said he did so simply to set a good example. He was called a faddist by one committee member. Marshall Stimson suggested that Hutchinson had some personal interest in mask propaganda. Except for Hutchinson, those attending the conference were "strongly against the masks." An assertion that San Francisco had brought the disease under control through the general wearing of masks was quickly refuted by statistics supplied by the state and city boards of health.[116]

A mass meeting was held in January, attended by some 700 physicians and "prominent citizens," who adopted a resolution recommending the immediate passage of a rigid mask ordinance. Despite that meeting, the Los Angeles City Council announced on January 22, 1919, that city citizens would not be forced to wear flu masks. All the council members, except for Frank H. True, declared themselves against passing any such law. Two of the council members said they deferred to the advice of Dr. Powers, the city health commissioner. Powers said, "I shall not recommend the passage of a flu mask ordinance today."[117]

Dr. John R. Haynes, representing the Citizens' League of Los Angeles, appeared before the finance committee to urge the enactment of mandatory masking regulations and provide funds to make compulsory vaccination possible. Haynes said, "There is no reasonable doubt but that the wearing of masks is efficacious in preventing the spread of influenza, and that vaccination with any one of a number of anti-influenza and anti-pneumonia vaccines is an additional aid." In his plea, he begged, "Gentlemen, you should order every person in the city to wear masks when on the street or outside of their own homes, you should establish stations all over the city for free distribution of masks and free vaccination."[118]

Dr. E.J. Banzhaf, assistant director of the Department of Preventive Medicines of the New York Health Department, stated on February 1, 1919, "It is foolish to have a law in a city requiring the wearing of flu masks. The order can't be thoroughly carried out as only a few persons know anything at all about wearing them correctly." He added, "The mask tends to keep people at home when they need to be out in the sunlight.... When a city gets frightened enough to use masks, the necessity for the mask is passed."[119]

A report on February 9, 1919, summarized data from the California Board of Health, which declared, "The very complete records at the disposal of the board indicate conclusively that the compulsory wearing of masks does not affect the progress of the epidemic.... There is nothing to indicate that the masks did any good whatever. Many doctors say they are harmful to health, except worn by people who thoroughly understand how to use them. In any event, they undoubtedly depress the spirits of the people and have a deterrent effect on business."[120]

Petaluma, California, was one of many, many communities in that state that imposed a masking ordinance on its residents. The town's police chief declared on November 1 that driving or riding in automobiles inside the city limits did not exempt the people from wearing their masks. He ruled that people riding in or driving cars had to wear their masks while inside the limits of the city. He asserted that he would enforce the law.[121]

In Napa, California, at the same time, violators of the community's mask ordinance were being sent to jail instead of being fined. Abel Erickson and Joe Rodgers, arrested for violating that law, were each sent to the county jail for ten days by Judge James M. Power. No alternative in the way of a fine was presented to the pair.[122]

In Hanford, Sherman Hutcheson, an employee at a lumberyard, was stopped by Charles Boyd, a sanitary inspector, because Hutcheson was not wearing a mask. When Boyd suggested that the man should be wearing a mask, Hutcheson replied, "To hell with a mask, and you too." One thing led to another; an altercation of some kind broke out, and the sanitary inspector shot Hutcheson in the leg. Boyd kept himself busy in Hanford, and four days later, he arrested five unmasked offenders from a local cigar store. In court, all were found guilty; each was fined $25, which they paid. Boyd stated he intended to enforce the ordinance rigidly and would arrest anyone he found unmasked in a public place.[123]

In December, Hanford voted to allow the mask rule to remain in place. But the city did say that the existing fine for violating the ordinance was "excessive" and thus ordered it reduced by 90 percent, from $25 to $2.50. Those who had already paid the higher fine were entitled to a refund. It was also explained that the arresting officers were inclined to display leniency toward the offenders because of the excessive fine. Hanford thus reasoned that if they lowered the fine, they could increase the number of arrests. Dr. Torrens, chair of the Hanford Health Board, declared, "Arrests should be made whenever the ordinance is violated or it becomes a mere farce. The mask is the greatest safety-first measure known at this time. Even limited meetings might be permitted with safety providing the mask restriction was enforced." Mayor Hammel admitted he did not have "any too much faith in the efficacy of the wearing of masks," but he had promised to back the health board in whatever restrictive measures they might see fit to impose. Several merchants submitted a petition asking for the repeal of the mask law. The law, explained W.C. Tarr, who presented the petition, was working a hardship on Hanford merchants because surrounding towns did not require a mask, and Hanford was losing business as residents did their Christmas shopping elsewhere. Tarr said of the mask, "It is more of a fad than a panacea and is not as effective as claimed for it."[124]

The City of Modesto, California, removed its masking ordinance on November 21. People were compelled to wear masks everywhere except at home. Less than one month later, on December 14, Modesto reimposed the mask rule on its citizens. No ban was placed on the holding of public meetings. Weeks later, the mask law was again repealed. Then it was reimposed for the third time on January 16, 1919.[125]

In Oakland, California, from November 1 through November 4, the courts collected $7,000 in fines from people caught not wearing their masks. A total of 709 citizens had been arrested over that period, with 610 having appeared in court, been convicted, and paid their fines. All had their particular alibis, but none were accepted by either of the two judges hearing the cases.[126]

One of those caught was Oakland Mayor John L. Davie, arrested in the lobby of a hotel in Sacramento on the evening of January 16. He was taken to the police station, where he was fined five dollars for not wearing his mask correctly. He paid the fine. Davie explained that he had the mask on but only hanging from his ear as he smoked a cigar.[127]

The first Oakland masking ordinance was repealed, but then there was an increase in cases with another wave of the disease, and the desire for masking was reborn. However, this time, when the city ordinance came up for final passage by the city council on January 21, it was turned down, with the vote being to lay the ordinance on the table to be called up in case of emergency.[128] That meant it was dead. Protests against another mask mandate came from Christian Scientists, members of labor unions, and others. Mayor John Davie attacked the ordinance. He recounted how he had been arrested in Sacramento for not wearing a mask and how he had to wait in jail until the police arrested someone else who had bail money so that they could get change for the mayor's $20 bill. Then Davie read from a report by the California Board of Health that indicated "conclusively that wearing masks does not affect the progress of the epidemic." Dr. Daniel Crosby, the health officer, was the only person in the crowded room who wore a mask.[129]

Escondido was another California community that reimposed the masking requirement. It did so on January 12, 1919. The new order mandated the wearing of masks in all public places where there was a gathering of more than five people. Churches could open, but all who attended had to wear masks, except the preacher and the teachers in Sunday schools. The same rule applied to public schools. The closing order applied to cinemas, with no exceptions for wearing masks.[130]

Later in January, in Pasadena, petitions calling upon the city commission to repeal the influenza mask law circulated. A reporter said, "They are being largely signed." The petition claimed the ordinance's purpose had utterly failed and that it was only an experimental measure. That morning in Pasadena, ten people had been fined amounts ranging from two to five dollars for mask ordinance violations. John Lambert, described as a prominent businessperson from the East who had just arrived in Pasadena to stay at his winter home, said, "Eastern people went through a great deal worse epidemic than has been experienced here in Southern California, but they had no experience with masks, except in a very few isolated instances. When they hear of a whole city masking, they are badly frightened and will not listen to argument.... Pasadena will lose an immense amount of tourist business so long as the ordinance remains effective."[131]

In San Francisco, the city's health board issued an order on October 19 that all barbers had to wear masks during the influenza epidemic. The masks had to be made with a double thickness of gauze with absorbent cotton in between. It was all part of an urgent appeal made by city Health Officer William C. Hassler that all men and boys in San Francisco should wear the gauze mask wherever they went. All women and girls should wear double-chiffon veils. Hassler explained, "If the public will do these things we are confident that we can master the epidemic within a week and that places of amusement might safely be re-opened." When he made that appeal, Hassler was with city and state health officers and Dr. Woods Hutchinson.[132]

A day later, a public relations piece by a bylined journalist, Fay King, appeared on page one of a San Francisco newspaper, hyping the mask. "THE BOARD OF HEALTH wants EVERY PERSON in San Francisco to wear a GAUZE MASK—and it's up to YOU to get one at Red Cross Headquarters, and wear it." She added, "You have to wear a mask, and thereby help to check it." King implored her female readers, "Oh, girls, you needn't pucker up your nose and giggle; you've taken to the hobble skirt, barber-pole, stockings, knee-length dress, and backless gown without a blush—you needn't shy at the Flu Mask.... Take it from me, it's just as becoming as a thousand other freak fashions we have fallen for, and now it's up to US to do what the Board of Health requests. If you are a REAL SAN FRANCISCAN—PROVE IT, by wearing a mask. We should ridicule those who DON'T wear them, because it's a matter of life and death. Every one in *The Examiner* office has his 'flu fence' on." King concluded, "EVERYBODY—On with the MASK!"[133]

Also on page one of the same newspaper issue, Dr. Woods Hutchinson warned that San Francisco would experience at least 50,000 cases of the Spanish flu. In a third article, also on page one, Dr. William Hassler, when asked about a slight decrease in the number of cases, denied it was a decrease at all, blaming it

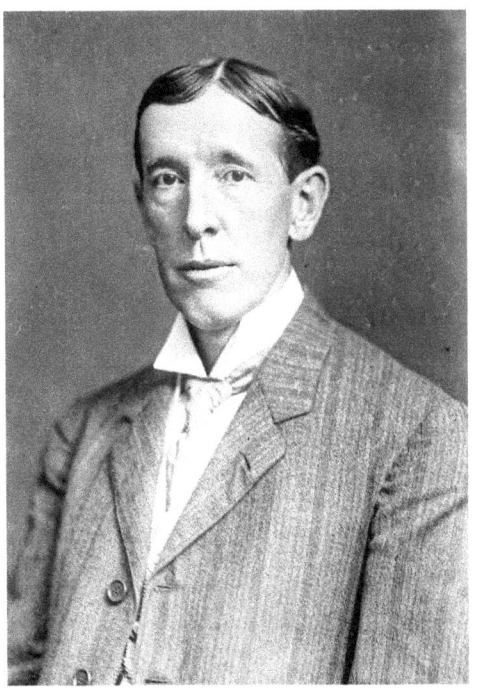

Dr. Woods Hutchinson, no date.

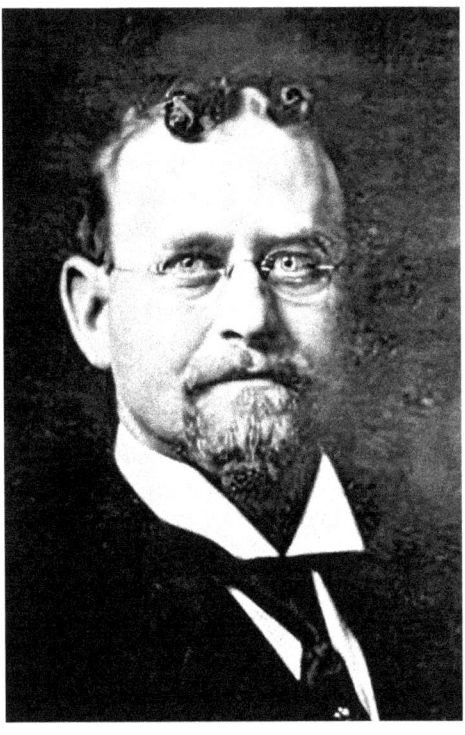

Dr. William C. Hassler of San Francisco, 1915.

SAN FRANCISCO HOLDS ITS CHURCH SERVICES IN OPEN AIR TO AVOID CONTAGION

AT TOP IS SHOWN BISHOP NICHOLS conducting the services of Grace Episcopal Cathedral on the lawn fronting the Divinity School. Below are shown the worshipers on the steps of St. Mary's Catholic Cathedral, a vast crowd, some of them kneeling in the street. The insert shows three of the women congregation assembled in a picturesque setting under the oak trees of Calvary Cemetery to attend mass.—Photo by International Film Service.

INFLUENZA IS NOT ABATINE

There was a slight decrease in th number of Spanish influenza cases i San Francisco yesterday, but, ac cording to health officers in charg of the epidemic, there are no direc indications of an abatement of th disease.

Dr. William C. Hassler, publi health officer, stated yesterday tha the decrease was due to the failur of a number of physicians to mak reports because of the Sabbath.

Two hundred and seventy-six nev cases were reported to the Healt Department up to an early hour las

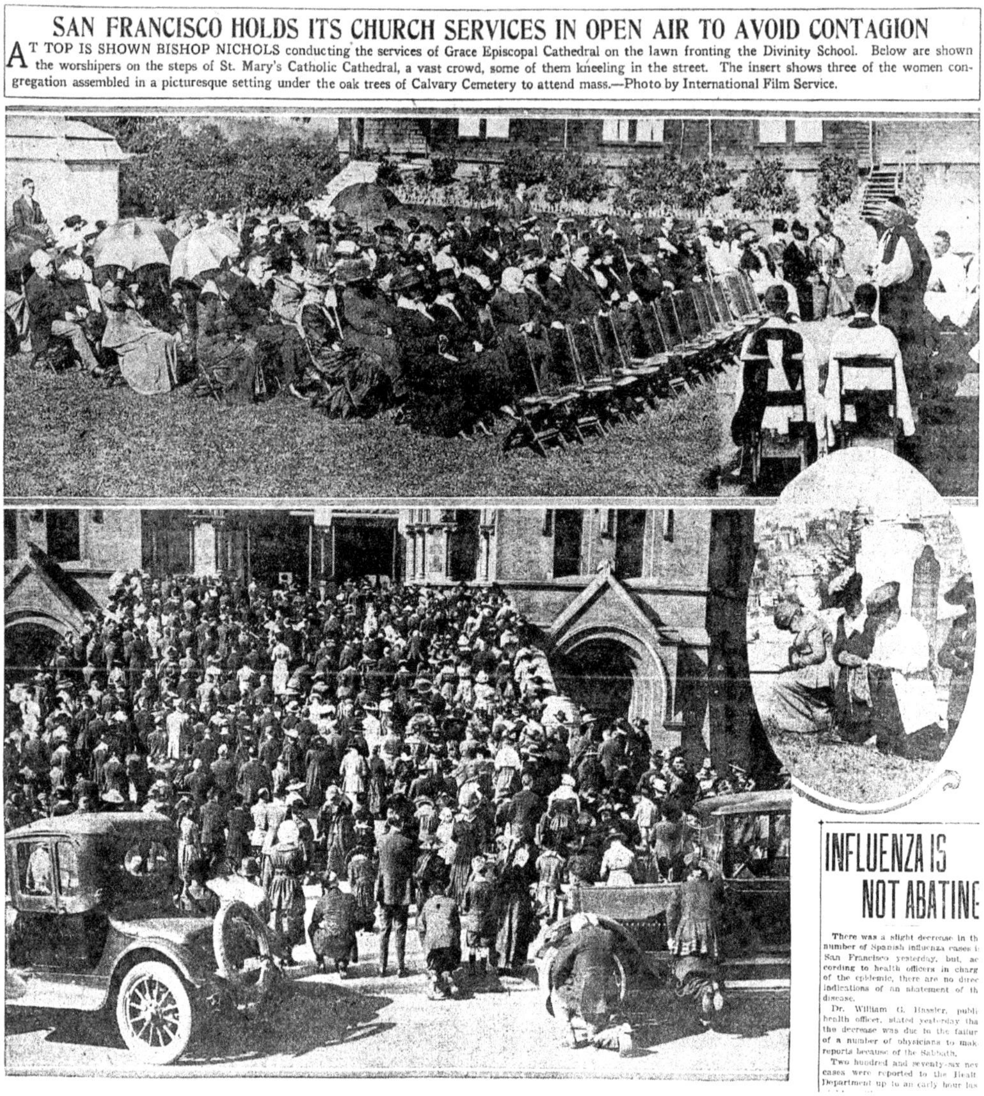

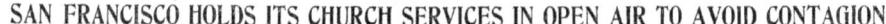

During its shutdowns involving the Rupert Blue Protocols, San Francisco closed the churches but did allow, as many places did, outdoor church services to be held.

on physicians who were laggards at making their legally required daily report of caseload. Hassler issued the following warning: "The Board of Health herewith calls upon every employer to impress upon those who are in his employ to wear the prescribed gauze mask both at their employment and on their way to and from their homes. Every citizen of San Francisco should wear a gauze mask when on the public street. This is imperative. So far the public is not demonstrating its willingness to cooperate in checking this epidemic. If the citizens continue to display their present lack of precaution we can look for a tremendous increase in the number of influenza cases and in the total of deaths." Hassler added, "Let us make the gauze mask popular. Make it a fad to wear them upon the streets. Instead of the person wearing one being an object of curiosity, let us shame those who refuse to take this necessary precaution into objects of scorn. If the citizens realized that it is possible to contract the influenza from a person whom you pass ten feet distant on the sidewalk they would immediately take this step of precaution. Every housewife should refuse to do her trading with a firm whose employees do not wear the masks. This same spirit should animate every avenue of business transaction." If all that did not inspire fear and panic in the citizenry, what would?[134]

San Francisco delayed for some days before passing an order mandating wearing masks. The likely reason was the difficulty of obtaining one of the face coverings. The local Red Cross chapter was swamped, as the group was everywhere. When masking was mandated, it took effect in a day or two, thus exacerbating the supply problem. Area newspapers published detailed instructions several times on how to make your own. One such piece remarked, "Those who are able to handle a needle and thread are requested to make their own." Meanwhile, Hassler continued his hyping, alternately hectoring the masses and praising them for their cooperation, real or imagined. He said, on October 23, "The citizens are only now awakening to the appeals issued by the Board of Health. If the precautions they are taking now were in force a week ago the present record would have been cut nearly in two." He hectored on, "Wear your gauze masks at all times and ridicule the person who refuses to wear one.... It was noticeable, the response of the patriotic citizens in wearing the masks, but I estimate only 25 percent have adopted the precaution so far. We must have 100 per cent in this mask campaign and the citizens should take the necessary steps to compel those with whom they associate to don the shields." Descending into hysteria, Hassler concluded, "The citizens must refrain from hysteria but follow the precautions. Wear the masks in the home as well as in the office and upon the street. That is the best precaution." Increasing the hysteria that was started and increased by Hassler and company, it was noted that San Francisco Police Chief D.A. White had given orders to the police officers to wear their masks at all times and to caution all pedestrians and drivers of vehicles to don the masks. Those officers were also instructed to visit every rooming house, hotel, apartment house, store, and other place of business on their beats and to advise all people to obtain a gauze mask and wear it until the epidemic had passed.[135]

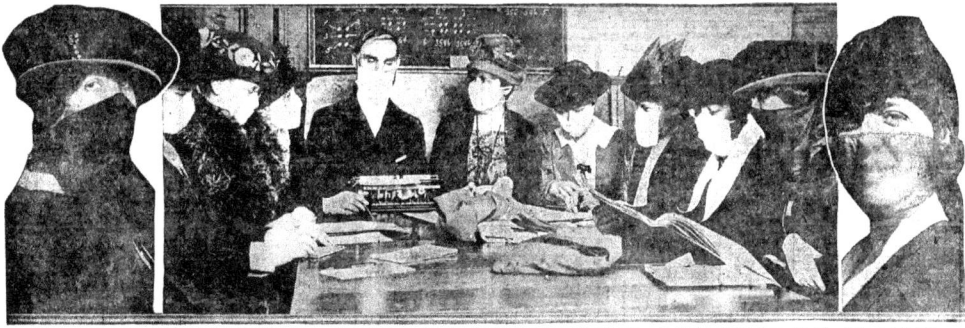

Society women meet in San Francisco to tirelessly continue to do good works. Lucille Stein, (*right*), is wearing a chiffon veil "that serves the same purpose" as the flu mask.

The hectoring by Hassler became an order to "wear your mask!" as of October 25. The board of supervisors passed the order as an emergency measure, and it took effect five days later. It required all people to wear a mask on the street, in public areas, and in all places "where two or more persons are together." Except for the necessary time at meals, masks had to be worn continuously. Those masks had to be made of four thicknesses of material and be not less than five inches wide by seven inches long. Failure to wear a mask made every person liable to a fine of $5 to $100 or imprisonment for ten days when the law took effect. In the intervening five days, the board of health relied on a resolution passed by the board of supervisors calling upon every person appearing outside the home to wear a mask. Hassler threatened that anybody found unmasked during those five days might be taken into quarantine. Hassler also issued a recommendation that "all persons who employed Chinese or Japanese servants would do well to keep them at home and not permit them to visit in Chinatown." The rule applied everywhere that two or more people gathered, except in homes where only two members of the family were present. That meant that in a household of three people—say, a husband, wife, and child—all three people had to be masked in their own home.[136]

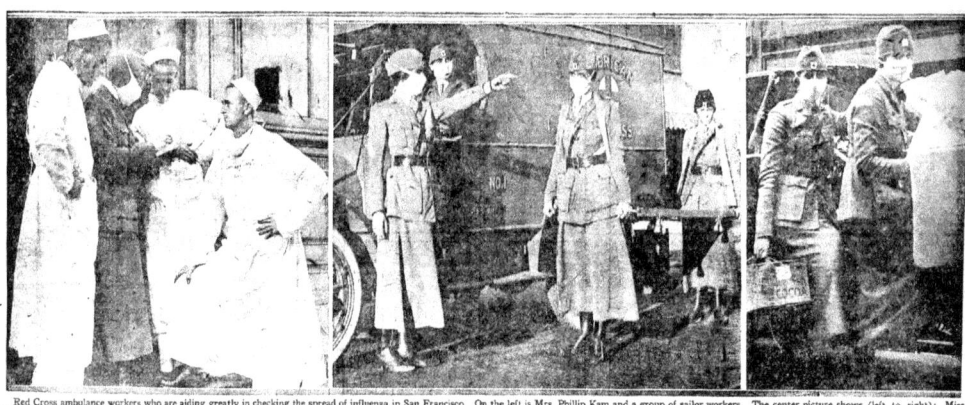

Red Cross ambulance workers who are aiding greatly in checking the spread of influenza in San Francisco. On the left is Mrs. Phillip Kam and a group of sailor workers. The center picture shows (left to right): Miss Helen Garrett, Miss Helen Son, Miss Aileen Treat and Miss Marjorie Levin, beside the Red Cross motor ambulance. In the photo on the right are: Miss Marjorie Levin (left) and Miss Helen St. Goar handling packages of "flu masks," which are to be distributed among the public.

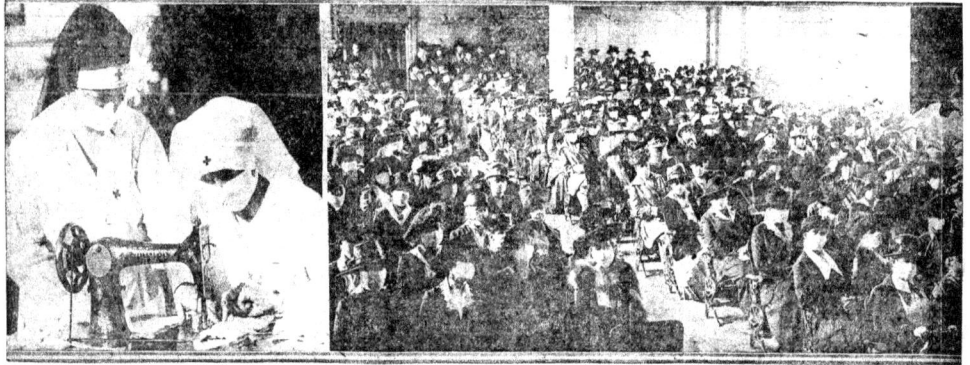

(Left) Mrs. James Rolph Jr. and her daughter, Miss Annette Rolph, aiding the Red Cross by making influenza masks. (Right) Assembly in the auditorium of Girls' High School, where about 750 teachers met in order to lend their services in the war being waged to check the influenza epidemic. All wore masks, as well as the speakers.

A composite shot of Red Cross workers in San Francisco. *Bottom left* are the wife and daughter of San Francisco mayor James Rolph, "doing good," reinforcing the old idea that a politician never lets anything go to waste, especially a crisis. *Bottom right* shows a large meeting of 750 teachers, all masked. The reader was informed that even the speakers at the event were masked.

On October 27 in San Francisco, police made 110 arrests of men charged with failure to wear influenza masks. All except a dozen were released on bail of ten dollars each. Those who remained in jail lacked the money for bail. The arrests were made all over the city. Some had their masks on their person or dangling from an ear or under their chin and claimed they had only lowered the mask briefly to smoke, but the police accepted no excuse.[137]

On the next day, another 100 men were arrested for failing to don their masks. In one violent incident, two men and a woman were shot at Powell and Market Streets when Henry D. Miller, an inspector in the city health department, discharged his revolver in a battle with James Wisser, a blacksmith who refused to don a gauze mask at the order of the health officer. Wisser was one of the wounded, shot in the arm and leg. Henry Appleton, a bystander, was shot in the leg by one of the four bullets fired by Miller, as was a woman bystander whose name was unavailable. According to the police, Miller found Wisser standing at the corner, waving his arms, and urging a crowd to dispense with the masks. "They are the bunk," he was alleged to have said. Miller tried to lead him toward a drugstore, insisting he buy a mask. At the door, Wisser allegedly struck Miller with a sack containing some silver dollars and then knocked him to the ground. Miller then drew his gun and fired four times. Wisser and Appleton were both taken to the hospital. The blacksmith was then charged with disturbing the peace, resisting an officer, and assault. Miller was taken to a police station, and a charge of assault with a deadly weapon was filed. No outcome of the case was reported.[138]

Up until midnight on November 1, 175 "mask slackers" were arrested in San Francisco. Those arrested on earlier days before the ordinance took effect were arrested on a charge of "disturbing the peace." Jail sentences were handed out to 33 people that day. Most of the violators received ten days of incarceration. Separately, that same day, the police stood guard at the ferry building and detained

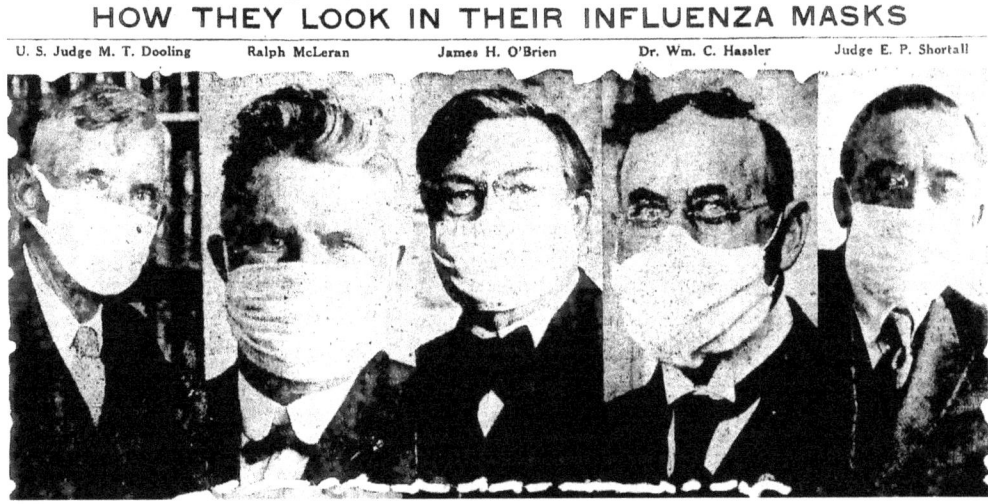

A group of famous San Francisco people in their masks setting that ubiquitous good example. Dr. William C. Hassler is *second from the right*.

incoming passengers without masks. Over 100 violators were detained in the crackdown. The detained people were taken in batches of 20 to the Harbor Police Station, where police Captain Patrick Shea lectured them on civic obligations. Except for a couple of drunks and one "anarchist," all those detained were dismissed with a reprimand.[139]

Then, on November 21 at noon, all of San Francisco could unmask. Hassler urged people not to destroy their masks but to personally deliver them to their nearest drug store. The stores would undertake to deliver the gauze to the Red Cross, which would sterilize it and use it for surgical dressings. All restrictions were lifted, and it was announced by the blowing of factory whistles and sirens. Public schools would reopen the following Monday. The only restriction remaining prohibited public dancing until December 1. As a final word, the city board of health made a few recommendations. One was that the disease existed elsewhere, and travelers entering the city could cause a new infection. Therefore, the board recommended that employers see that their employees, especially those in downtown stores and hotels, continue to wear masks.[140]

On November 16, a major fight was held in the auditorium in San Francisco that featured Meehan versus Fulton. George Blum, a police photographer, took a picture at the event, which police Captain Daniel O'Brien took to Dr. Hassler. The doctor said, "Now, it is possible that I may have lowered or raised my mask to take a puff at a cigar. At any rate I am willing to abide by the law. I shall send to the Police

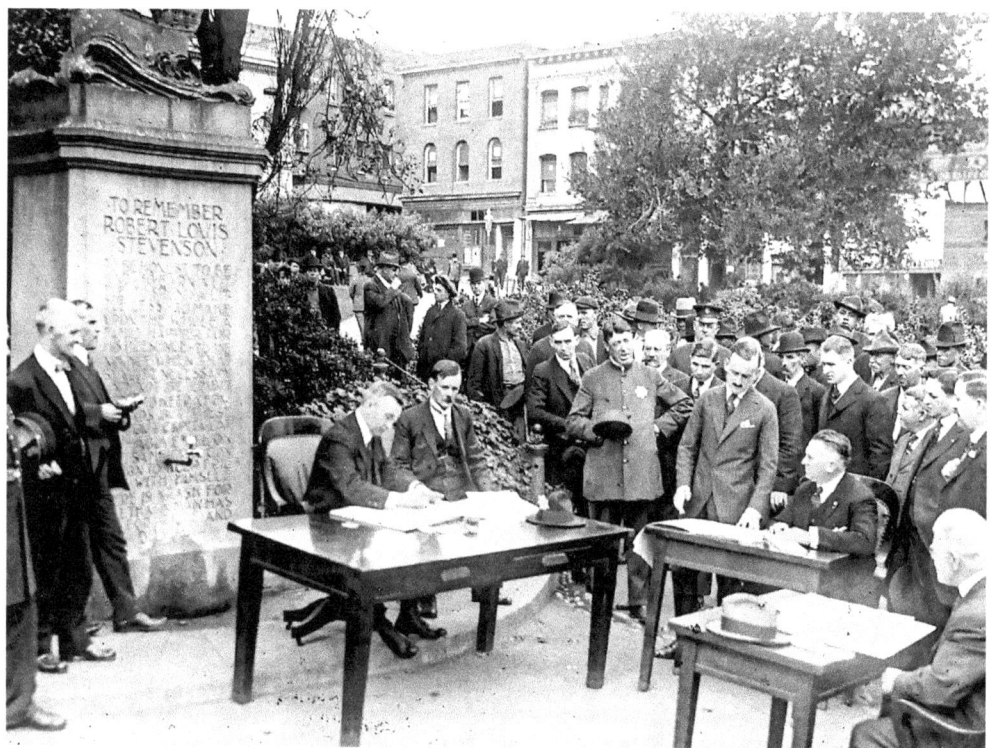

A session of a San Francisco court was held outdoors in the open air as panic gripped the city.

Department a check for $25 by way of a fine." He did so later that day. With his mask over one ear, San Francisco Mayor James Rolph also appeared in the picture, as did the unmasked features of city Supervisor Joseph Mulvihill. Each promised to pay a fine.[141]

The sirens and horns that signaled the end of masking in San Francisco were greeted with much enthusiasm. According to one reporter, 95 percent of the people had gotten rid of their face coverings five minutes after the hour. "A few minutes later few masks were to be seen save those which littered the sidewalks or had been hung up in conspicuous places." Columnist Annie Laurie wrote, "Whew—isn't it good to breathe again! … Didn't you hate your mask? Wasn't it a nuisance—didn't you feel smothered and breathless—and shut up and tied down with a mask on? And now they're gone—forever let's hope."[142]

Agitation to reimpose masking in San Francisco began on December 7, when the city board of health, at a meeting that day, requested that the general and universal wearing of masks be resumed immediately. After the meeting, Mayor Rolph issued a proclamation asking that mask wearing be resumed immediately. He was expected to ask the board of supervisors to revive the recently rescinded masking ordinance. Cases of the flu had reportedly increased dramatically.[143]

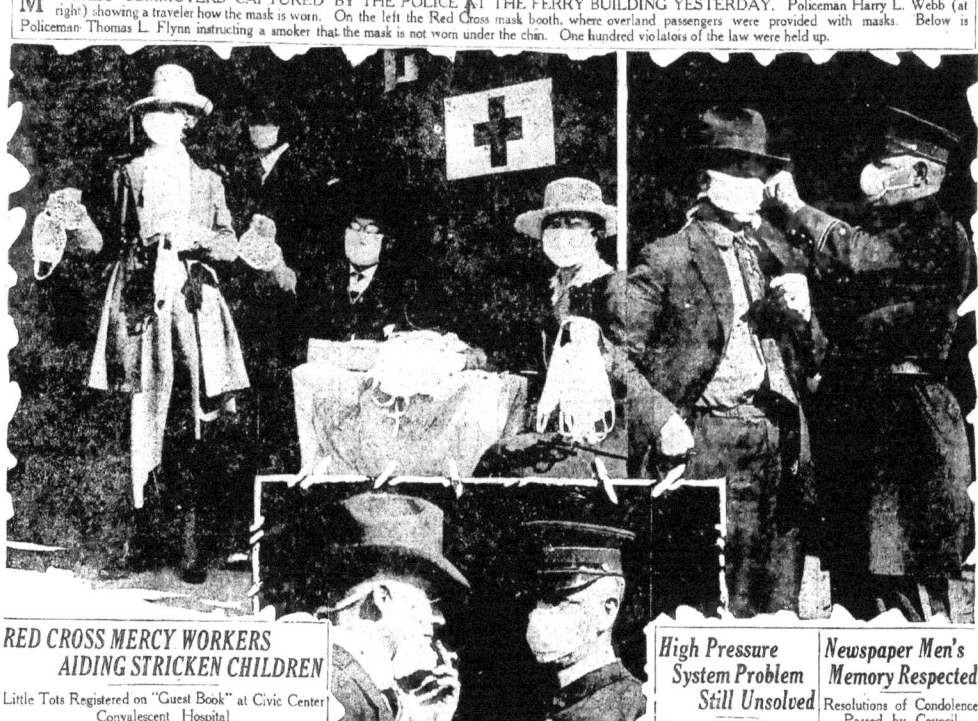

San Francisco police arrest passengers alighting from ferries for not being masked. Note the man smoking in the bottom photograph. He has slipped the mask under his chin while smoking and is herein admonished for his sins. In an era where a higher proportion of people smoked, this was a regularly occurring problem.

A few days later, at a meeting, the board of supervisors decided to postpone, for several days, action on the request submitted by Hassler, asking the board to invoke the mandatory masking law. Hassler agreed to the postponement but insisted that mask wearing was the only solution to the problem.[144]

A week after that, Hassler issued a special appeal to the people of San Francisco to don influenza masks immediately instead of waiting for the board of supervisors to take action and make their use compulsory. Hassler declared, "Those who wish to safeguard their health and stall off possible death should wear masks. Influenza again is epidemic in the city and the mask is the only known preventive of any worth."[145]

Nothing much happened in San Francisco until January 10, 1919, when Mayor Rolph issued a proclamation calling on the city's men, women, and children to wear influenza masks. The board of supervisors had just passed an ordinance requiring the universal wearing of masks.[146]

Wearing gauze masks became compulsory in San Francisco for the second time on January 20, 1919. The police were given orders to arrest all who were unmasked. The police had been out on the streets the day before to warn people about the mandatory mask-wearing order that was going into effect.[147]

When the ordinance was voted on for the second time on January 17, the board of supervisors voted 12 to 2 in favor of the law, with four members absent. In the wake of the vote, Mrs. C.E. Grosjean, who had opposed the mask ordinance on every occasion that it had been before the board of supervisors, announced, after the meeting, that an anti-mask league had been formed. She said the league's object was to "oppose by lawful means the compulsory wearing of masks. Mrs. E.C. Harrington, a local attorney, was elected league president." A mass meeting was to be held early in the next week when the support of the public would be sought in a test case that the new association proposed to bring into the court system.[148]

On January 20, the first masking day, the police had made 186 arrests for ordinance violations by 10 p.m. that first night. Most of those arrested were released on five-dollar bail. Meanwhile, a mass meeting of the Anti-Mask League of San Francisco was slated for January 25. At the meeting, it was expected that petitions would be circulated demanding the firing of Hassler and threatening the mayor with recall if he did not rescind the order.[149]

The police were even more active in San Francisco concerning the mandatory masking laws. On that day, they arrested 483 offenders, with the majority released on five-dollar bail. One place in San Francisco where the flu masks did not have to be worn was the city prison.[150]

At the Anti-Mask League meeting on January 25, a reporter estimated the crowd at 2,000. Resolutions were passed denouncing the mask ordinance as contrary to the desires of a majority of the people. City Supervisor Eugene Schmitz was advertised as the principal speaker of the evening, but he failed to appear at the gathering.[151]

The California Board of Health published a report at this time noting that flu masks did little good in curbing influenza. The board issued a bulletin stating masks were "inefficacious." It added that they were worn on the streets but not in offices where they were needed and that the majority were improperly made. Many masks, it was reported, were worn under the chin in San Francisco, even by pedestrians. The report appeared in a few newspapers in America, not as many as might have been expected, but not in any San Francisco newspapers.[152]

On January 28, it was announced that Hassler was prepared to make a recommendation to the board of health at their meeting on January 30 to remove the mask requirement one day later, on January 31. During the meeting of the board of supervisors, members of the Anti-Mask League were sharply rebuked by Mayor Rolph when they hissed Supervisor Andrew J. Gallagher, author of the mask law, and applauded Supervisors Schmitz and Nelson, who opposed the ordinance.[153]

The Anti-Mask League of San Francisco held a meeting on January 31, coinciding with the end of mandatory masking in the city. The meeting itself came to an abrupt end as factions fought over what direction the group should follow. One faction wanted to fight to recall Hassler, while the other group favored going after Mayor Rolph with a petition signed by voters. More squabbling took place, and there was a refusal to hold a vote on one resolution. And then it was lights out on the meeting.[154]

One newspaper in California that did print the state board of health's findings was in Pomona. Dr. N.J. Rice summarized the results of their study of the issue: "The report shows that many, or rather most, of the precautions such as wearing flu masks, rigid closing of schools, theaters, churches, etc., have been of no avail in checking the epidemic ... it was learned by actual figures that those cities which did not take strict precautions, as New York, had a lower death rate than cities like San Francisco, which took nearly every kind of precaution.... It also appears that the flu mask was of very little, if any, advantage." It was also learned that in the San Francisco hospitals where the nurses all wore masks, 75 percent of the nurses contracted influenza.[155]

A report released by California giving yearly arrest totals showed that in the fiscal year July 1, 1918, to June 30, 1919, there were more than 3,000 arrests made in San Francisco for violation of the influenza masking ordinance.[156]

Hawaii

Hawaii was barely touched by influenza during the entire year of 1918. The press on the islands often mentioned the epidemic and its ravages on the mainland, but there was little effect in Hawaii. Kirk B. Porter, executive officer on the board of health, was, as of October 22, 1918, sending out notices to the government physicians in the territory informing them of the action taken a day earlier concerning influenza. Since the illness seemed to be prevalent in Oahu only, it was only there that precautions would be implemented. Porter stated that he did not feel that there was any occasion for alarm, provided that people afflicted with the disease cooperated with the health authorities to the extent of not coming into contact with others while passing through the infectious stage of the illness.[157]

At a meeting of the Board of Trade in Hilo, Hawaii, in mid–January 1919, Dr.

L.L. Sexton told his audience that it was time for Hilo to organize against the entry of Spanish influenza. Only two cases had been reported in Hilo, both in passengers arriving on ships. The Board of Trade went on to appoint a committee on prevention. As everywhere else in America, the local chapter of the Red Cross put itself to work making masks.[158]

The steps taken in Hilo to combat the flu consisted mainly of a public education campaign and a more vigorous inspection of passengers arriving on ships. Dr. Sexton said using flu masks was not advisable, as they "were not pleasant to wear, and people rebelled against them unless they were known to be a positive necessity." When needed, their wearing had to be enforced by law because "one or two carriers going about for a few hours without masks would nullify all the good effects of the masking."[159]

On January 21, a reporter observed that the first flu mask was seen that day on the streets of Hilo when a middle-sized boy walked down the street wearing one. "He looked proud of himself, and seemed to think he had reason to be, as he was protecting both others and himself. Now that the ice has been broken, masks will probably occur sporadically with more and more frequency, until they either become compulsory or the need of them vanishes entirely."[160]

An editorial in a Hilo newspaper on March 5 stated, "I cannot, indeed, think of anything more conducive to influenza, or any other living or throat disease, than this absurd practice. To rebreathe the carbolic acid and other impurities of the lungs, while carrying around impurities from without, caught on the moist meshes of a mask, through which millions of germs may easily penetrate, is monumental folly." He then cited a circular that had been issued a couple of weeks earlier in which the California Board of Health declared that "investigations made by the board's trained workers show that the compulsory use of the mask upon the general public has no effect whatever in the control of the outbreak in any of the cities where this measure has been adopted."[161]

In Honolulu, as of October 30, 1918, the city had recorded just eight official cases of Spanish influenza but was also undertaking its action plan. A committee of women began an inspection of schools in the area to monitor the children. A plan in the works to have local physicians visit area theaters to give four-minute talks explaining the best methods of avoiding the disease was abandoned when physicians rebelled against the idea.[162]

In mid- to late January, the number of cases in Honolulu increased, but not enough to let mindless panic drive the situation. Some advocated the immediate closure of the usual suspects. Colonel Hathaway, collector of internal revenue, stated, "It has been proved, and doctors all agree now, that a serum is not a cure for the disease and that the flu masks do not prevent it." He argued that preventing large gatherings and isolating the sick were the only means of checking the disease.[163]

Then, on January 25, 1919, the usual suspects in Honolulu were closed. The schools were allowed to remain open but were placed under a daily inspection carried out by the Nurses' Association. The rules were applied across the territory. But there was no mention of masks.

A brief news item in a Honolulu newspaper on March 1, 1919, indicated how alien the face mask was to residents of Hawaii. It was reported that the mask came to town when the sailors from a U.S. Navy vessel came into port to visit Honolulu. According to the story, "much amusement was caused by the masks, which were new to many of the Honolulans, and among the Asiatic population when the boys appeared with their faces covered and nothing but their eyes showing, there was consternation mixed with wonder." The story added that "a flu mask is not a thing of beauty nor a joy forever, it being averred by those who have worn them that they are more provocative of profanity than anything that has yet been invented…. Honolulans after seeing the sailor boys' masks are hoping they won't have to wear them."

Chapter Notes

Chapter 1

1. "No influenza in U.S." *Alexandria Gazette* (VA), Jul 16, 1918.
2. Ibid.
3. "Spanish influenza widespread but not severe." *Sun* (NY), Aug 4, 1918.
4. "Fear of epidemic from Spanish grip scouted by officials." *New York Tribune*, Aug 17, 1918.
5. "Influenza patients are quarantined." *Brownsville Herald* (TX), Sep 10, 1918.
6. "Spanish influenza here officials fear." *New York Tribune*, Sep 12, 1918.
7. "Influenza finds Camp Lee alert." *Evening Public Ledger* (Philadelphia), Sep 17, 1918.
8. "Influenza in nine camps." *Bisbee Review* (AZ), Sep 21, 1918.
9. "19 die of influenza in nearby camps." *Sun* (NY), Sep 22, 1918.
10. "Spanish flu much like grip." *Evening Times-Republican* (Marshalltown, IA), Sep 30, 1918.
11. https://chroniclingamerica.loc.gov. Accessed Dec 1, 2022.
12. "Plague spreading over a large area." *Sun* (NY), Oct 5, 1918; "District churches and playgrounds ordered closed." *Washington Times* (Washington, D.C.), Oct 5, 1918.
13. "Uncle Sam's advice." *Rathdrum Tribune* (ID), Oct 18, 1918.
14. "Speed up flu law." *Topeka State Journal* (KS), Sep 15, 1919; "While Congress snores." *Seattle Star*, Oct 2, 1919.
15. "Interesting health questions." *Richmond Times-Dispatch* (VA), Mar 16, 1919.
16. "Facts on influenza." Ogden Standard (UT), Feb 3, 1920.
17. "Scots in France wearing gas masks." *Meridian Times* (ID), Jun 2, 1916.
18. "Exclusive pictures of stricken Rheims." *Sun* (NY), Feb 27, 1916.
19. "Children wear masks." *Chariton Courier* (Keytesville, MO), Dec 1, 1916.
20. "Where the gas mask originated." *Richmond Palladium* (IN), Mar 23, 1917.
21. "The girl in the gas mask." *Richmond Palladium* (IN), Jan 17, 1918.
22. "Poison gas in warfare." *Ogden Standard* (UT), Jan 26, 1918.
23. "Gas will win the war." *Evening Star* (Washington, D.C.), May 10, 1918.
24. "German gas visits Swiss." *Evening Star* (Washington, D.C.), May 13, 1918.
25. "Wear masks to escape plague." *Shoshone Journal* (ID), Jun 14, 1918.
26. "Meade men must wear gas masks during routine." *Washington Times* (Washington, D.C.), Jun 14, 1918.
27. "29,002 cases Spanish flu army's report." *Washington Herald* (Washington, D.C.), Sep 26, 1918.
28. "Gas masks used as influenza preventive." *New York Tribune*, Sep 27, 1918.
29. "Gas masks on phones to ward off influenza." *Evening Star* (Washington, D.C.), Oct 8, 1918.
30. "Kentuckians don masks." *Chattanooga News* (TN), Oct 2, 1918; "Clippings of capital coupons." *Evening Capital* (Annapolis, MD), Oct 28, 1918.
31. "Uncle Sam has gas mask which would get Hun." *Ogden Standard* (UT), Dec 14, 1918.
32. Ad. *Evening Star* (Washington, D.C.), Nov 5, 1918.

Chapter 2

1. "Epidemic fought by New England." *Evening Star* (Washington), Sep 26, 1918.
2. "Open clinic to check influenza spread." *Evening Journal* (Wilmington, DE), Oct 1, 1918.
3. "Anti-influenza serum made in tests here." *New York Tribune*, Oct 2, 1918.
4. "Influenza serum now discovered." *Wheeling Intelligencer* (WV), Oct 2, 1918.
5. "Influenza serum a success." *Carson City Appeal* (NV), Oct 8, 1918.
6. "Successful influenza vaccine is not found." *Tulsa World* (OK), Oct 11, 1918.
7. "Dr. Mayo tells of influenza serum." *Evening Missourian* (Columbia), Oct 14, 1918.
8. "Works on serum." *Topeka State Journal* (KS), Oct 16, 1918.
9. "Spanish influenza vaccine is provided." *Capital Journal* (Salem, OR), Oct 17, 1918.
10. "Mayo Brothers have flu serum." *Evening Times-Republican* (Marshalltown, IA), Oct 17, 1918.

11. "Few new cases of influenza are reported." *Grand Forks Herald* (ND), Oct 17, 1918.
12. "Decrease here shown in new grippe cases." *New York Tribune*, Oct 18, 1918.
13. Ad. *Parisian* (Paris, TN), Oct 18, 1918; Ad. *El Paso Herald* (TX), Oct 19, 1918.
14. "Mayo influenza vaccine is offered." *Evening World* (NY), Oct 19, 1918.
15. "100,000 shots of anti-flu serum set for each day." *Rock Island Argus* (IL), Oct 21, 1918.
16. "But one death reported today from influenza." *Bismarck Tribune* (ND), Oct 23, 1918.
17. "Influenza here burning out Copeland says." *New York Tribune*, Oct 22, 1918.
18. "New influenza serum." *Brattleboro Reformer* (VT), Oct 23, 1918.
19. "Influenza serum shot into Gary and steel forces." *Evening World* (NY), Oct 23, 1918.
20. "Vaccinate class one." *Gate City* (Keokuk, IA), Oct 23, 1918.
21. "Slight improvement in the influenza epidemic." *Wheeling Intelligencer* (WV), Oct 23, 1918.
22. "Physicians give anti-flu vaccine." *West Virginian* (Fairmont), Oct 23, 1918.
23. Ibid.
24. "Six deaths today's toll." *Bismarck Tribune* (ND), Oct 24, 1918.
25. "Employees will all be shot." *Lake County Times* (Hammond, IN), Oct 24, 1918.
26. "Vaccine used to curb spread of influenza." *Rogue River Courier* (Grants Pass, OR), Oct 24, 1918.
27. "Influenza serum is being made in Tulsa." *Tulsa World* (OK), Oct 24, 1918.
28. "A sure cure for the flu." *Middletown Transcript* (DE), Oct 26, 1918.
29. "Vaccine given R&V workers." *Rock Island Argus* (IL), Oct 26, 1918.
30. "Advise vaccine as preventive of influenza." *Arizona Republican* (Phoenix), Oct 26, 1918.
31. Ibid.
32. "Influenza vaccine still experiment." *Sun* (NY), Oct 27, 1918.
33. "What eminent authorities say." *Morgan City Review* (LA), Oct 28, 1918.
34. "Influenza serums." *Bridgeport Times* (CT), Oct 28, 1918.
35. "Influenza serums." *Shoshone Journal* (ID), Nov 1, 1918.
36. Ad. *Seattle Star*. Nov 5, 1918.
37. "Flu serum in hands of all doctors here." *Bismarck Tribune* (ND), Nov 7, 1918.
38. "Vaccination against pneumonia." *Topeka State Journal* (KS), Nov 12, 1918.
39. Ibid.
40. "Conference is held to discuss matter of reopening." *Arizona Republican* (Phoenix), Nov 14, 1918.
41. "Schools open Monday." *Diamond Drill* (Crystal Falls, MI), Nov 16, 1918.
42. "Value of vaccination against influenza." *Arizona Republican* (Phoenix), Nov 17, 1918.
43. "People take action, make regulations." *Arizona Republican* (Phoenix), Nov 19, 1918.
44. "El Paso doctors get Rosenow's flu vaccine." *El Paso Herald* (TX), Nov 26, 1918.
45. "Consignment of flu vaccine arrives." *Payne Field Zooms* (West Point, MS), Nov 27, 1918.
46. Ad. *Audubon Journal* (Exira, IA), Nov 28, 1918.
47. "Influenza ban is taken off." *Alma Record* (MI), Nov 28, 1918.
48. "Influenza vaccine to check epidemic." *Iron County Record* (Cedar City, IA), Nov 29, 1918.
49. Ad. *Albuquerque Morning Journal* (NM), Nov 29, 1918.
50. Ad. *Ogden Standard* (UT), Dec 3, 1918.
51. "Vaccination station here." *Gate City* (Keokuk, IA), Dec 4, 1918.
52. "U.S. Health warns against flu vaccines." *Eureka Sentinel* (NV), Dec 7, 1918.
53. "Vaccine for flu." *Topeka Stat Journal* (KS), Dec 10, 1918.
54. "Flu vaccine used successfully here." *Idaho Springs Sifting-News* (CO), Dec 13, 1918.
55. "Flu hysteria not warranted." *Bismarck Tribune* (ND), Dec 12, 1918.
56. "New flu vaccine produced at University of Missouri." *Omaha Bee*, Dec 14, 1918.
57. "Free vaccine to all people." *Webster City Freeman* (IA), Dec 16, 1918.
58. "Vaccine for school is not recommended." *Ogden Standard* (UT), Dec 17, 1918.
59. "Make flu serum." *Topeka State Journal* (KS), Dec 17, 1918.
60. "Flu serum no good, says Ohio newspaper." *Public Ledger* (Maysville, KY), Dec 19, 1918.
61. "Board of health modifies flu ban." *Canon City Record* (CO), Dec 19, 1918.
62. "Inoculated against the danger of influenza." *L'Anse Sentinel* (MI), Dec 20, 1918.
63. "More about vaccination." *Albuquerque Morning Journal* (NM), Jan 2, 1919.
64. "Doctor says flu serum has no effect." *Seattle Star*, Jan 13, 1919.
65. "Flu serum useless." *Elk Mountain Pilot* (Irwin, CO), Feb 27, 1919.
66. "Free vaccine for flu prevention." *Glasgow Courier* (MT), Aug 29, 1919.
67. "Two new cases of influenza in this city today." *Topeka State Journal* (KS), Sep 17, 1919.
68. "Influenza for poor of state." *Morning Tulsa World* (OK), Oct 11, 1919.
69. "Cultivating anti-influenza vaccine." *Hartford Republican* (KY), Oct 31, 1919.
70. "Bar use of serum." *Rock Island Argus* (IL), Jan 21, 1920.
71. "1,332 new case spur flu fight." *Sun* (NY), Jan 24, 1920.
72. "Influenza again." *Crittenden Press* (Marion, KY), Feb 6, 1920.
73. "Flu ban continues in effect." *Parisian* (Paris, TN), Mar 5, 1920.
74. "Influenza vaccine free." *Ardmoreite* (Ardmore, OK), Oct 3, 1920.

Chapter 3

1. "Physicians wear masks to avoid the infection." *Bridgeport Times* (CT), Sep 27, 1918.
2. "Masks for doctors and nurses in epidemics." *Norwich Bulletin* (CT), Oct 10, 1918.
3. "Influenza cases here total 939." *Bridgeport Telegram* (CT), Oct 12, 1918.
4. "Influenza vaccine to be used." *Bridgeport Telegram* (CT), Oct 16, 1918.
5. "Flying squadron of speakers." *Bridgeport Telegram* (CT), Oct 17, 1918.
6. "Fairfield doctors at odds." *Bridgeport Telegram* (CT), Oct 21, 1918.
7. "Wear a muslin mask to balk influenza." *New Britain Herald* (CT), Sep 30, 1918.
8. "Westerly." *Norwich Bulletin* (CT), Oct 5, 1918.
9. "Gauze face masks." *New Britain Herald* (CT), Oct 11, 1918.
10. "Anniversary of the epidemic." *New Britain Herald* (CT), Sep 19, 1919.
11. "Schools, churches and entertainment." *Burlington Free Press* (VT), Oct 5, 1918.
12. "No convention no platform." *Richford Gazette* (VT), Oct 18, 1918; "Until November three." *Richford Gazette* (VT), Oct 25, 1918; "Quarantine is off." *Richford Gazette* (VT), Nov 1, 1918; "Ban declared off." *News and Citizen* (Morrisville, VT), Nov 6, 1918.
13. "Send the children to school." *Richford Gazette* (VT), Nov 22, 1918.
14. "East Fairfield." *Richford Gazette* (VT), Dec 13, 1918; "Fairfax." *Richford Gazette* (VT), Feb 21, 1919.
15. "Influenza in fifty more homes here." *Rutland Daily Herald* (VT), Oct 7, 1918.
16. "Uncle Sam's advice on flu." *Rutland Daily Herald* (VT), Oct 14, 1918.
17. "Predicts return of flu." *Burlington Free Press* (VT), Sep 17, 1919.
18. "The influenza epidemic." *Newport Mercury* (RI), Oct 5, 1918; "Influenza improving." *Newport Mercury* (RI), Oct 19, 1918.
19. "Uncle Sam's advice on flu." *Newport Mercury* (RI), Oct 12, 1918.
20. "Bangor's battle with the grip." *Bangor Daily News* (ME), Oct 5, 1918.
21. "Many cases of influenza in Lewiston and Auburn." *Lewiston Daily Sun* (ME), Sep 28, 1918.
22. "How grip spreads and how to dodge it." *Bangor Daily News* (ME), Oct 7, 1918.
23. "Belfast has masks for influenza cases." *Bangor Daily News* (ME), Oct 12, 1918.
24. "Influenza preventives split health meeting." *Bangor Daily News* (ME), Dec 13, 1918.
25. "Brands rumors of closing ban here as false." *Portland Evening Express* (ME), Dec 26, 1918.
26. "Predicts return of flu epidemic." *Bangor Daily News* (ME), Sep 17, 1919.
27. "Closing order to hold over another week." *Portsmouth Herald* (NH), Oct 17, 1918.
28. "Ayer." *Hollis Times* (NH), Sep 20, 1918.
29. "How Boston fights spread of epidemic." *Des Moines Register* (IA), Oct 12, 1918.
30. "Physicians use influenza masks." *Winona Daily News* (MN), Sep 28, 1918.
31. "Charlie Chaplin stopped the flu." *Fall River Daily Globe* (MA), Sep 5, 1919.
32. "Influenza masks." *Holyoke Daily Transcript* (MA), Oct 2, 1918.
33. "Common sense about the epidemic." *Boston Globe*, Sep 18, 1918.
34. "Influenza deaths in Boston fewer." *Boston Globe*, Sep 28, 1918.
35. "Hospital grew in a night." *Boston Globe*, Sep 29, 1918.
36. "Headway of the epidemic checked." *Boston Globe*, Oct 2, 1918.
37. "Gauze masks to every policeman." *Boston Globe*, Oct 5, 1918.
38. "Dr. Woodward's advice to coughers and sneezers." *Boston Globe*, Dec 29, 1918.

Chapter 4

1. Ads. *Hopewell Herald* (NJ), Oct 9, 1918.
2. "Church services will again be held tomorrow." *Daily Home News* (New Brunswick, NJ), Oct 26, 1918.
3. "All dentists and barbers to wear masks in Clifton." *Passaic Daily News* (NJ), Oct 16, 1918.
4. "Uncle Sam's advice on flu." *Asbury Park Press* (NJ), Oct 12, 1918.
5. "Spanish influenza here." *New York Sun*, Sep 12, 1918.
6. "Quarantine order is essential as disease spreads." *Buffalo Enquirer* (NY), Oct 12, 1918; "Those exposed to flue should wear masks." *Buffalo Enquirer* (NY), Oct 12, 1918.
7. "Quarantine to be raised Monday." *Buffalo Times* (NY), Nov 1, 1918; "Quarantine raised." *Buffalo Times* (NY), Nov 1, 1918; "Ban effective another week." *Buffalo Times* (NY), Nov 1, 1918; "Closing ban has been lifted." *Buffalo Times* (NY), Nov 1, 1918.
8. "Quarantine again at Niagara Falls." *Buffalo Enquirer* (NY), Nov 18, 1918.
9. "Elmira placed under strict quarantine." *Star-Gazette* (Elmira, NY), Oct 15, 1918.
10. "Barbers adopt flu masks while at work." *Star-Gazette* (Elmira, NY), Oct 17, 1918.
11. "May close all public places to check flu." *Buffalo Enquirer* (NY), Oct 7, 1918.
12. "City authorities decide against general closing." *Buffalo Morning Express* (NY), Oct 8, 1918.
13. "1,726 new cases." *Buffalo Courier* (NY), Oct 13, 1918.
14. "Influenza spreads, need for doctors and nurses urgent." *Buffalo Courier* (NY), Oct 13, 1918.
15. "Health authorities every resource to check disease." *Buffalo Enquirer* (NY), Oct 14, 1918.
16. "Influenza being held in check by determined fight." *Buffalo Enquirer* (NY), Oct 15, 1918.

17. "Keep down spread of influenza." *Buffalo Evening News* (NY), Oct 16, 1918.
18. "Teachers to help combat influenza among children." *Buffalo Courier* (NY), Oct 17, 1918.
19. "Influenza cases show sharp drop." *Buffalo Evening News* (NY), Oct 18, 1918.
20. "Kings Co. hospital bars flu masks; called dangerous." *Brooklyn Eagle* (NY), Oct 4, 1918.
21. "The influenza epidemic." *Brooklyn Eagle* (NY), Oct 13, 1918.
22. "The influenza quarantine." *New York Times*, Oct 1, 1918.
23. "Copeland says theatres must obey or close." *New York Tribune*, Oct 10, 1918.
24. "Grip crisis in N.Y. over, but fight goes on." *New York Sun*, Oct 13, 1918.
25. Ad. *Brooklyn Eagle* (NY), Oct 15, 1918; "New York health boss says chiffon veil is safe mask against flu." *Des Moines Register* (IA), Oct 16, 1918.
26. "Quarantine on influenza is observed here." *Harrisburg Telegraph* (PA), Oct 4, 1918.
27. "City accepts quarantine on influenza in good spirits." *Harrisburg Telegraph* (PA), Oct 5, 1918.
28. "Tent hospitals as last resort." *Harrisburg Telegraph* (PA), Oct 7, 1918.
29. "Saloonman is arrested by city." *Harrisburg Telegraph* (PA), Oct 8, 1918.
30. "Crest of influenza." *Harrisburg Telegraph* (PA), Oct 10, 1918.
31. Ad. *Harrisburg Telegraph* (PA), Oct 11, 1918.
32. "City closed tight tonight." *Harrisburg Telegraph* (PA), Oct 12, 1918.
33. "Everybody his own quarantine officer, Dr. Raunick." *Harrisburg Telegraph* (PA), Oct 15, 1918.
34. "All stores to close Saturday evening at 6:30." *Harrisburg Telegraph* (PA), Oct 16, 1918.
35. "Why certainly! It's safe and sane to wear gas mask." *Harrisburg Telegraph* (PA), Oct 17, 1918.
36. "Free whiskey for those who need stimulant." *Harrisburg Telegraph* (PA), Oct 18, 1918.
37. "8,000 influenza cases developed." *Harrisburg Telegraph* (PA), Oct 18, 1918.
38. "Worst of grip epidemic has passed city." *Harrisburg Telegraph* (PA), Oct 21, 1918; "The city's splendid emergency hospital." *Harrisburg Telegraph* (PA), Oct 23, 1918.
39. "Third Saturday night closing is ordered at 6:30." *Harrisburg Telegraph* (PA), Oct 26, 1918.
40. "City's streets must be quiet on Halloween." *Harrisburg Telegraph* (PA), Oct 29, 1918.
41. "Quarantine in Harrisburg to be off Tuesday." *Harrisburg Telegraph* (PA), Oct 30, 1918; "Ban on church services is not to be lifted." *Harrisburg Telegraph* (PA), Nov 1, 1918.
42. "Dr. Royer tells Judge Landis he has no power." *Harrisburg Telegraph* (PA), Nov 4, 1918.
43. "No thirsty rush as lid lifted." *Evening Public Ledger* (Philadelphia), Oct 30, 1918.
44. "Royer's order isolates city of Lancaster." *Harrisburg Telegraph* (PA), Nov 2, 1918.
45. "Ban on business lifted at noon; theaters open." *Harrisburg Telegraph* (PA), Nov 5, 1918.
46. "Politics in Pennsylvania." *Harrisburg Telegraph* (PA), Nov 5, 1918.
47. "Saturday night ban is removed." *Harrisburg Telegraph* (PA), Nov 8, 1918; "Influenza ban raised at last." *Harrisburg Telegraph* (PA), Nov 9, 1918.
48. "Quarantine for influenza not favored by city." *Harrisburg Telegraph* (PA), Dec 10, 1918.
49. "Flu flares up in many places throughout PA." *Harrisburg Telegraph* (PA), Nov 20, 1918.
50. "Recurrence of influenza is not at danger point." *Harrisburg Telegraph* (PA), Jan 24, 1919.
51. "Teachers call for more pay." *Evening Public Ledger* (Philadelphia), Jan 3, 1919.
52. "Sweeping quarantine against influenza." *Banner* (Cambridge, MD), Oct 4, 1918; "Philadelphia is bone dry." *Sun* (NY), Oct 5, 1918.
53. "Rigid grip test as schools open." *Evening Public Ledger* (Philadelphia), Oct 26, 1918.
54. "Barber will wear flu mask." *New Castle Herald* (PA), Oct 30, 1918.
55. "Fewer new cases reported for day." *Scranton Republican* (PA), Oct 24, 1918.
56. "Help control the epidemic." *Scranton Republican* (PA), Oct 26, 1918.
57. "Newsboys plead for gauze masks." *Scranton Republican* (PA), Oct 28, 1918.
58. "Needs in fight on epidemic supplied." *Pittsburgh Post-Gazette*, Oct 8, 1918.
59. "Many flareups of influenza in state." *Pittsburgh Post-Gazette*, Nov 21, 1918.
60. "Views on cure for influenza differ widely." *Pittsburgh Post-Gazette*, Dec 13, 1918; "Branding influenza mask as fake splits conference." *Pittsburgh Daily Post*, Dec 13, 1918.

Chapter 5

1. "May close all public places." *Evening Journal* (Wilmington, DE), Oct 1, 1918; "Churches, schools, saloons." *Evening Journal* (Wilmington, DE), Oct 2, 1918; "200 deaths in city." *Evening Journal* (Wilmington, DE), Oct 4, 1918.
2. "Influenza grip on city." *Evening Journal* (Wilmington, DE), Oct 9, 1918.
3. "Quarantine lifted." *Middletown Transcript* (DE), Oct 26, 1918.
4. "Police restrict liquor business." *Evening Journal* (Wilmington, DE), Oct 31, 1918.
5. "Schools closed by the influenza." *Morning News* (Wilmington, DE), Nov 23, 1918.
6. "A matter of life and death." *Evening Journal* (Wilmington, DE), Jul 31, 1919.
7. "Flu causes the public schools to be closed." *Maryland Gazette* (Annapolis), Oct 3, 1918; "County schools closed today." *Maryland Gazette* (Annapolis), Oct 9, 1918.
8. "Drastic action is taken today." *Maryland Gazette* (Annapolis), Oct 11, 1918; "No church tomorrow." *Baltimore Sun* (MD), Oct 12, 1918; "Flu cuts store hours." *Baltimore Sun* (MD), Oct 10, 1918.

9. "Dr. Welch may lift ban by week's end." *Maryland Gazette* (Annapolis), Oct 23, 1918; "The ban is lifted." *Maryland Gazette* (Annapolis), Oct 24, 1918; "Schools do not open on Monday." *Maryland Gazette* (Annapolis), Oct 26, 1918.
10. "Wear a mask against the flu." *Evening Capital* (Annapolis, MD), Sep 30, 1918.
11. "Twenty thousand influenza masks wanted." *Baltimore Sun* (MD), Oct 2, 1918.
12. "Flu prevention and treatment." *Evening Sun* (Baltimore, MD), Oct 8, 1918.
13. "Flu cuts store hours." *Baltimore Sun* (MD), Oct 10, 1918.
14. "Saloons restricted; Laurel races to end." *Baltimore Sun* (MD), Oct 12, 1918.
15. "Blake lifts last of influenza bans." *Evening Sun* (Baltimore, MD), Nov 6, 1918.
16. "Warns of Spanish flu." *Baltimore Sun* (MD), Sep 14, 1918.
17. "Combat influenza by use of masks." *Evening Star* (Washington, D.C.), Sep 25, 1918.
18. "29,002 cases Spanish flu army's report." *Washington Herald* (Washington, D.C.), Sep 26, 1918.
19. "Gas masks on phones to ward off influenza." *Evening Star* (Washington, D.C.), Oct 8, 1918.
20. "Outdoor meetings barred in effort to stop influenza." *Evening Star* (Washington, D.C.), Oct 9, 1918.
21. "Churchless and gasolineless." *Evening Star* (Washington, D.C.), Oct 11, 1918.
22. "D.C. deaths fall to 65 in today's influenza report." *Evening Star* (Washington, D.C.), Oct 12, 1918; "65 die of influenza here." *Washington Herald* (Washington, D.C.), Oct 13, 1918.
23. "Influenza deaths 78 in 24 hours." *Evening Star* (Washington, D.C.), Oct 15, 1918.
24. "Postmaster Chance among mask-wearers." *Evening Star* (Washington, D.C.), Oct 15, 1918.
25. "83 deaths in day from influenza." *Evening Star* (Washington, D.C.), Oct 16, 1918.
26. "All at capital don influenza masks." *New York Sun*, Oct 16, 1918.
27. Ad. *Evening Star* (Washington, D.C.), Oct 18, 1918.
28. "The Ku Klux Klan comes to town." *Brooklyn Eagle* (NY), Oct 20, 1918.
29. "Epidemic forces drastic action." *Times-Dispatch* (Richmond, VA); Oct 6, 1918.
30. "Close all fairs during epidemic." *Times-Dispatch* (Richmond, VA), Oct 9, 1918.
31. "Close warehouses to curb influenza." *Times-Dispatch* (Richmond, VA), Oct 15, 1918.
32. "Boards of health advise." *Times-Dispatch* (Richmond, VA), Oct 31, 1918; "Medical men protest lifting epidemic ban." *Times-Dispatch* (Richmond, VA), Nov 1, 1918.
33. "Will quarantine city tomorrow." *Alexandria Gazette* (VA), Oct 3, 1918.
34. "To check disease." *Alexandria Gazette* (VA), Oct 5, 1918.
35. "Masks against flu." *Alexandria Gazette* (VA), Oct 18, 1918.
36. "Epidemic is over." *Alexandria Gazette* (VA), Oct 31, 1918.
37. "Grippe situation now well in hand." *Times-Dispatch* (Richmond, VA), Oct 11, 1918.
38. "Influenza toll may be swelled by bad weather." *Virginian Pilot* (Norfolk), Oct 4, 1918.
39. "Soda fountains will be closed." *Virginian Pilot* (Norfolk), Oct 8, 1918.
40. "Urges use of masks to curb influenza." *Times-Dispatch* (Richmond, VA), Oct 9, 1918.
41. "Members of board must wear gauze masks." *Times-Dispatch* (Richmond, VA), Oct 11, 1918.
42. "Face masks worn in office of local draft board." *Daily News Leader* (Staunton, VA), Oct 12, 1918.
43. "Flu defense is up before state health officers." *Virginian Pilot* (Norfolk), Sep 14, 1919.
44. "Jepson issues order." *Wheeling Intelligencer* (WV), Oct 7, 1918.
45. "Health board acts." *West Virginian* (Fairmont), Oct 7, 1918; "Closing order complied with." *West Virginian* (Fairmont), Oct 8, 1918.
46. "Must quarantine influenza cases." *West Virginian* (Fairmont), Oct 9, 1918.
47. "Lid to be shut tighter." *West Virginian* (Fairmont), Oct 28, 1918; "Flu quarantine will be lifted." *West Virginian* (Fairmont), Nov 6, 1918.
48. "Charleston people wear gauze masks." *West Virginian* (Fairmont), Oct 17, 1918.
49. "The influenza still with us." *Shepherdstown Register* (WV), Oct 24, 1918.
50. "Charlotte streets take on Sabbath appearance." *Charlotte Observer* (NC), Oct 5, 1918.
51. "Lumberton lifts flu quarantine." *Wilmington Morning Star* (NC), Oct 16, 1918.
52. "Spanish influenza quarantine." *Lenoir Topic* (NC), Oct 18, 1918; "County is quarantined against Spanish flu." *Lenoir Topic* (NC), Oct 25, 1918.
53. "Influenza quarantine air tight here." *Kings Mountain Herald* (NC), Oct 24, 1918.
54. "Resolution in favor of influenza quarantine." *Winston-Salem Journal* (NC), Oct 29, 1918.
55. "Influenza quarantine to be lifted Thursday." *Charlotte Observer* (NC), Nov 4, 1918.
56. "Flu quarantine." *News of Henderson County* (Hendersonville, NC), Dec 24, 1918.
57. "Flu quarantine on again at Statesville." *News and Observer* (Raleigh, NC), Jan 13, 1919; "Flu ban at Statesville." *Charlotte Observer* (NC), Feb 14, 1919; "Asheville influenza quarantine raised." *Journal and Tribune* (Knoxville, TN), Feb 13, 1919.
58. "Over 175 cases of influenza." *Charlotte News* (NC), Oct 3, 1918.
59. "Influenza masks made for the local doctors." *Greensboro Daily News* (NC), Oct 10, 1918.
60. "Albemarle citizens may be forced to wear masks." *Charlotte Observer* (NC), Oct 13, 1918.
61. "Flu masks for bond captains." *Charlotte Observer* (NC), Oct 15, 1918.
62. "Local and otherwise." *Concord Tribune* (NC), Oct 16, 1918.

63. "Decrease in flu is noted." *Charlotte News* (NC), Oct 16, 1918.
64. "Adult appearances suggest Halloween." *Asheville Citizen-Times* (NC), Oct 16, 1918.
65. "Ten commandments for the prevention of flu." *News and Observer* (Raleigh, NC), Oct 21, 1918.
66. "Mask against influenza." *Daily Free Press* (Kinston, NC), Nov 4, 1918.
67. "Quarantine over state is ordered." *Greenville News* (SC), Oct 8, 1918.
68. "State board put quarantine on city and county." *Greenville News* (SC), Oct 8, 1918.
69. "Extends flu quarantine." *Watchman & Southron* (Sumter, SC), "Epidemic in Marion." *Sumter Item* (SC), Jan 20, 1919; "Flu quarantine is lifted at Woodruff." *Greenville News* (SC), Feb 7, 1918.
70. "Request to all ladies." *Sumter Daily Item* (SC), Oct 5, 1918.
71. "Influenza situation has improved notably, cases on decrease." *Greenville News* (SC), Oct 12, 1918.
72. "Spartanburg folk wearing face masks." *The State* (Columbia, SC), Oct 16, 1918.
73. "Must change face mask." *Evening Herald* (Rock Hill, SC), Oct 17, 1918.
74. "Hooded Terrors." *Abbeville Press and Banner* (SC), Oct 18, 1918.
75. "Flu epidemic spreads." *Watchman & Southron* (Sumter, SC), Oct 19, 1918.
76. "The flu situation serious." *Keowee Courier* (Pickens, SC), Oct 23, 1918.
77. "Weapons against influenza." *Greenville Daily News* (SC), Dec 7, 1918.
78. "What made the epidemic of Spanish influenza so deadly." *Columbia Record* (SC), Dec 14, 1918.
79. "Influenza cards on many homes." *The State* (Columbia, SC), Jan 26, 1919.
80. "Public gathering places closed." *Atlanta Constitution* (GA), Oct 8, 1918.
81. "Reports on flu in state received." *Atlanta Constitution* (GA), Oct 20, 1918.
82. "Happy Atlantans throng theaters." *Atlanta Constitution* (GA), Oct 27, 1918.
83. "Flu quarantine in Augusta." *Washington Herald* (Washington, D.C.), Jan 12, 1918; "Augusta to lift flu ban Saturday." *Atlanta Constitution* (GA), Jan 30, 1919.
84. "Gauze masks to be worn by people as safeguard." *Americus Times-Recorder* (GA), Oct 15, 1918.
85. "More steps to down the flu." *Columbus Ledger* (GA), Oct 20, 1918.
86. "Wear masks—keep off the flu." *Columbus Enquirer-Sun* (GA), Oct 20, 1918.
87. "Reports on flu in state received." *Atlanta Constitution* (GA), Oct 20, 1918.
88. "Flu mask order for Georgia fairs." *Macon Daily Telegraph* (GA), Oct 15, 1918.
89. "Nurses are wanted to help fight flu." *Macon Daily Telegraph* (GA), Oct 15, 1918.
90. "Flu masks in use by local firm." *Macon News* (GA), Oct 15, 1918.
91. "Theaters to come under mask order." *Macon Daily Telegraph* (GA), Oct 17, 1918.
92. "No federal court account of flu." *Macon Daily Telegraph* (GA), Oct 18, 1918.
93. "Children in schools to wear flu masks." *Atlanta Constitution* (GA), Oct 19, 1918.
94. "Hello girls wearing masks." *Macon Daily Telegraph* (GA), Oct 20, 1918.
95. "Flu masks scorned by councilmen, but session is brief." *Macon News* (GA), Oct 23, 1918.
96. "Slight increase in new flu cases." *Macon Daily Telegraph* (GA), Oct 30, 1918.
97. "Inspector asks suspension of flu mask fines." *Macon News* (GA), Nov 6, 1918.
98. "Macon discards masks Wednesday." *Macon News* (GA), Nov 6, 1918.
99. "Camilla lifts influenza ban." *Macon News* (GA), Dec 29, 1918; "Sandersville to re-open schools." *Macon News* (GA), Dec 29, 1918.
100. "100,000 influenza masks are needed." *Atlanta Constitution*, Oct 4, 1918.
101. "Spanish influenza not epidemic here." *Atlanta Constitution*, Oct 10, 1918.
102. "Awards announced at great exhibits at Lakewood Fair." *Atlanta Constitution*, Oct 16, 1918.
103. "Grand jury to hold sessions in flu masks." *Atlanta Constitution*, Oct 24, 1918.
104. "A.B. & A. mechanics strike because flu mask rule." *Atlanta Constitution*, Oct 27, 1918.
105. "As precaution close all public places." *Orlando Sentinel* (FL), Oct 8, 1918.
106. "Influenza checked." *Orlando Sentinel* (FL), Oct 18, 1918.
107. "Tampa acts to head off epidemic here." *Tampa Times* (FL), Oct 8, 1918.
108. "Nurses needed to handle flu." *Tampa Times* (FL), Oct 19, 1918; "Tampa schools open Monday." *Orlando Evening Star* (FL), Nov 7, 1918.
109. "Influenza is waning here." *Miami Herald* (FL), Oct 9, 1918.
110. "Mandatory order issued by city board of health." *Miami Herald* (FL), Oct 10, 1918.
111. "Mayor issues a drastic order." *Miami Herald* (FL), Oct 22, 1918.
112. "Normal hours of business be observed." *Miami Herald* (FL), Oct 27, 1918.
113. "The lid will be lifted Friday." *Miami Herald* (FL), Oct 31, 1918.
114. "Winter Park news item." *Orlando Sentinel* (FL), Oct 11, 1918.
115. "Jacksonville is much improved." *Tampa Bay Times* (St. Petersburg, FL), Oct 25, 1918.
116. "Influenza mask worn by Boston police." *Miami News* (FL), Oct 18, 1918.
117. "Tampa Electric Co., take precautions." *Tampa Times* (FL), Oct 19, 1918.
118. "Deaths fewer but number of new cases grows." *Tampa Tribune* (FL), Oct 20, 1918.
119. "Spanish influenza cases have jumped." *Tampa Tribune* (FL), Oct 21, 1918.

120. "Rotarians are enforcing rules." *Tampa Tribune* (FL), Oct 22, 1918.
121. "Safety first!" *Tampa Times* (FL), Nov 5, 1918.
122. "Plan a program for flu fight." *Tampa Times* (FL), Dec 12, 1918.
123. "Quarantine and use of masks ridiculed as flu preventives." *Tampa Tribune* (FL), Dec 13, 1918.
124. "Influenza precepts reviewed by the State Board of Health." *Tampa Times* (FL), Jan 17, 1919.

Chapter 6

1. "All public places in Selma to be closed." *Montgomery Advertiser* (AL), Oct 10, 1918; "Teachers may be paid during the epidemic." *Montgomery Advertiser* (AL), Oct 26, 1918.
2. "Violates flu rule, pays fine." *Montgomery Advertiser* (AL), Oct 29, 1918.
3. "Ban lifted and shows will open." *Birmingham News* (AL), Oct 29, 1918.
4. "Gypsy Smith from trenches." *Montgomery Advertiser* (AL), Nov 1, 1918; "Many schools in state re-opened." *Montgomery Advertiser* (AL), Nov 5, 1918.
5. "Mass meeting is urged." *Montgomery Advertiser* (AL), Dec 7, 1918; "Further agitation of flu ban." *Montgomery Advertiser* (AL), Dec 10, 1918.
6. "Steps taken to check disease." *Roanoke Leader* (AL), Oct 23, 1918.
7. "Dr. Grote makes statement." *Huntsville Times* (AL), Dec 15, 1918.
8. "Death claims 10 more influenza victims in city." *Birmingham News* (AL), Oct 10, 1918.
9. "Mask precautions advised for city." *Birmingham News* (AL), Dec 6, 1918.
10. "Schools should not be closed." *Birmingham News* (AL), Dec 7, 1918.
11. "Bound and gagged?—No, she is warding off influenza." *Birmingham News* (AL), Dec 8, 1918.
12. "Compulsory wearing of masks considered." *Birmingham News* (AL), Dec 10, 1918.
13. "Medicos vote to back health man." *Birmingham News* (AL), Dec 10, 1918.
14. "Hornady declares that masks must be worn for protection." *Birmingham News* (AL), Dec 15, 1918.
15. "Jackson closes churches." *Jackson News* (MS), Oct 8, 1918.
16. "No occasion for alarm." *Star Herald* (Kosciusko, MS), Oct 18, 1918.
17. "Flu quarantine may be lifted in 10 days." *Jackson News* (MS), Oct 21, 1918.
18. "Jackson to remain closed for a week." *Jackson News* (MS), Oct 25, 1918; "Flu ban wholly lifted in county." *Jackson News* (MS), Oct 8, 1918.
19. "Must wear flu masks." *Natchez Democrat* (MS), Oct 19, 1918.
20. "Uncle Sam's advice on flu." *Daily Herald* (Biloxi, MS), Oct 15, 1918.
21. "No cause for alarm." *Jackson Daily News* (MS), Dec 13, 1918.
22. "State board's influenza advice." *Greenville Sun* (TN), Oct 8, 1918.
23. "Flu epidemic is spreading here." *Knoxville Sentinel* (TN), Oct 9, 1918.
24. "Sanitary campaign on to stop influenza." *Chattanooga News* (TN), Oct 9, 1918.
25. "Nashville ban lifted." *Knoxville Sentinel* (TN), Oct 30, 1918; "Flu quarantine proves failure." *Tennessean* (Nashville, TN), Dec 8, 1918.
26. "Flu ban is lifted." *Knoxville Sentinel* (TN), Feb 3, 1919.
27. "Influenza masks have appeared in Knoxville." *Journal and Tribune* (Knoxville, TN), Oct 16, 1918.
28. "Four simple rules for combating influenza." *Knoxville Sentinel* (TN), Mar 21, 1919.
29. "How well do you know friends." *Knoxville Sentinel* (TN), Jan 18, 1919.
30. "Look like gas masks." *Chattanooga News* (TN), Oct 10, 1918.
31. "Thousands of gauze masks doing service." *Chattanooga News* (TN), Oct 11, 1918.
32. "Three thousand masks needed immediately." *Chattanooga News* (TN), Oct 11, 1918.
33. "Day off for the barbers." *Chattanooga Daily Times* (TN), Oct 12, 1918.
34. Ad. *Chattanooga News* (TN), Oct 16, 1918.
35. "Influenza is subsiding." *Chattanooga Daily Times* (TN), Oct 17, 1918.
36. "Market house merchants shy at gauze masks." *Chattanooga Daily Times* (TN), Oct 18, 1918.
37. "Combating influenza." *Chattanooga Daily Times* (TN), Dec 11, 1918.
38. "Must close." *Kentucky Advocate* (Danville, KY), Oct 7, 1918.
39. "Flu quarantine is modified." *Public Ledger* (Maysville, KY), Nov 7, 1918.
40. "Influenza quarantine." *Courier-Journal* (Louisville, KY), Dec 2, 1918.
41. "Heard about town." *Richmond Register* (KY), Jan 7, 1919.
42. "Fine Taylor $100." *Paducah Sun-Democrat* (KY), Jan 29, 1919.
43. "Influenza situation looks unpromising." *Bourbon News* (Paris, KY), Oct 22, 1918.
44. "Timely warning given by health officer Locke." *Public Ledger* (Maysville, KY), Oct 23, 1918.
45. "When doctors disagree." *Messenger-Inquirer* (Owensboro, KY), Dec 15, 1918.
46. "The influenza mask." *Courier-Journal* (Louisville, KY), Oct 29, 1918.
47. "Many are wearing influenza masks." *Vicksburg Evening Post* (MS), Oct 1, 1918.
48. "4 more deaths, 17 new cases." *Lexington Herald* (KY), Nov 2, 1918; "3,000 wear masks at football game." *Birmingham News* (KY), Nov 3, 1918.

Chapter 7

1. "Clamp lid on Orleans." *Shreveport Times* (LA), Oct 10, 1918; "Take steps to halt influenza." *Shreveport Times* (LA), Oct 8, 1918.
2. No title. *Shreveport Journal* (LA), Nov 5, 1918.

3. "Ban on all public meetings." *Shreveport Journal* (LA), Nov 7, 1918.
4. "Phone operators now wear masks on job." *Shreveport Times* (LA), Oct 24, 1918.
5. "Women urged to wear masks." *Shreveport Times* (LA), Oct 21, 1918.
6. "Modify store closing orders at Monroe." *Shreveport Times* (LA), Oct 22, 1918.
7. "Flu masks are doomed." *Town Talk* (Alexandria, LA), Oct 29, 1918.
8. "Flu masks go on what-not shelf." *Shreveport Times* (LA), Nov 15, 1918.
9. "Drastic statewide quarantine order." *Arkansas Democrat* (Little Rock), Oct 7, 1918.
10. "City put under strict quarantine." *Fayetteville Democrat* (AR), October 9, 1918.
11. "Quarantine rules to be lifted here Monday." *Arkansas Democrat* (Little Rock), Oct 30, 1918; "All quarantine rules to be lifted Sunday." *Arkansas Democrat* (Little Rock), Oct 31, 1918.
12. "State will not be quarantine for flu." *Arkansas Democrat* (Little Rock), Jan 20, 1919.
13. "Flu under control." *Daily Arkansas Gazette* (Little Rock), Oct 21, 1918.
14. "Warns against needless travel." *Daily Arkansas Gazette* (Little Rock), Nov 27, 1918.
15. "More influenza cases in state." *Daily Arkansas Gazette* (Little Rock), Jan 20, 1919.
16. "Statewide quarantine ordered by Dr. Duke." *Guthrie Leader* (OK), Oct 10, 1918.
17. "Picture shows ordered closed." *Ardmoreite* (Ardmore, OK), Oct 10, 1918.
18. "Teachers will get full pay." *Chickasha Express* (OK), Oct 24, 1918.
19. "Nov 11 date of opening." *Oklahoma News* (Oklahoma City), Nov 2, 1918; "Influenza quarantine to continue." *Woodward News-Bulletin* (OK), Oct 25, 1918; "Influenza quarantine to be raised Saturday." *Chandler Tribune* (OK), Nov 7, 1918.
20. "Wear ward masks." *Muskogee Times-Democrat* (OK), Oct 9, 1918.
21. "Spanish influenza—three-day fever, the flu." *Muskogee Times-Democrat* (OK), Oct 17, 1918.
22. "Dr. Clinton tells about best mask." *Tulsa Democrat* (OK), Nov 3, 1918.
23. "Not to close city says mayor." *Tulsa Daily World* (OK), Dec 14, 1918.
24. "Donnelly advises using flu masks." *Oklahoma City Times*, Nov 21, 1918.
25. "To the citizenship of Clinton." *Custer County Chronicle* (Clinton, OK), Dec 5, 1918.
26. No title. *Clinton Messenger* (OK), Dec 12, 1918.
27. "Flu masks abolished." *Clinton Messenger* (OK), Dec 19, 1918.
28. "Combating influenza." *Laredo Times* (TX), Oct 12, 1918.
29. "Austin shuts all its public places." *Austin American* (TX), Oct 9, 1918; "City puts ban on funerals." *El Paso Times* (TX), Oct 9, 1918; "Influenza closes Travis County." *Austin American* (TX), Oct 12, 1918; https://www.statista.com/statistics/189959/housing-units-with-telephones. Accessed Jan 11, 2023.
30. "Close schools another week." *El Paso Herald* (TX), Oct 12, 1918.
31. "Influenza quarantine ended." *Houston Post* (TX), Oct 26, 1918; "School attendance is 10 per cent less." *Fort Worth Star Telegram* (TX), Oct 30, 1918.
32. "Amarillo quarantines against influenza." *Fort Worth Star Telegram* (TX), Oct 23, 1918.
33. "Influenza encyclopedia. San Antonio." https://influenzaarchive.org. Accessed Dec 20, 2023.
34. "They're wearing gas masks in El Paso." *El Paso Times* (TX), Oct 6, 1918.
35. "Barbers may wear flu masks." *Marshall Messenger* (TX), Dec 20, 1918.
36. "Hutchinson says wearing masks is way to curb flu." *Fort Worth Star Telegram* (TX), Dec 11, 1918.

Chapter 8

1. "Shows to run, churches open." *Detroit Free Press*, Oct 13, 1918.
2. "Public places not to be closed yet." *Detroit Free Press*, Oct 16, 1918.
3. "State grip decree closes up Detroit." *Detroit Free Press*, Oct 19, 1918.
4. "Detroit obeys influenza ban." *Detroit Free Press*, Oct 21, 1918; "Schools close as influenza plague gains." *Detroit Free Press*, Oct 22, 1918.
5. "City extends closing hour." *Detroit Free Press*, Oct 23, 1918; "All schools will reopen Monday." *Detroit Free Press*, Oct 30, 1918.
6. "Drastic steps are taken by officials." *Port Huron Times-Herald* (MI), Oct 22, 1918.
7. "Quarantine against flu." *Herald-Press* (St. Joseph, MI), Dec 10, 1918; "Influenza quarantine is in effect." *Herald-Press* (St. Joseph, MI), Dec 11, 1918.
8. "Ban is lifted." *Diamond Drill* (Crystal Falls, MI), Jan 11, 1919.
9. "City extends closing order." *Detroit Free Press*, Oct 23, 1918; "Drastic steps are taken by officials." *Port Huron Times-Herald* (MI), Oct 22, 1918.
10. "To confer on state closing." *Lansing State Journal* (MI), Oct 18, 1918.
11. "Control is near here." *Lansing State Journal* (MI), Oct 23, 1918.
12. "Four maskless men are nipped." *Escanaba Morning Press* (MI), Dec 8, 1918; "Masks off Wednesday." *Escanaba Morning Press* (MI), Dec 10, 1918.
13. "Influenza masks now popular in Kalamazoo." *Battle Creek Enquirer* (MI), Dec 15, 1918.
14. "Some doctors question the efficacy of closing." *Battle Creek Enquirer* (MI), Dec 13, 1918.
15. "Chiffon veil gas mask for sneeze." *Detroit Free Press*, Oct 16, 1918.
16. "Face masks worn by draft board." *Detroit Free Press*, Oct 19, 1918.

17. "Face mask need urged on women." *Detroit Free Press*, Oct 22, 1918.
18. Ad. *Detroit Free Press*, Oct 25, 1918.
19. "Sterilize mask every two hours." *Detroit Free Press*, Oct 27, 1918.
20. "Influenza gain not alarming." *Detroit Free Press*, Dec 7, 1918.
21. "Health board issues rigid closing order." *Mansfield News* (OH), Oct 7, 1918.
22. "The exercise of vigilance." *Mansfield News* (OH), Oct 8, 1918.
23. "One as dangerous as other." *Mansfield News* (OH), Oct 9, 1918.
24. "A wide-spread closing order." *Mansfield News* (OH), Oct 11, 1918.
25. "Cleveland is now under quarantine." *Akron Beacon Journal* (OH), Oct 14, 1918.
26. "City enforces closing order." *Evening Review* (East Liverpool, OH), Oct 21, 1918.
27. "Police prosecutor gets names." *Akron Beacon Journal* (OH), Oct 22, 1918.
28. "Restrictions on the flu quarantine tightened." *Chillicothe Gazette* (OH), Oct 24, 1918.
29. "Toledo lifts quarantine." *Cincinnati Enquirer* (OH), Nov 2, 1918.
30. "Springfield lifts the influenza ban." *Mansfield News* (OH), Nov 1, 1918.
31. "Cleveland's influenza." *Mansfield News* (OH), Nov 5, 1918; "Youngstown lifts ban." *Mansfield News* (OH), Nov 14, 1918.
32. "Lift flu ban soon is plan." *News Journal* (Mansfield, OH), Nov 6, 1918.
33. "Cincinnati schools." *Mansfield News* (OH), Dec 2, 1918; "Marion may wear masks." *Mansfield News* (OH), Dec 16, 1918; "All Marion people at sixes and sevens." *Mansfield News* (OH), Dec 20, 1918.
34. "Possibly flu ban lifted next week." *Bucyrus Evening Telegraph* (OH), Dec 18, 1918; "Ohio happenings." *Marysville Journal Tribune* (OH), Dec 19, 1918.
35. "Crowding banned by health board." *Lima Republican Gazette* (OH), Dec 19, 1918.
36. "Dame rumor." *Coshocton Tribune* (OH), Nov 17, 1918; "Plague holds entire county in its grip." *Coshocton Tribune* (OH), Nov 17, 1918.
37. "Post office clerks wearing flu masks." *Coshocton Tribune* (OH), Nov 18, 1918.
38. "Flu situation is not yet improved." *Coshocton Tribune* (OH), Nov 19, 1918.
39. "Keep will!" *Cincinnati Enquirer* (OH), Oct 4, 1918.
40. "Burton advises influenza mask." *Lima Republican Gazette* (OH), Nov 5, 1918.
41. "Quarantine will not stop flu, doctor declares." *Lima Republican Gazette* (OH), Dec 11, 1918.
42. "Lima to wear muzzles." *Lima Republican Gazette* (OH), Dec 12, 1918.
43. "City in disguise ventures abroad in gauze masks." *Lima Republican Gazette* (OH), Dec 13, 1918.
44. "Masks in church Sunday program." *Lima Republican Gazette* (OH), Dec 13, 1918.
45. "Make it universal." *Lima Times Democrat* (OH), Dec 13, 1918.
46. "Board of health changes mask order." *Lima Times Democrat* (OH), Dec 13, 1918.
47. "Masked nabobs dine and smoke at club." *Lima Republican Gazette* (OH), Dec 14, 1918.
48. "Forty-six violators of flu mask order." *Lima Times Democrat* (OH), Dec 16, 1918.
49. "Flu mask order stands." *Lima Republican Gazette* (OH), Dec 17, 1918.
50. "Doctors oppose wearing of flu masks in public." *Lima Republican Gazette* (OH), Dec 18, 1918.
51. "Dance ban must stay, says board." *Lima Republican Gazette* (OH), Dec 22, 1918.
52. "Epidemic closes public places." *Indianapolis Star*, Oct 7, 1918.
53. "Health rule on flue likely for 10 days." *Indianapolis Star*, Oct 9, 1918.
54. "Ban placed on state." *Indianapolis Star*, Oct 10, 1918.
55. "New hours for retail stores." *Indianapolis Star*, Oct 14, 1918.
56. "City flu order off tomorrow." *Indianapolis Star*, Oct 30, 1918.
57. "State flu ban will be lifted." *Indianapolis Star*, Nov 1, 1918.
58. "Strict influenza quarantine." *Bedford Mail* (IN), Nov 21, 1918.
59. "14 theater men arrested at Terre Haute." *Indianapolis Star*, Nov 29, 1918.
60. "Flu masks must be worn here." *Brazil Times* (IN), Nov 19, 1918.
61. "Flu mask order now effective." *Brazil Times* (IN), Nov 20, 1918.
62. "Flu masks must be worn by all." *Brazil Times* (IN), Nov 25, 1918.
63. "Flu masks must be worn." *Indianapolis Star*, Nov 19, 1918.
64. "Opposes waring of flu masks by public." *South Bend Tribune* (IN), Nov 20, 1918.
65. "Parents urged to keep their children home." *Republic* (Columbus, IN), Nov 20, 1918.
66. "Newcastle to don masks." *Star Press* (Muncie, IN), Nov 21, 1918.
67. "Linthicum advises influenza masks." *Evansville Press* (IN), Nov 22, 1918.
68. "Health board discusses flu." *Evansville Press* (IN), Nov 22, 1918.
69. "More flu masks worn." *Tribune* (Seymour, IN), Nov 23, 1918.
70. Ad. *Fort Wayne Journal Gazette* (IN), Oct 16, 1918.
71. "Must wear flu masks." *Fort Wayne Sentinel* (IN), Dec 3, 1918.
72. "Increase of influenza brings appeal to public." *Fort Wayne Journal Gazette* (IN), Dec 5, 1918.
73. "Mask order is issued." *Huntington Herald* (IN), Dec 10, 1918.
74. "A proclamation by the mayor." *Muncie Evening Press* (IN), Oct 24, 1918.
75. "The influenza masks and treatment." *Muncie Evening Press* (IN), Nov 22, 1918.

76. "The saving grace of common sense." *Muncie Evening News* (IN), Dec 16, 1918.
77. "Doctors disagree on influenza issue." *Logansport Pharos-Tribune* (IN), Dec 17, 1918.
78. "Theaters join fight on flu infection." *Indianapolis Star*, Sep 29, 1918.
79. "Flu masks must be worn." *Indianapolis Star*, Nov 19, 1918.
80. "Board prepares to enforce flu mask wearing." *Indianapolis Star*, Nov 20, 1918.
81. "Order to close schools stands." *Indianapolis News*, Nov 20, 1918.
82. "No mask; pinched." *Indianapolis Star*, Nov 21, 1918.
83. "Flu drops off." *Indianapolis Star*, Nov 21, 1918.
84. "Co-operation, not criticism, needed." *Indianapolis Star*, Nov 22, 1918.
85. "Few churches plan services." *Indianapolis Star*, Nov 23, 1918.
86. "249 new cases show increase." *Indianapolis Star*, Nov 23, 1918.
87. "Mask order will remain in effect." *Indianapolis News*, Nov 23, 1918.
88. "Flu mask order stands." *Indianapolis Star*, Nov 24, 1918.
89. "Board rescinds the mask order." *Indianapolis Star*, Nov 25, 1918.
90. "Health rules." *Indianapolis News*, Nov 25, 1918.
91. "Wear masks at Bedford." *Indianapolis News*, Nov 1, 1918; "Masks off at Newcastle." *Indianapolis News*, Nov 22, 1918; "Flu mask order is off." *Indianapolis Star*, Nov 24, 1918.
92. "All flu cases quarantined." *Chicago Tribune*, Oct 1, 1918.
93. "Theaters and movies closed." *Chicago Tribune*, Oct 15, 1918.
94. "Flu quarantine to become stricter." *Journal Gazette* (Mattoon, IL), Oct 16, 1918.
95. "Theaters downstate warned not to open." *Decatur Herald* (IL), Nov 1, 1918.
96. "Flu lid come entirely off in city tomorrow." *Chicago Tribune*, Nov 3, 1918.
97. "Quarantine ends here late Friday." *Decatur Herald* (IL), Nov 7, 1918.
98. "Quarantine rules are slackened here." *Streator Times* (IL), Dec 13, 1918.
99. "Influenza mask is proposed in Chicago." *Champaign News* (IL), Sep 27, 1918.
100. "Masks are worn." *Oshkosh Northwestern* (WI), Oct 2, 1918.
101. "Wearing gas masks in Chicago." *Chicago Tribune*, Oct 2, 1918; "Germ screen." *Chicago Tribune*, Oct 6, 1918.
102. "Reynolds calls face mask best epidemic check." *Chicago Tribune*, Oct 18, 1918.
103. "Health experts plan great war on influenza." *Chicago Tribune*, Dec 11, 1918.
104. "Jury to pass on masks and lid in fighting flu." *Chicago Tribune*, Dec 13, 1918.
105. "Experts tell how to combat flu." *Chicago Tribune*, Dec 14, 1918.

106. "Schools, churches, theaters and dance halls." *Racine Journal-News* (WI), Oct 5, 1918.
107. "Business not to be disturbed." *Racine Journal-News* (WI), Oct 7, 1918.
108. "Philipp may issue sweeping order." *Racine Journal-News* (WI), Oct 10, 1918.
109. "Closing order is extended." *Racine Journal-News* (WI), Oct 18, 1918.
110. "Doctors ask board to close saloons." *Racine Journal-News* (WI), Oct 19, 1918.
111. "Health board decides not to shut saloon." *Racine Journal-News* (WI), Oct 21, 1918.
112. "Schools, churches and theaters to be freed." *Racine Journal-News* (WI), Nov 1, 1918.
113. "Schools, churches, theaters closed." *La Crosse Tribune* (WI), Oct 10, 1918; "1,000 flu cases in Madison." *Wisconsin State Journal* (Madison), Oct 10, 1918; "La Crosse closed up." *Green Bay Press Gazette* (WI), Oct 23, 1918.
114. "Quarantine on epidemic." *Green Bay Press Gazette* (WI), Dec 2, 1918.
115. "Madison adopts flu quarantine." *La Crosse Tribune* (WI), Dec 3, 1918.
116. "Quarantine to be strict." *Stevens Point Journal* (WI), Dec 4, 1918.
117. "Ask that flu masks be used." *Journal Times* (Racine, WI), Oct 8, 1918.
118. "Influenza jump due to exposures threaten masks." *Journal Times* (Racine, WI), Nov 21, 1918.
119. "Quarantine to be strict." *Stevens Point Journal* (WI), Dec 4, 1918.
120. "Wear flu masks board suggests." *Kenosha Evening News* (WI), Dec 7, 1918.
121. "Laundry and factory girls to be masked." *Leader-Telegram* (Eau Claire, WI), Oct 13, 1918.
122. "Flu puts 9 more to bed." *Leader-Telegram* (Eau Claire, WI), Oct 15, 1918.
123. "Health board recommends anti-flu mask." *Leader-Telegram* (Eau Claire, WI), Oct 29, 1918.
124. "Masks as sensible as gum shoes." *Leader-Telegram* (Eau Claire, WI), Oct 30, 1918.
125. "Week begins with fewer flu cases." *Leader-Telegram* (Eau Clair, WI), Nov 19, 1918.

Chapter 9

1. "8 deaths from influenza here." *Star Tribune* (Minneapolis), Oct 9, 1918; "Influenza gains among civilians." *Star Tribune* (Minneapolis), Oct 9, 1918; "Influenza gains slowly in city." *Star Tribune* (Minneapolis), Oct 10, 1918.
2. "Doctors propose drastic lid." *Star Tribune* (Minneapolis), Oct 11, 1918.
3. "City closed to end wave of influenza." *Star Tribune* (Minneapolis), Oct 12, 1918.
4. "Business hours may be changed." *Star Tribune* (Minneapolis), Oct 15, 1918.
5. "Guilford wins fight to keep schools shut." *Star Tribune* (Minneapolis), Oct 22, 1918.
6. "City laughs once more as movies open." *Star Tribune* (Minneapolis), Nov 16, 1918.

7. "Draft boards use masks." Minneapolis Morning Tribune, October 17, 1918.
8. "Winona barbers don flu masks." *Winona News* (MN), Oct 17, 1918; "Nurses wear flu masks." *Winona News* (MN), Oct 24, 1918.
9. "Wear cheese cloth mask." *Winona News* (MN), Oct 17, 1918.
10. "Nurses are masked against influenza." *Minneapolis Journal*, Oct 3, 1918.
11. "Influenza is waning." *Star Tribune* (Minneapolis), Oct 17, 1918.
12. "Opening with masks rejected by movies." *Star Tribune* (Minneapolis), Nov 2, 1918.
13. "St. Paul closed by influenza spread." *Minneapolis Journal*, Nov 4, 1918.
14. "Everything is closed tight by the flu." *Bismarck Tribune* (ND), Oct 9, 1918.
15. "Flu epidemic in Fargo." *Fargo Forum* (ND), Oct 7, 1918; "Fargo is closed tight." *Fargo Forum* (ND), Oct 9, 1918.
16. "Everything is closed tight by the flu." *Bismarck Tribune* (ND), Oct 9, 1918.
17. "Stay at home." *Bismarck Tribune* (ND), Oct 14, 1918.
18. "All Fargo wants a Red Cross face mask." *Fargo Forum* (ND), Oct 9, 1918.
19. "Flu coming back." *Jamestown Alert* (ND), Nov 14, 1918.
20. "Public gatherings in city." *Rapid City Journal* (SD), Oct 8, 1918.
21. "Close all public places but schools." *Argus Leader* (Sioux Falls, SD), Oct 12, 1918.
22. "Holding city well in hand." *Argus Leader* (Sioux Falls, SD), Oct 14, 1918.
23. "Keystone takes drastic measures of prevention." *Rapid City Journal* (SD), Oct 24, 1918.
24. "Quarantine placed in the city." *Rapid City Journal* (SD), Oct 25, 1918.
25. "Town quarantined." *Custer Chronicle* (Custer City, SD), Oct 26, 1918.
26. "All closed places but schools opened." *Rapid City Journal* (SD), Nov 5, 1918; "Quarantine at Gregory lifted." *Rapid City Journal* (SD), Nov 7, 1918.
27. "Remove lid on meetings." *Argus Leader* (Sioux Falls, SD), Nov 27, 1918.
28. "Hot Springs holds up the flu with masks." *Argus Leader* (Sioux Falls, SD), Nov 5, 1918.
29. "Aberdeen people must wear flu masks." *Citizen-Republican* (Scotland, SD), Dec 19, 1918.
30. "Aberdeen debates value flu war." *Argus Leader* (Sioux Falls, SD), Dec 26, 1918.
31. "Influenza conditions better at Aberdeen." *Argus Leader* (Sioux Falls, SD), Dec 30, 1918.
32. "The flu mask." *Weekly Pioneer Times* (Deadwood, SD), Feb 13, 1919.
33. "Quarantine lid goes on at 9 o'clock." *Des Moines Tribune* (IA), Oct 10, 1918.
34. "City placed under plague restrictions." *Muscatine Journal* (IA), Oct 18, 1918.
35. "City closed till state lid lifted." *Des Moines Tribune* (IA), Oct 21, 1918; "Up to each city." *Gate City* (Keokuk, IA), Oct 24, 1918; "Resumes normal activity." *Des Moines Register* (IA), Oct 29, 1918.
36. "Flu quarantine imposed." *Muscatine Journal* (IA), Nov 28, 1918.
37. "Davenport puts on real lid." *Courier* (Waterloo, IA), Dec 11, 1918; "Hampton again puts on influenza quarantine." *Courier* (Waterloo, IA), Dec 21, 1918; "Lid goes on again in Keota." *Times* (Davenport, IA), Dec 21, 1918.
38. "Flu quarantine ordered by state." *Des Moines Register* (IA), Sep 30, 1919.
39. "Barbers wear masks to stop spread of flu." *Daily Times* (Davenport, IA), Oct 18, 1918.
40. "Gauze masks to ward off influenza." *Quad City Times* (Davenport, IA), Oct 18, 1918.
41. "Many flu masks are being worn." *Daily Times* (Davenport, IA), Dec 2, 1918.
42. "Public and parochial schools are ordered closed." *Daily Times* (Davenport, IA), Dec 2, 1918.
43. "Masks become more popular." *Daily Times* (Davenport, IA), Dec 3, 1918.
44. "Wearing flu masks made compulsory." *Quad City Times* (Davenport, IA), Dec 4, 1918.
45. "Immune to influenza." *Sioux City Journal* (IA), Dec 4, 1918.
46. "Use thermometer at M.S." *Sioux City Journal* (IA), Dec 10, 1918.
47. "Flu mask scare is false alarm." *Gate City* (Keokuk, IA). Nov 15, 1918.
48. "Health board orders wearing of flu masks." *Muscatine Journal* (IA), Dec 12, 1918.
49. "Des Moines board of health." *Courier* (Waterloo, IA), Nov 27, 1918.
50. "Flu masks ordered by health board." *Des Moines Register* (IA), Nov 29, 1918.
51. "Flu mask order is modified." *Des Moines Tribune* (IA), Nov 30, 1918.
52. Ibid.
53. "Say flu masks handicap." *Des Moines Register* (IA), Nov 30, 1918.
54. "The face mask." *Des Moines Tribune* (IA), Nov 30, 1918.
55. "Flu mask order is effective tonight." *Des Moines Tribune* (IA), Dec 2, 1918.
56. "Flu mask order is rescinded." *Des Moines Tribune* (IA), Dec 3, 1918.
57. "Theater men to resist mask rule." *Logansport Pharos-Tribune* (IA), Dec 7, 1918.
58. "Wrangle on flu in Des Moines." *Quad City Times* (Davenport, IA), Dec 9, 1918.
59. "Says barbers and dentists should wear flu masks." *Gazette* (Cedar Rapids, IA), Dec 25, 1918.
60. "Schools to be shut because of influenza." *St. Louis Star* (MO), Oct 7, 1918.
61. "Closing order in effect." *St. Louis Star* (M), Oct 8, 1918.
62. "192 new cases of influenza." *St. Louis Star* (MO), Oct 9, 1918.
63. "Limit on trade hours downtown." *St. Louis Star* (MO), Oct 23, 1918; "Officials again refuse to lift influenza ban." *St. Louis Star* (MO), Nov 1, 1918.
64. "Flu closing ban is made more drastic." *St. Louis Star* (MO), Nov 9, 1918; "Flu ban on theaters is to be lifted." *St. Louis Star* (MO), Nov 12, 1918.

65. "760 new flu cases sets high record." *St. Louis Star* (MO), Nov 28, 1918; "Decline in cases." *St. Louis Star* (MO), Dec 20, 1918.
66. "Stop gatherings." *Kansas City Star* (MO), Oct 7, 1918.
67. "Block car crowd order." *Kansas City Star* (MO), Oct 8, 1918.
68. "Lift ban under protest." *Kansas City Star* (MO), Oct 14, 1918.
69. "A drastic ban is on." *Kansas City Star* (MO), Oct 17, 1918.
70. "Epidemic fight goes on." *Kansas City Star* (MO), Oct 20, 1918.
71. "Mayor will lift the ban." *Kansas City Star* (MO), Nov 8, 1918.
72. "Using flu masks." *Daily Democrat Forum* (Maryville, MO), Oct 31, 1918.
73. "May wear masks." *St. Joseph Gazette* (MO), Dec 1, 1918.
74. "Masks on street." *Evening Missourian* (Columbia), Oct 17, 1918.
75. "To re-open Thursday." *Evening Missourian* (Columbia), Oct 28, 1918; "University women make masks." *Evening Missourian* (Columbia), Oct 30, 1918.
76. "Now the influenza mask." *Kansas City Times* (MO), Oct 22, 1918.
77. "Big plants adopt masks." *Kansas City Star* (MO), Oct 22, 1918.
78. "Progress in mask drive." *Kansas City Star* (MO), Oct 23, 1918.
79. "Says physicians regard flu masks as absurd." *St. Louis Star* (MO), Dec 13, 1918.
80. F.H. Collier. "Echoes of the street." *St. Louis Globe Democrat* (MO), Dec 17, 1918.
81. "Flu masks to be worn." *St. Louis Post-Dispatch* (MO), Jan 9, 1919.
82. "Use mask and avoid all crowds, they say." *Evening Missourian* (Columbia), Dec 23, 1918.
83. "No need to close things in Lincoln." *Lincoln Journal Star* (NE), Oct 8, 1918.
84. "Closing order in force in Lincoln." *Lincoln Journal Star* (NE), Oct 12, 1918.
85. "May be necessary to re-establish flu quarantine." *Lincoln Star* (NE), Nov 27, 1918; "Revise flu quarantine." *Albion News* (NE), Nov 28, 1918.
86. "Beatrice business men resent order." *Lincoln Star* (NE), Dec 1, 1918; "New order closes stores and plants." *Beatrice Sun* (NE), Nov 30, 1918.
87. "Board to reconsider drastic order." *Beatrice Sun* (NE), Dec 1, 1918; "Beatrice health board." *Lincoln Star* (NE), Dec 2, 1918.
88. "Short state notes." *Bennet Sun* (NE), Nov 7, 1918; "Flu quarantine to be raised here Friday." *Alliance Herald* (NE), Nov 14, 1918.
89. "Norfolk officials decide on strict flu quarantine." *Lincoln Star* (NE), Dec 14, 1918.
90. "Strict quarantine ordered for flu." *Clearwater Record* (NE), Jan 3, 1919.
91. "Flu quarantine useless." *Lincoln Star* (NE), Dec 27, 1918.
92. "Masks voted out by council." *Custer County Republican* (Broken Bow, NE), Nov 14, 1918.
93. "Manning advises use of influenza masks." *Evening World-Herald* (Omaha, NE), Oct 17, 1918.
94. "Telephone flu mask is latest stroke." *Omaha Evening Bee* (NE), Oct 19, 1918.
95. "Pneumonia wards filled." *Lincoln Journal Star* (NE), Oct 19, 1918.
96. "Epidemic problem puzzling experts." *Lincoln Journal Star* (NE), Dec 17, 1918.
97. "Board advise extreme care." *Elgin Review* (NE), Dec 20, 1918.
98. "Lincoln flu death rate low." *Lincoln Star* (NE), Feb 18, 1919.
99. "Flu is serious." *Topeka State Journal* (KS), Oct 9, 1918.
100. "Flu is spreading." *Topeka State Journal* (KS), Oct 10, 1918; "Close next week." *Topeka State Journal* (KS), Oct 24, 1918; "To lift the lid." *Topeka State Journal* (KS), Oct 30, 1918; "Ends the influenza ban." *Kansas City Star* (MO), Nov 14, 1918.
101. "Courts to pass on validity." *Wichita Eagle* (KS), Nov 30, 1918.
102. "Flu ban on again." *Wichita Eagle* (KS), Dec 1, 1918.
103. "Wichita's flu ban unlawful." *Wichita Eagle* (KS), Dec 1, 1918.
104. "Limit shoppers." *Salina Evening Journal* (KS), Dec 6, 1918.
105. "Wearing anti-flu masks." *Salina Evening Journal* (KS), Oct 31, 1918; No title. *Junction City Union* (KS), Dec 4, 1918.
106. "Fight flu wear a mask." *Concordia Empire* (KS), Dec 5, 1918.
107. "Barbers must wear flu masks." *Lawrence Journal World* (KS), Oct 22, 1918.
108. "K.U. doctor says many flu masks defective." *Topeka Capital* (KS), Oct 29, 1918.
109. "Workers wear flu masks." *Guard* (Council Grove, KS), Oct 22, 1918.
110. "Fair closed." *Wichita Beacon* (KS), Oct 10, 1918.
111. "Must make bids thru a flu mask." *Wichita Beacon* (KS), Oct 22, 1918.
112. "Topeka to wear masks." *Topeka Daily Capital* (KS), Oct 19, 1918.
113. "Closing order to remain in effect." *Topeka Daily Capital* (KS), Oct 25, 1918.
114. "Use more masks." *Topeka State Journal* (KS), Oct 30, 1918; "Influenza ban lifted." *Topeka Capital* (KS), Nov 9, 1918.
115. "Close up again." *Topeka State Journal* (KS), Nov 26, 1918.

Chapter 10

1. "Regulation for control of influenza." *Helena Independent* (MT), Oct 8, 1918.
2. "Flu here and at Bozeman." *Helena Independent* (MT), Oct 17, 1918.
3. "Bozeman saloons get orders to close doors." *Butte Miner* (MT), Oct 26, 1918.
4. "Influenza quarantine in Butte lifted." *Missoulian* (Missoula, MT), Nov 9, 1918; "Missoula

quarantine partly lifted today." *Butte Miner* (MT), Nov 20, 1918; "Butte lifts flu ban on ads." *Great Falls Tribune* (MT), Nov 29, 1918.

5. "Flu epidemic far from over." *Billings Gazette* (MT), Dec 12, 1918.

6. "Little disease prevalent in city." *Billings Gazette* (MT), Dec 14, 1918.

7. "Helena board keeps lid on flu." *Billings Gazette* (MT), Dec 17, 1918.

8. "Flu lid lifted here." *Helena Independent* (MT), Dec 22, 1918; "Influenza quarantine is lifted at Helena." *Great Falls Tribune* (MT), Jan 10, 1919.

9. "Anti-flu masks prove popularity." *Missoulian* (MT), Oct 25, 1918.

10. "Wearing masks grows common." *Great Falls Tribune* (MT), Oct 26, 1918.

11. "Gauze masks not street essential." *Great Falls Tribune* (MT), Oct 29, 1918.

12. "Can go to church and shows if masks are worn." *Great Falls Tribune* (MT), Dec 9, 1918.

13. "Wearing of masks forced upon the residents of Havre." *Great Falls Tribune* (MT), Nov 19, 1918.

14. "Influenza lid is shut down tight in city of Havre." *Great Falls Tribune* (MT), Nov 20, 1918.

15. "Force vaccination upon Havre people." *Great Falls Tribune* (MT), Dec 2, 1918.

16. "Influenza still spreading in county and city." *Butte Miner* (MT), Oct 18, 1918.

17. "Order barbers and clerks to wear flu masks." *Billings Gazette* (MT), Oct 22, 1918; "Closing the penalty for non-compliance." *Butte Miner* (MT), Oct 27, 1918.

18. "City shut down to ward off spread of flu." *Butte Miner* (MT), Nov 30, 1918.

19. "San Francisco and the masks." *Butte Miner* (MT), Dec 1, 1918.

20. Ad. *Independent Record* (Helena, MT), Oct 9, 1918.

21. "Two thousand cases develop at Billings." *Great Falls Tribune* (MT), Oct 24, 1918.

22. "Order extended on places that must be closed." *Independent Record* (Helena, MT), Oct 24, 1918.

23. "Not yet over the flu peak in Helena." *Independent Record* (Helena, MT), Oct 25, 1918.

24. "Flu cases are on increase in Helena." *Independent Record* (Helena, MT), Oct 27, 1918.

25. "Spread of flu in Helena is unabated." *Independent Record* (Helena, MT), Oct 29, 1918.

26. "State flu ban to be lifted." *Independent Record* (Helena, MT), Dec 16, 1918.

27. "Facing hazards bravely." *Independent Record* (Helena, MT), Dec 16, 1918.

28. "Doctors at Chicago meet." *Independent Record* (Helena, MT), Dec 17, 1918.

29. "Influenza closes the university." *Daily Star-Mirror* (Moscow, ID), Oct 21, 1918; "Five victims of Spanish influenza." *Idaho Daily Statesman* (Boise, ID), Oct 27, 1918.

30. "Epidemic gain causes anxiety among officers." *Idaho Daily Statesman* (Boise), Oct 29, 1918; "Everybody must wear flu masks." *Daily Star-Mirror* (Moscow, ID), Oct 30, 1918.

31. Notice. *Idaho Republican* (Blackfoot, ID), Nov 1, 1918; "Further modification of quarantine proclamation." *Idaho Republican* (Blackfoot, ID), Dec 13, 1918.

32. "Flu quarantine is raised in Pocatello." *Salt Lake Tribune*, Dec 22, 1918; "Reopen in January." *Rathdrum Tribune* (ID), Dec 13, 1918; "Idaho state news items." *Rathdrum Tribune* (ID), Jan 3, 1919.

33. "Red Cross asks city officials to warn public." *Idaho Daily Statesman* (Boise), Jan 4, 1919.

34. "Controversy over flu quarantine." *Idaho Republican* (Blackfoot), Jan 14, 1919.

35. "Only two new cases of influenza in Burley." *Herald-Bulletin* (Burley, ID), Jan 31, 1919.

36. "Town board of health rules and regulations." *Northern Herald* (Cody, WY), Oct 23, 1918.

37. "Health officer over zealous." *Wyoming State Journal* (Lander, WY), Oct 25, 1918; "Lander business men refuse to close for influenza quarantine." *Billings Gazette* (MT), Oct 27, 1918.

38. "Influenza quarantine modified at Kemmerer." *Sheridan Enterprise* (WY), Dec 30, 1918; "Stringent rules against epidemic." *Casper Press* (WY), Dec 7, 1918; "Health officer's bulletin." *Wyoming State Journal* (Laramie), Dec 13, 1918; "Schools closed." *Kemmerer Camera* (WY), Mar 26, 1919.

39. "Health officer condemns masks." *Sheridan Post* (WY), Nov 3, 1918.

40. "How you would look in a flu mask." *Wyoming State Tribune* (Cheyenne), Nov 26, 1918.

41. Ad. *Casper Star-Tribune* (WY), Apr 23, 1919.

42. "Order of health dept." *Labor Bulletin* (CO), Oct 12, 1918.

43. "Spanish flu rigid quarantine." *Sentinel* (Grand Junction, CO), Nov 5, 1918.

44. "Teachers will dray pay for flu period." *Sentinel* (Grand Junction, CO), Nov 21, 1918.

45. "Emergency hospital is needed." *Courier* (Fort Collins, CO), Dec 6, 1918.

46. "Local news." *Sentinel* (Grand Junction, CO), Jan 22, 1919.

47. "Vote early." *Sentinel* (Grand Junction, CO), Nov 4, 1918.

48. "Loveland physician dies of influenza." *Sentinel* (Grand Junction, CO), Oct 30, 1918.

49. "Quarantine unnecessary if influenza masks are used." *Arizona Star* (Tucson), Nov 24, 1918; "Flu masks are now ordered to be worn." *Santa Fe New Mexican*, Nov 22, 1918.

50. "Denver wrathy at violations of flu mask order." *Santa Fe New Mexican*, Nov 25, 1918.

51. "Denver theatres and the flu." *Goodwin's Weekly* (Salt Lake City, UT), Nov 30, 1918.

52. "Denver to enforce influenza mask." *El Paso Times* (TX), Nov 27, 1918.

53. "Flu in Denver becomes more alarming." *Courier* (Fort Collins, CO), Nov 29, 1918; "Colorado state news." *Cheyenne Record* (WY), Dec 5, 1918.

54. "Denver fails to obey order." *Star* (Marion, OH), Dec 21, 1918.

55. "Public places closed." *Albuquerque Morning Journal* (NM), Oct 6, 1918.

56. "Not to restore quarantine." *Albuquerque Morning Journal* (NM), Dec 13, 1918.
57. "Quarantine on Spanish flu to be more rigid." *Albuquerque Morning Journal* (NM), Oct 24, 1918.
58. "Flu situation is clearing up." *Albuquerque Morning Journal* (NM), Nov 23, 1918.
59. "Influenza quarantine here ordered raised." *Evening Herald* (Albuquerque, NM), Nov 28, 1918; "Albuquerque Thanksgiving." *Albuquerque Morning Journal* (NM), Dec 1, 1918.
60. No title. *Mountainair Independent* (NM), Nov 7, 1918; "Spanish influenza." *Mountainair Independent* (NM), Nov 7, 1918.
61. "For not wearing masks." *Mountainair Independent* (NM), Nov 14, 1918.
62. "Nation and state gets ready." *Santa Fe New Mexican*, Sep 18, 1919.
63. "Masks, sprays, drugs and vaccines useless." *Santa Fe New Mexican*, Sep 20, 1919.
64. "Des Moines under flu quarantine." *Seattle Star*, Oct 10, 1918.
65. "Condition of influenza in Cache County." *Logan Republican* (UT), Oct 22, 1918.
66. "Influenza regulations which must be obeyed." *Ogden Standard* (UT), Nov 27, 1918.
67. "Salt Lake takes off quarantine." *Ogden Standard* (UT), Dec 7, 1918.
68. "Guards placed to protect Ogden." *Ogden Standard* (UT), Dec 7, 1918.
69. "Jim Chinaman fails to wear a mask and is fined." *Ogden Standard* (UT), Dec 9, 1918.
70. Ad. *Ogden Standard* (UT), Dec 19, 1918.
71. "Flu situation reported today." *Journal* (Logan, UT), Nov 18, 1918.
72. "Flu situation." *Journal* (Logan, UT), Dec 24, 1918.
73. "Influenza epidemic worse at Brigham." *Salt Lake Tribune*, Dec 12, 1918.
74. "Health regulations." *Vernal Express* (UT), Jan 17, 1919.
75. "Wearing flu masks mandatory in Provo." *Salt Lake Telegram*, Oct 19, 1918; "Wearing influenza masks to be made mandatory in Provo." *Salt Lake Telegram*, Nov 19, 1918.
76. "Californians doubt flu mask efficacy." *Salt Lake Telegram*, Nov 23, 1918.
77. "Provo will partially lift flu mask ban." *Provo Post* (UT), Dec 17, 1918.
78. "Utah County lifts ban Dec 27." *Provo Post* (UT), Dec 20, 1918; "Gauze mask order in Provo modified." *Sentinel* (Grand Junction, CO), Dec 20, 1918.
79. "Society girls busy making flu masks." *Deseret News* (Salt Lake City), Oct 18, 1918.
80. "Scouts do good work." *Deseret News* (Salt Lake City), Oct 21, 1918.
81. "Everybody may have to wear mask in fight on influenza." *Deseret News* (Salt Lake City), Oct 24, 1918.
82. "Asks government for 12 nurses." *Salt Lake Tribune*, Oct 25, 1918.
83. "Doctors advise immediate order." *Deseret News* (Salt Lake City), Nov 22, 1918.
84. "Malady continues on the wan in Salt Lake." *Deseret News* (Salt Lake City), Nov 26, 1918.
85. "Flu mask issue up to board of health." *Salt Lake Tribune*, Nov 30, 1918.
86. "Influenza mask menace, Salt Lake experts say." *Salt Lake Tribune*, Dec 3, 1918.
87. "Gauze muzzle is opposed by doctors." *Salt Lake Tribune*, Dec 3, 1918.
88. "This is last day of wearing the mask in Salt Lake City." *Deseret News* (Salt Lake City), Dec 17, 1918.
89. "Influenza." *Ogden Standard* (UT), Oct 14, 1918.
90. "Masks should be seen on streets." *Ogden Standard* (UT), Oct 17, 1918.
91. "Wearing of gauze masks." *Ogden Standard* (UT), Oct 17, 1918.
92. "Checking the influenza." *Ogden Standard* (UT), Oct 23, 1918.
93. "Face masks must be worn by those afflicted." *Ogden Standard* (UT), Oct 26, 1918.
94. "Inspector again advises use of gauze masks." *Ogden Standard* (UT), Nov 19, 1918.
95. "Spanish influenza." *Ogden Standard* (UT), Nov 23, 1918.
96. "Barber forfeits $10 for refusing to wear mask." *Ogden Standard* (UT), Nov 26, 1918.
97. "Influenza regulations." *Ogden Standard* (UT), Nov 28, 1918.
98. "Store people called on to make their own masks." *Ogden Standard* (UT), Nov 29, 1918.
99. "Warning." *Ogden Standard* (UT), Nov 30, 1918.
100. "Clerks in stores, failing to wear masks." *Ogden Standard* (UT), Dec 6, 1918.
101. "This mask bunk." *Goodwin's Weekly* (Salt Lake City), Dec 7, 1918.
102. "Second arrest influenza law." *Arizona Republican* (Phoenix), Oct 27, 1918.
103. "Flu may last all winter." *Arizona Republican* (Phoenix), Oct 28, 1918.
104. No title. *Bisbee Review* (AZ), Nov 1, 1918.
105. No title. *Bisbee Review* (AZ), Nov 6, 1918.
106. "Condition of the quarantine still unsettled." *Bisbee Review* (AZ), Nov 14, 1918.
107. "May close city tight as means to end epidemic." *Arizona Republican* (Phoenix), Nov 18, 1918.
108. "Good effect is noted in fight against flu." *Arizona Republican* (Phoenix), Nov 21, 1918.
109. "Anti-flu rules displease hunter." *Arizona Republican* (Phoenix), Nov 21, 1918.
110. "Flu ban off Friday." *Arizona Republican* (Phoenix), Dec 9, 1918.
111. "Schools are closed." *Arizona Republican* (Phoenix), Jan 6, 1919.
112. "Quarantine goes to dances here." *Bisbee Review* (AZ), Jan 9, 1919.
113. "Masks on people brave influenza." *Bisbee Review* (AZ), Oct 30, 1918.
114. "Grasping for a straw." *Bisbee Review* (AZ), Nov 19, 1918.
115. "Anti-germ mask order." *Arizona Star* (Tucson), Nov 19, 1918.

116. "Let us be consistent." *Tucson Citizen* (AZ), Nov 19, 1918.
117. "Masks de rigeur in public places." *Tucson Citizen* (AZ), Nov 19, 1918.
118. "What is the limit?" *Tucson Citizen* (AZ), Nov 28, 1918.
119. "Masks still required in stores, shows." *Tucson Citizen* (AZ), Dec 3, 1918.
120. "Scores of arrests follow flu mask ordinance." *Arizona Star* (Tucson), Dec 17, 1918.
121. "An exploded theory." *Tucson Citizen* (AZ), Dec 20, 1918.
122. "No decrease in influenza here figures show." *Arizona Republican* (Phoenix), Oct 30, 1918.
123. "May close city tight as means to end epidemic." *Arizona Republican* (Phoenix), Nov 18, 1918.
124. "Must tell why you are on the streets today." *Arizona Republican* (Phoenix), Nov 20, 1918; "Start fight to stamp out the influenza here." *Arizona Republican* (Phoenix), Nov 20, 1918.
125. "Begin manana everyone must wear flu mask." *Arizona Republican* (Phoenix), Nov 26, 1918.
126. "Mask order was obeyed in city by 95 per cent." *Arizona Republican* (Phoenix), Nov 28, 1918; "Thanksgiving offer." *Arizona Republican* (Phoenix), Nov 28, 1918.
127. "First arrests made for not wearing masks." *Arizona Republican* (Phoenix), Nov 30, 1918.
128. "No flu masks need be worn on streets of city." *Arizona Republican* (Phoenix), Dec 3, 1918.
129. "A long visit." *Arizona Republican* (Phoenix), Dec 4, 1918.
130. "To return single no-flu mask fine." *Arizona Republican* (Phoenix), Dec 4, 1918.
131. "Closing ban is barbarism says Dr. Hutchinson." *Arizona Republican* (Phoenix), Dec 11, 1918.
132. "Flu likely to return says health service." *Arizona Republican* (Phoenix), Sep 17, 1919.
133. "Douglas council decides to lift quarantine." *Bisbee Review* (AZ), Dec 15, 1918; "Flu mask enforcement." *Arizona Star* (Tucson), Dec 22, 1918; "Douglas lifts quarantine." *Coconino Sun* (Flagstaff), Jan 3, 1919.
134. "Quarantine to prevent spread of influenza." *Reno Gazette* (NV), Oct 11, 1918.
135. "Influenza ban is lifted here." *Reno Gazette* (NV), Nov 15, 1918.
136. "Flu ordinance will be enforced." *Goldfield News* (NV), Dec 14, 1918.
137. "Raising the embargo on wearing masks." *Tonopah Bonanza* (NV), Jan 7, 1919.
138. "Governor orders inspection of trains." *Reno Gazette* (NV), Oct 23, 1918.
139. "Must wear masks." *Reno Gazette* (NV), Oct 28, 1918; "Fined for no mask." *Reno Gazette* (NV), Nov 5, 1918.
140. "Influenza situation becomes more serious." *Las Vegas Age* (NV), Nov 9, 1918.
141. "Influenza not bad in Reno now; care needed." *Reno Gazette* (NV), Oct 22, 1918.
142. No title. *Reno Gazette* (NV), Oct 23, 1918.
143. "Masks may be ordered for Reno." *Reno Gazette* (NV), Dec 3, 1918.
144. "Health officer favors masks." *Reno Gazette* (NV), Dec 12, 1918.

Chapter 11

1. "Wick tries to pull meeting against law." *Alaska Empire* (Juneau), Nov 1, 1918.
2. "Influenza quarantine is declared against Juneau." *Alaska Empire* (Juneau), Dec 18, 1918.
3. "Safety measures being taken." *Douglas Island News* (Douglas, AK), Nov 15, 1918.
4. "Regulations for flu modified." *Douglas Island News* (Douglas, AK), Dec 6, 1918.
5. "Off again on again worse again." *Douglas Island News* (Douglas, AK), Dec 20, 1918.
6. "Masks are here for influenza." *Alaska Empire* (Juneau), Nov 1, 1918.
7. "Safety first is slogan of Juneau people." *Alaska Empire* (Juneau), Nov 5, 1918.
8. "Wear your mask." *Alaska Empire* (Juneau), Nov 14, 1918.
9. "Get your mask or your money will be needed." *Alaska Empire* (Juneau), Nov 16, 1918.
10. "Flu ban lifted in Juneau by order of mayor." *Alaska Empire* (Juneau), Nov 27, 1918; "Juneauites to take off masks at midnight." *Alaska Empire* (Juneau), Nov 30, 1918.
11. "Influenza quarantine is declared against Juneau." *Alaska Empire* (Juneau), Dec 18, 1918.
12. "Flu masks can now be discarded while out in open air." *Alaska Empire* (Juneau), Dec 28, 1918.
13. "Influenza ban is raised by city officers." *Alaska Empire* (Juneau), Dec 30, 1918.
14. "Flu quarantine clamped down again." *Kennewick Courier-Reporter* (WA), Oct 24, 1918.
15. "Flu regulations are pulled tight." *Seattle Star*, Oct 26, 1918.
16. Ibid.
17. Ad. *Seattle Star*, Nov 11, 1918.
18. Ad. *Pullman Herald* (WA), Nov 15, 1918.
19. "Extend the quarantine." *Bisbee Review* (AZ), Dec 5, 1918.
20. "Spanish flu has Boston in tragic grip." *Seattle Star*, Sep 26, 1918.
21. "Flu again on the ascendancy here." *Seattle Star*, Oct 25, 1918.
22. "Thousands hit by flu mask order Monday." *Seattle Star*, Oct 28, 1918.
23. "City takes over distribution of all flu masks." *Seattle Star*, Oct 29, 1918.
24. "Wear a gauze mask and smile; help the fight against influenza." *Seattle Star*, Oct 30, 1918.
25. "Arrest seven for ignoring mask orders." *Seattle Star*, Oct 30, 1918.
26. "All stores are closed by Hanson." *Seattle Star*, Oct 31, 1918.
27. "Influenza on decline." *Seattle Star*, Nov 4, 1918.

28. "Flu ban is off except the masks." *Seattle Star*, Nov 11, 1918.
29. "Vaccination first rule against flu." *Seattle Star*, Dec 13, 1918.
30. "Masks proposed for car riders." *Tacoma Ledger* (WA), Oct 11, 1918.
31. "Influenza here now on decrease." *Tacoma Ledger* (WA), Oct 24, 1918.
32. "Day's deaths 9; week's total 47." *Tacoma Ledger* (WA), Oct 27, 1918.
33. "Influenza worst it has been here." *Tacoma Ledger* (WA), Oct 28, 1918.
34. "90 new cases of influenza here." *Tacoma Ledger* (WA), Oct 30, 1918.
35. "New cases of flu drop down to 36." *Tacoma Ledger* (WA), Nov 3, 1918.
36. Ad. *Spokane Chronicle* (WA), Oct 22, 1918.
37. "Soldier boys in Spokane must don masks now." *Spokane Chronicle* (WA), Oct 26, 1918.
38. "Bankers shed the flu masks." *Spokane Chronicle* (WA), Oct 29, 1918.
39. "State health officials order wearing of masks." *Spokane Chronicle* (WA), Nov 7, 1918.
40. "Abolish flu mask rule." *Spokesman-Review* (Spokane, WA), Nov 12, 1918.
41. "Opposing wearing influenza masks." *Spokesman-Review* (WA), Nov 7, 1918.
42. "Test case of flu mask order." *Spokesman-Review* (Spokane, WA), Nov 9, 1918; "Yakima judge upholds edict." *Spokesman-Review* (Spokane, WA), Nov 9, 1918.
43. "Win suit against gauze mask order." *Tacoma Ledger* (WA), Nov 10, 1918.
44. "Makes denial of flu story." *Seattle Star*, Nov 12, 1918.
45. "Health officers instruct public." *Oregon Journal* (Portland), Oct 8, 1918.
46. "Influenza patients now in quarantine." *Evening Herald* (Klamath Falls, OR), Dec 13, 1918.
47. "New ordinance being drafted." *East Oregonian* (Pendleton), Jan 3, 1919.
48. "Here are terms of new flu ordinance." *East Oregonian* (Pendleton), Jan 4, 1919.
49. "Four feet or flu mask is dictum here." *East Oregonian* (Pendleton), Jan 6, 1919.
50. "Flu masks appear in Pendleton today." *East Oregonian* (Pendleton), Jan 7, 1919.
51. "Charged with violating flu ordinance." *East Oregonian* (Pendleton), Jan 9, 1919.
52. "Barbers et al no need face ornament." *East Oregonian* (Pendleton), Jan 10, 1919.
53. "Nine new families reported for influenza." *East Oregonian* (Pendleton), Jan 29, 1920.
54. "Masks ordered worn to guard against the flu." *Medford Mail Tribune* (OR), Dec 9, 1918.
55. "5 arrested for not observing flu regulation." *Medford Mail Tribune* (OR), Dec 11, 1918.
56. "Storm council, demand repeal flu mask edict." *Medford Mail Tribune* (OR), Dec 18, 1918.
57. "Flu masks no longer required on the streets." *Medford Mail Tribune* (OR), Dec 23, 1918.
58. "Health condition in Portland is almost normal." *Oregon Journal* (Portland), Oct 20, 1918.
59. "Thousands take anti-flu serum as a precaution." *Oregon Journal* (Portland), Oct 27, 1918.
60. "Calls for serum exceed supplies." *Oregon Journal* (Portland), Oct 28, 1918.
61. "Flu epidemic is not yet at peak." *Oregon Journal* (Portland), Nov 1, 1918.
62. "Cooperation is asked in battle against the flu." *Oregon Journal* (Portland), Jan 11, 1919.
63. "Masks will be worn as influenza safeguards." *Oregon Journal* (Portland), Jan 12, 1919.
64. "Laws compelling wearing of masks are recommended." *Oregon Journal* (Portland), Jan 13, 1919.
65. "Influenza mask measure drawn." *Oregon Journal* (Portland), Jan 14, 1919.
66. "Decline in flu cases expected." *Oregon Journal* (Portland), Jan 16, 1919.
67. "Flu and masks." *Oregon Journal* (Portland), Jan 17, 1919.
68. "Officials say flu epidemic is over; masks not needed." *Oregon Journal* (Portland), Feb 10, 1919.
69. "Death toll of flu 13 in week." *Statesman Journal* (Salem, OR), Jan 15, 1919.
70. "Cooperation in stamping out epidemic asked." *Statesman Journal* (Salem, OR), Jan 23, 1919.
71. "Influenza ban is raised by proclamation." *Statesman Journal* (Salem, OR), Jan 26, 1919.
72. "Must report influenza." *Los Angeles Times*, Oct 6, 1918.
73. "Spanish influenza and how to combat it." *Daily Telegram* (Long Beach, CA), Oct 12, 1918.
74. "State board urges masks." *Sacramento Bee* (CA), Oct 21, 1918.
75. "To lift lid Saturday night." *Times Advocate* (Escondido, CA), Nov 9, 1918; "Ban replaced here by the city trustees." *Times Advocate* (Escondido, CA), Nov 30, 1918.
76. "Flu lid on again in Southern Cal cities." *Santa Ana Register* (CA), Nov 27, 1918.
77. "Los Angeles lifted the flu quarantine." *Modesto Morning Herald* (CA), Dec 3, 1918.
78. "All flu cases in quarantine." *Los Angeles Times*, Dec 10, 1918.
79. "Woman sought as flu quarantine violator." *Los Angeles Evening Express*, Dec 20, 1918.
80. "Flu law violations charged in warrants." *Los Angeles Evening Express*, Dec 23, 1918.
81. "Spray is ordered as guard against spread of disease." *San Diego Union*, Oct 17, 1918.
82. "Influenza fight must be real, official warning." *San Diego Union*, Oct 19, 1918.
83. "Board asks rulings be mandatory." *San Diego Tribune*, Oct 24, 1918.
84. "Want ordinance to penalize violators." *Evening Tribune* (San Diego), Oct 24, 1918.
85. "All who appear in public required by health board." *San Diego Union*, Oct 25, 1918.
86. "Proposed quarantine of entire city." *Evening Tribune* (San Diego), Oct 31, 1918.
87. "San Diego removes flu restrictions." *Long Beach Press* (CA), Nov 15, 1918.
88. "Council postpones quarantine action until

afternoon." *Evening Tribune* (San Diego), Dec 5, 1918.
89. "Flu ban on; to run four days." *San Diego Union*, Dec 6, 1918.
90. "Flu mask violators go to police court." *Evening Tribune* (San Diego), Dec 7, 1918.
91. "Ordinance requires all in San Diego to wear masks." *Evening Tribune* (San Diego), Dec 10, 1918.
92. "Flu cases reach low mark; masks doffed at midnight." *San Diego Union*, Dec 24, 1918.
93. "Trains to be met by committee." *Morning Union* (Grass Valley, CA), Oct 25, 1918.
94. "Influenza mask hides faces in Fresno crowds?" *Fresno Morning Republican* (CA), Oct 19, 1918.
95. "All are ordered to wear flu masks today." *Fresno Morning Republican* (CA), Oct 24, 1918.
96. "Mask violators fined by Smith." *Fresno Morning Republican* (CA), Nov 1, 1918.
97. "Flu masks come off today." *Fresno Morning Republican* (CA), Feb 3, 1919.
98. "Influenza masks worn in Sacramento." *Sacramento Bee* (CA), Oct 23, 1918.
99. "Wearing of flu masks now requested." *San Bernardino County Sun* (CA), Oct 23, 1918.
100. "Flu mask ordinance meets with defeat." *Sacramento Star* (CA), Oct 24, 1918.
101. "Haynes blocks all efforts to compel wearing of flu masks." *Sacramento Star* (CA), Oct 28, 1918.
102. "Flu mask ordinance is passed." *Sacramento Star* (CA), Oct 29, 1918.
103. "State health board doubts efficacy of influenza masks." *Sacramento Bee* (CA), Nov 14, 1918.
104. "Must wear masks in lobbies." *Sacramento Bee* (CA), Nov 19, 1918.
105. "Discard influenza masks at Sacramento." *San Diego Union*, Nov 27, 1918.
106. "Sacramento puts ban on flu mask." *Santa Barbara Daily News* (CA), Dec 17, 1918.
107. "Simmons urges state influenza mask law." *Sacramento Bee* (CA), Jan 25, 1919.
108. "Barbers hard hit by influenza mask." *Stockton Evening Record* (CA), Nov 1, 1918.
109. "Twenty-five special officers." *Stockton Evening Record* (CA), Nov 15, 1918.
110. "Flu masks come off tomorrow at hour of twelve." *Stockton Evening Record* (CA), Nov 27, 1918.
111. "Flu masks to aid in city fight." *Los Angeles Record*, Oct 24, 1918.
112. "May reopen schools soon." *Los Angeles Times*, Oct 24, 1918.
113. "Los Angeles will not wear flu masks." *Pomona Progress* (CA), Oct 25, 1918.
114. "Compulsory masking, business ban asked." *Los Angeles Evening Express* (CA), Nov 9, 1918.
115. "Swat flu mask; also Hutchinson." *Los Angeles Times*, Nov 8, 1918.
116. "Mask law is refused by council." *Los Angeles Record*, Jan 22, 1919.
117. "Flu masks, forced vaccination urged." *Los Angeles Evening Express*, Jan 23, 1919.
118. "Expert flays flu mask." *Los Angeles Times*, Feb 1, 1919.
119. "See end of influenza scourge." *Los Angeles Times*, Feb 9, 1919.
120. "Must wear masks in town even if riding in autos." *Petaluma Argus Courier* (CA), Nov 5, 1918.
121. "Jail terms given mask slackers by Napa judge." *Sacramento Bee* (CA), Nov 1, 1918.
122. "Refused to don flu mask." *Hanford Sentinel* (CA), Nov 24, 1918; "Violated flu mask ordinance." *Hanford Sentinel* (CA), Nov 28, 1918.
123. "Flu masks are to stay." *Hanford Sentinel* (CA), Dec 17, 1918.
124. "Modesto is to discard influenza mask." *Fresno Morning Republican* (CA), Nov 20, 1918; "Modesto orders wearing of influenza masks." *Sacramento Bee*, Dec 14, 1918; "Modesto again wearing masks." *Hanford Sentinel* (CA), Jan 16, 1919.
125. "$7000 fines paid in flu mask cases." *Oakland Tribune* (CA), Nov 4, 1918.
126. "Oakland mayor pays influenza mask fine." *Stockton Evening Record* (CA), Jan 17, 1919.
127. "Escondido wears flu masks again." *San Diego Union*, Jan 13, 1919.
128. "Flu masking ordinance is turned down." *Oakland Tribune* (CA), Jan 21, 1919.
129. "Flu ordinance is repugnant." *Los Angeles Times*, Jan 24, 1919.
130. "Barbers muzzled under new rule." *San Francisco Examiner*, Oct 20, 1918; "People urged to wear masks everywhere." *San Francisco Examiner*, Oct 20, 1918.
131. Fay King. "Ward of influenza by wearing mask on street." *San Francisco Examiner*, Oct 21, 1918.
132. "50,000 cases foreseen by Dr. Hutchinson." *San Francisco Examiner*, Oct 21, 1918; "Influenza is not abating." *San Francisco Examiner*, Oct 21, 1918.
133. "S.F. dons gas mask to stop flu ravages." *San Francisco Examiner*, Oct 23, 1918.
134. "Emergency measure hits all persons." *San Francisco Chronicle*, Oct 25, 1918.
135. "110 arrested for not wearing flu masks." *San Francisco Examiner*, Oct 28, 1918.
136. "Three shot in struggle with mask slacker." *San Francisco Chronicle*, Oct 29, 1918.
137. "175 mask slackers arrested in city." *San Francisco Chronicle*, Nov 2, 1918; "Maskless folk are taught lesson by health sleuths." *San Francisco Chronicle*, Nov 2, 1918.
138. "All S.F. to unmask at noon today." *San Francisco Examiner*, Nov 21, 1918.
139. "Author of flu masks voluntarily pays fine." *San Francisco Examiner*, Nov 21, 1918.
140. "Flu mask wearers get bawling out." *San Francisco Examiner*, Nov 22, 1918; Annie Laurie. "S.F. feels good without mask." *San Francisco Examiner*, Nov 22, 1918.
141. "Flu masks in San Francisco be resumed." *San Bernardino County Sun* (CA), Dec 8, 1918.

142. "San Francisco waits go give decision." *Modesto Morning Herald* (CA), Dec 12, 1918.
143. "Hassler urges people of city to wear masks." *San Francisco Chronicle*, Dec 18, 1918.
144. "Don flu masks at once, mayor advises citizens." *San Francisco Examiner*, Jan 12, 1919.
145. "Flu mask or jail is choice in S.F. today." *San Francisco Examiner*, Jan 20, 1919.
146. "San Francisco again puts on health masks." *San Francisco Chronicle*, Jan 18, 1919.
147. "186 arrests on first mask day." *San Francisco Chronicle*, Jan 21, 1919; "Anti-Mask League calls mass meeting to protest." *San Francisco Chronicle*, Jan 21, 1919.
148. "Influenza on wane, Tuesday reports show." *San Francisco Chronicle*, Jan 22, 1919.
149. "New cases of influenza at low record." *San Francisco Examiner*, Jan 26, 1919.
150. "Flu masks do little good, says health board." *Oregon Daily Journal* (Portland), Jan 27, 1919.
151. "S.F. may doff flu masks Friday morning." *San Francisco Examiner*, Jan 28, 1919.
152. "Anti-Mask League mass meeting ends in battle royal." *San Francisco Chronicle*, Feb 1, 1919.
153. "Flu mask and many other precautions failed." *The Bulletin* (Pomona, CA), Jan 28, 1919.
154. "San Francisco's first dry year." *Bakersfield Morning Echo* (CA), Oct 9, 1920.
155. "Government physicians advised of influenza quarantine." *Honolulu Star-Bulletin*, Oct 22, 1918.
156. "Time to act now if Hilo hopes to escape the flu." *Hilo Tribune*, Jan 15, 1919.
157. "Flu campaign to begin with wide publicity drive." *Hilo Tribune*, Jan 16, 1919.
158. "Flu appears both here and at Olaa." *Hilo Tribune*, Jan 21, 1919.
159. "Masks." *Hawaii Tribune-Herald* (Hilo), Mar 5, 1919.
160. "Spanish influenza strikes two more residents of city." *Honolulu Advertiser*, Oct 30, 1918.
161. "Publicity is found to be aid in fight against influenza." *Honolulu Advertiser*, Jan 18, 1919.
162. "Public gatherings forbidden." *Honolulu Advertiser*, Jan 24, 1918.
163. "The flu mask." *Honolulu Star-Bulletin*, Mar 1, 1919.

Bibliography

"A.B. & A. mechanics strike because flu mask rule." *Atlanta Constitution*, Oct 27, 1918.
"Aberdeen debates value flu war." *Argus Leader* (Sioux Falls, SD), Dec 26, 1918.
"Aberdeen people must wear flu masks." *Citizen-Republican* (Scotland, SD), Dec 19, 1918.
"Abolish flu mask rule." *Spokesman-Review* (Spokane, WA), Nov 12, 1918.
Ad. *Albuquerque Morning Journal* (NM), Nov 29, 1918.
Ad. *Audubon Journal* (Exira, IA), Nov 28, 1918.
Ad. *Brooklyn Eagle* (NY), Oct 15, 1918.
Ad. *Chattanooga News* (TN), Oct 16, 1918.
Ad. *Detroit Free Press*, Oct 25, 1918.
Ad. *El Paso Herald* (TX), Oct 19, 1918.
Ad. *Evening Star* (Washington, D.C.), Nov 5, 1918.
Ad. *Evening Star* (Washington, D.C.), Oct 18, 1918.
Ad. *Fort Wayne Journal Gazette* (IN), Oct 16, 1918.
Ad. *Harrisburg Telegraph* (PA), Oct 11, 1918.
Ad. *Independent Record* (Helena, MT), Oct 9, 1918.
Ad. *Ogden Standard* (UT), Dec 19, 1918.
Ad. *Ogden Standard* (UT), Dec 3, 1918.
Ad. *Parisian* (Paris, TN), Oct 18, 1918.
Ad. *Pullman Herald* (WA), Nov 15, 1918.
Ad. *Seattle Star*, Nov 11, 1918.
Ad. *Seattle Star*, Nov 5, 1918.
Ad. *Spokane Chronicle* (WA), Oct 22, 1918.
Ads. *Hopewell Herald* (NJ), Oct 9, 1918.
"Advise vaccine as preventive of influenza." *Arizona Republican* (Phoenix), Oct 26, 1918.
"Albemarle citizens may be forced to wear masks." *Charlotte Observer* (NC), Oct 13, 1918.
"Albuquerque Thanksgiving." *Albuquerque Morning Journal* (NM), Dec 1, 1918.
"All Fargo wants a Red Cross face mask." *Fargo Forum* (ND), Oct 9, 1918.
"All are ordered to wear flu masks today." *Fresno Morning Republican* (CA), Oct 24, 1918.
"All at capital don influenza masks." *New York Sun*, Oct 16, 1918.
"All closed places but schools opened." *Rapid City Journal* (SD), Nov 5, 1918.
"All dentists and barbers to wear masks in Clifton." *Passaic Daily News* (NJ), Oct 16, 1918.
"All flu cases in quarantine." *Los Angeles Times*, Dec 10, 1918.
"All flu cases quarantined." *Chicago Tribune*, Oct 1, 1918.
"All Marion people at sixes and sevens." *Mansfield News* (OH), Dec 20, 1918.
"All public places in Selma to be closed." *Montgomery Advertiser* (AL), Oct 10, 1918.
"All quarantine rules to be lifted Sunday." *Arkansas Democrat* (Little Rock, AR), Oct 31, 1918.
"All S.F. to unmask at noon today." *San Francisco Examiner*, Nov 21, 1918.
"All schools will reopen Monday." *Detroit Free Press*, Oct 30, 1918.
"All stores are closed by Hanson." *Seattle Star*, Oct 31, 1918.
"All stores to close Saturday evening at 6:30." *Harrisburg Telegraph* (PA), Oct 16, 1918.
"All who appear in public required by health board." *San Diego Union*, Oct 25, 1918.
"Amarillo quarantines against influenza." *Fort Worth Star Telegram* (TX), Oct 23, 1918.
"Anniversary of the epidemic." *New Britain Herald* (CT), Sep 19, 1919.
"Anti-flu masks prove popularity." *Missoulian* (MT), Oct 25, 1918.
"Anti-flu rules displease hunter." *Arizona Republican* (Phoenix), Nov 21, 1918.
"Anti-germ mask order." *Arizona Star* (Tucson), Nov 19, 1918.
"Anti-influenza serum made in tests here." *New York Tribune*, Oct 2, 1918.
"Anti-Mask League calls mass meeting to protest." *San Francisco Chronicle*, Jan 21, 1919.
"Anti-Mask League mass meeting ends in battle royal." *San Francisco Chronicle*, Feb 1, 1919.
"Arrest seven for ignoring mask orders." *Seattle Star*, Oct 30, 1918.
"As precaution close all public places." *Orlando Sentinel* (FL), Oct 8, 1918.
"Asheville influenza quarantine raised." *Journal and Tribune* (Knoxville, TN), Feb 13, 1919.
"Ask that flu masks be used." *Journal Times* (Racine, WI), Oct 8, 1918.
"Asks government for 12 nurses." *Salt Lake Tribune*, Oct 25, 1918.
"Augusta to lift flu ban Saturday." *Atlanta Constitution* (GA), Jan 30, 1919.
"Austin shuts all its public places." *Austin American* (TX), Oct 9, 1918.
"Author of flu masks voluntarily pays fine." *San Francisco Examiner*, Nov 21, 1918.

"Awards announced at great exhibits at Lakewood Fair." *Atlanta Constitution*, Oct 16, 1918.
"Ayer." *Hollis Times* (NH), Sep 20, 1918.
"Ban declared off." *News and Citizen* (Morrisville, VT), Nov 6, 1918.
"Ban effective another week." *Buffalo Times* (NY), Nov 1, 1918.
"Ban is lifted." *Diamond Drill* (Crystal Falls, MI), Jan 11, 1919.
"The ban is lifted." *Maryland Gazette* (Annapolis), Oct 24, 1918.
"Ban lifted and shows will open." *Birmingham News* (AL), Oct 29, 1918.
"Ban on all public meetings." *Shreveport Journal* (LA), Nov 7, 1918.
"Ban on business lifted at noon; theaters open." *Harrisburg Telegraph* (PA), Nov 5, 1918.
"Ban on church services is not to be lifted." *Harrisburg Telegraph* (PA), Nov 1, 1918.
"Ban placed on state." *Indianapolis Star*, Oct 10, 1918.
"Ban replaced here by the city trustees." *Times Advocate* (Escondido, CA), Nov 30, 1918.
"Bangor's battle with the grip." *Bangor Daily News* (ME), Oct 5, 1918.
"Bankers shed the flu masks." *Spokane Chronicle* (WA), Oct 29, 1918.
"Bar use of serum." *Rock Island Argus* (IL), Jan 21, 1920.
"Barber forfeits $10 for refusing to wear mask." *Ogden Standard* (UT), Nov 26, 1918.
"Barbers hard hit by influenza mask." *Stockton Evening Record* (CA), Nov 1, 1918.
"Barber will wear flu mask." *New Castle Herald* (PA), Oct 30, 1918.
"Barbers adopt flu masks while at work." *Star-Gazette* (Elmira, NY), Oct 17, 1918.
"Barbers et al no need face ornament." *East Oregonian* (Pendleton), Jan 10, 1919.
"Barbers may wear flu masks." *Marshall Messenger* (TX), Dec 20, 1918.
"Barbers must wear flu masks." *Lawrence Journal World* (KS), Oct 22, 1918.
"Barbers muzzled under new rule." *San "Francisco Examiner*, Oct 20, 1918.
"Barbers wear masks to stop spread of flu." *Daily Times* (Davenport, IA), Oct 18, 1918.
"Beatrice business men resent order." *Lincoln Star* (NE), Dec 1, 1918.
"Beatrice health board." *Lincoln Star* (NE), Dec 2, 1918.
"Begin manana everyone must wear flu mask." *Arizona Republican* (Phoenix), Nov 26, 1918.
"Belfast has masks for influenza cases." *Bangor Daily News* (ME), Oct 12, 1918.
"Big plants adopt masks." *Kansas City Star* (MO), Oct 22, 1918.
"Blake lifts last of influenza bans." *Evening Sun* (Baltimore, MD), Nov 6, 1918.
"Block car crowd order." *Kansas City Star* (MO), Oct 8, 1918.
"Board advise extreme care." *Elgin Review* (NE), Dec 20, 1918.

"Board asks rulings be mandatory." *San Diego Tribune*, Oct 24, 1918.
"Board of health changes mask order." *Lima Times Democrat* (OH), Dec 13, 1918.
"Board of health modifies flu ban." *Canon City Record* (CO), Dec 19, 1918.
"Board prepares to enforce flu mask wearing." *Indianapolis Star*, Nov 20, 1918.
"Board rescinds the mask order." *Indianapolis Star*, Nov 25, 1918.
Board to reconsider drastic order." *Beatrice Sun* (NE), Dec 1, 1918.
"Boards of health advise." *Times-Dispatch* (Richmond, VA), Oct 31, 1918.
Bound and gagged?—No, she is warding off influenza." *Birmingham News* (AL), Dec 8, 1918.
"Bozeman saloons get orders to close doors." *Butte Miner* (MT), Oct 26, 1918.
"Branding influenza mask as fake splits conference." *Pittsburgh Daily Post*, Dec 13, 1918.
"Brands rumors of closing ban here as false." *Portland Evening Express* (ME), Dec 26, 1918.
"Burton advises influenza mask." *Lima Republican Gazette* (OH), Nov 5, 1918.
"Business hours may be changed." *Star Tribune* (Minneapolis), Oct 15, 1918.
"Business not to be disturbed." *Racine Journal-News* (WI), Oct 7, 1918.
"But one death reported today from influenza." *Bismarck Tribune* (ND), Oct 23, 1918.
"Butte lifts flu ban on ads." *Great Falls Tribune* (MT), Nov 29, 1918.
"Californians doubt flu mask efficacy." *Salt Lake Telegram*, Nov 23, 1918.
"Calls for serum exceed supplies." *Oregon Journal* (Portland), Oct 28, 1918.
"Camilla lifts influenza ban." *Macon News* (GA), Dec 29, 1918.
"Can go to church and shows if masks are worn." *Great Falls Tribune* (MT), Dec 9, 1918.
"Charged with violating flu ordinance." *East Oregonian* (Pendleton), Jan 9, 1919.
"Charleston people wear gauze masks." *West Virginian* (Fairmont), Oct 17, 1918.
"Charlie Chaplin stopped the flu." *Fall River Daily Globe* (MA), Sep 5, 1919.
"Charlotte streets take on Sabbath appearance." *Charlotte Observer* (NC), Oct 5, 1918.
"Checking the influenza." *Ogden Standard* (UT), Oct 23, 1918.
"Chiffon veil gas mask for sneeze." *Detroit Free Press*, Oct 16, 1918.
"Children in schools to wear flu masks." *Atlanta Constitution* (GA), Oct 19, 1918.
"Children wear masks." *Chariton Courier* (Keytesville, MO), Dec 1, 1916.
"Church services will again be held." *Daily Home News* (New Brunswick, NJ), Oct 26, 1918.
"Churches, schools, saloons." *Evening Journal* (Wilmington, DE), Oct 2, 1918.
"Churchless and gasolineless." *Evening Star* (Washington, D.C.), Oct 11, 1918.

"Cincinnati schools." *Mansfield News* (OH), Dec 2, 1918.
"City accepts quarantine on influenza in good spirits." *Harrisburg Telegraph* (PA), Oct 5, 1918.
"City authorities decide against general closing." *Buffalo Morning Express* (NY), Oct 8, 1918.
"City closed tight tonight." *Harrisburg Telegraph* (PA), Oct 12, 1918.
"City closed till state lid lifted." *Des Moines Tribune* (IA), Oct 21, 1918.
"City closed to end wave of influenza." *Star Tribune* (Minneapolis), Oct 12, 1918.
"City enforces closing order." *Evening Review* (East Liverpool, OH), Oct 21, 1918.
"City extends closing hour." *Detroit Free Press*, Oct 23, 1918.
"City extends closing order." *Detroit Free Press*, Oct 23, 1918.
"City flu order off tomorrow." *Indianapolis Star*, Oct 30, 1918.
"City in disguise ventures abroad in gauze masks." *Lima Republican Gazette* (OH), Dec 13, 1918.
"City laughs once more as movies open." *Star Tribune* (Minneapolis), Nov 16, 1918.
"City placed under plague restrictions." *Muscatine Journal* (IA), Oct 18, 1918.
"City put under strict quarantine." *Fayetteville Democrat* (AR), October 9, 1918.
"City puts ban on funerals." *El Paso Times* (TX), Oct 9, 1918.
"City shut down to ward off spread of flu." *Butte Miner* (MT), Nov 30, 1918.
"City takes over distribution of all flu masks." *Seattle Star*, Oct 29, 1918.
"The city's splendid emergency hospital." *Harrisburg Telegraph* (PA), Oct 23, 1918.
"City's streets must be quiet on Halloween." *Harrisburg Telegraph* (PA), Oct 29, 1918.
"Clamp lid on Orleans." *Shreveport Times* (LA), Oct 10, 1918.
"Clerks in stores, failing to wear masks." *Ogden Standard* (UT), Dec 6, 1918.
"Cleveland is now under quarantine." *Akron Beacon Journal* (OH), Oct 14, 1918.
"Cleveland's influenza." *Mansfield News* (OH), Nov 5, 1918.
"Clippings of capital coupons." *Evening Capital* (Annapolis, MD), Oct 28, 1918.
"Close all fairs during epidemic." *Times-Dispatch* (Richmond, VA), Oct 9, 1918.
"Close all public places but schools." *Argus-Leader* (Sioux Falls, SD), Oct 12, 1918.
"Close next week." *Topeka State Journal* (KS), Oct 24, 1918.
"Close schools another week." *El Paso Herald* (TX), Oct 12, 1918.
"Close up again." *Topeka State Journal* (KS), Nov 26, 1918.
"Close warehouses to curb influenza." *Times-Dispatch* (Richmond, VA), Oct 15, 1918.
"Closing ban has been lifted." *Buffalo Times* (NY), Nov 1, 1918.
"Closing ban is barbarism says Dr. Hutchinson." *Arizona Republican* (Phoenix), Dec 11, 1918.
"Closing order complied with." *West Virginian* (Fairmont), Oct 8, 1918.
"Closing order in effect." *St. Louis Star* (MO), Oct 8, 1918.
"Closing order in force in Lincoln." *Lincoln Journal-Star* (NE), Oct 12, 1918.
"Closing order is extended." *Racine Journal-News* (WI), Oct 18, 1918.
"Closing order to hold over another week." *Portsmouth Herald* (NH), Oct 17, 1918.
"Closing order to remain in effect." *Topeka Daily Capital* (KS), Oct 25, 1918.
"Closing the penalty for non-compliance." *Butte Miner* (MT), Oct 27, 1918.
"Co-operation, not criticism, needed." *Indianapolis Star*, Nov 22, 1918.
Collier, F.H. "Echoes of the street." *St. Louis Globe Democrat* (MO), Dec 17, 1918.
"Colorado state news." *Cheyenne Record* (WY), Dec 5, 1918.
"Combat influenza by use of masks." *Evening Star* (Washington, D.C.), Sep 25, 1918.
"Combating influenza." *Chattanooga Daily Times* (TN), Dec 11, 1918.
"Combating influenza." *Laredo Times* (TX), Oct 12, 1918.
"Common sense about the epidemic." *Boston Globe*, Sep 18, 1918.
"Compulsory masking, business ban asked." *Los Angeles Evening Express* (CA), Nov 9, 1918.
"Compulsory wearing of masks considered." *Birmingham News* (AL), Dec 10, 1918.
"Condition of influenza in Cache County." *Logan Republican* (UT), Oct 22, 1918.
"Condition of the quarantine still unsettled." *Bisbee Review* (AZ), Nov 14, 1918.
"Conference is held to discuss matter of reopening." *Arizona Republican* (Phoenix), Nov 14, 1918.
"Consignment of flu vaccine arrives." *Payne Field Zooms* (West Point, MS), Nov 27, 1918.
"Control is near here." *Lansing State Journal* (MI), Oct 23, 1918.
"Controversy over flu quarantine." *Idaho Republican* (Blackfoot), Jan 14, 1919.
"Cooperation in stamping out epidemic asked." *Statesman Journal* (Salem, OR), Jan 23, 1919.
"Cooperation is asked in battle against the flu." *Oregon Journal* (Portland), Jan 11, 1919.
"Copeland says theatres must obey or close." *New York Tribune*, Oct 10, 1918.
"Council postpones quarantine action until afternoon." *Evening Tribune* (San Diego), Dec 5, 1918.
"County is quarantined against Spanish flu." *Lenoir Topic* (NC), Oct 25, 1918.
"County schools closed today." *Maryland Gazette* (Annapolis), Oct 9, 1918.
"Courts to pass on validity." *Wichita Eagle* (KS), Nov 30, 1918.
"Crest of influenza." *Harrisburg Telegraph* (PA), Oct 10, 1918.

"Crowding banned by health board." *Lima Republican Gazette* (OH), Dec 19, 1918.
"Cultivating anti-influenza vaccine." *Hartford Republican* (KY), Oct 31, 1919.
"D.C. deaths fall to 65 in today's influenza report." *Evening Star* (Washington, D.C.), Oct 12, 1918.
"Dame rumor." *Coshocton Tribune* (OH), Nov 17, 1918.
"Dance Ban must stay, says board." *Lima Republican Gazette* (OH), Dec 22, 1918.
"Davenport puts on real lid." *Courier* (Waterloo, IA), Dec 11, 1918.
"Day off for the barbers." *Chattanooga Daily Times* (TN), Oct 12, 1918.
"Day's deaths 9; week's total 47." *Tacoma Ledger* (WA), Oct 27, 1918.
"Death claims 10 more influenza victims in city." *Birmingham News* (AL), Oct 10, 1918.
"Death toll of flu 13 in week." *Statesman Journal* (Salem, OR), Jan 15, 1919.
"Deaths fewer but number of new cases grows." *Tampa Tribune* (FL), Oct 20, 1918.
"Decline in cases." *St. Louis Star* (MO), Dec 20, 1918.
"Decline in flu cases expected." *Oregon Journal* (Portland), Jan 16, 1919.
"Decrease here shown in new grippe cases." *New York Tribune*, Oct 18, 1918.
"Decrease in flu is noted." *Charlotte News* (NC), Oct 16, 1918.
"Denver fails to obey order." *Star* (Marion, OH), Dec 21, 1918.
"Denver theatres and the flu." *Goodwin's Weekly* (Salt Lake City, UT), Nov 30, 1918.
"Denver to enforce influenza mask." *El Paso Times* (TX), Nov 27, 1918.
"Denver wrathy at violations of flu mask order." *Santa Fe New Mexican*, Nov 25, 1918.
"Des Moines board of health." *Courier* (Waterloo, IA), Nov 27, 1918.
"Des Moines under flu quarantine." *Seattle Star*, Oct 10, 1918.
"Detroit obeys influenza ban." *Detroit Free Press*, Oct 21, 1918;
"Discard influenza masks at Sacramento." *San Diego Union*, Nov 27, 1918.
"District churches and playgrounds ordered closed." *Washington Times* (Washington, D.C.), Oct 5, 1918.
"Doctor says flu serum has no effect." *Seattle Star*, Jan 13, 1919.
"Dr. Clinton tells about best mask." *Tulsa Democrat* (OK), Nov 3, 1918.
"Dr. Grote makes statement." *Huntsville Times* (AL), Dec 15, 1918.
"Dr. Mayo tells of influenza serum." *Evening Missourian* (Columbia), Oct 14, 1918.
"Dr. Royer tells Judge Landis he has no power." *Harrisburg Telegraph* (PA), Nov 4, 1918.
"Dr. Welch may lift ban by week's end." *Maryland Gazette* (Annapolis), Oct 23, 1918.
"Dr. Woodward's advice to coughers and sneezers." *Boston Globe*, Dec 29, 1918.

"Doctors advise immediate order." *Deseret News* (Salt Lake City), Nov 22, 1918.
"Doctors ask board to close saloons." *Racine Journal-News* (WI), Oct 19, 1918.
"Doctors at Chicago meet." *Independent Record* (Helena, MT), Dec 17, 1918.
"Doctors disagree on influenza issue." *Logansport Pharos-Tribune* (IN), Dec 17, 1918.
"Doctors oppose wearing of flu masks in public." *Lima Republican Gazette* (OH), Dec 18, 1918.
"Doctors propose drastic lid." *Star Tribune* (Minneapolis), Oct 11, 1918.
"Don flu masks at once, mayor advises citizens." *San Francisco Examiner*, Jan 12, 1919.
"Donnelly advises using flu masks." *Oklahoma City Times*, Nov 21, 1918.
"Douglas council decides to lift quarantine." *Bisbee Review* (AZ), Dec 15, 1918.
"Douglas lifts quarantine." *Coconino Sun* (Flagstaff), Jan 3, 1919.
"Draft boards use masks." *Minneapolis Morning Tribune*, Oct 17, 1918.
"Drastic action is taken today." *Maryland Gazette* (Annapolis), Oct 11, 1918.
"A drastic ban is on." *Kansas City Star* (MO), Oct 17, 1918.
"Drastic statewide quarantine order." *Arkansas Democrat* (Little Rock), Oct 7, 1918.
"Drastic steps are taken by officials." *Port Huron Times-Herald* (MI), Oct 22, 1918.
"East Fairfield." *Richford Gazette* (VT), Dec 13, 1918.
"8 deaths from influenza here." *Star Tribune* (Minneapolis), Oct 9, 1918.
"8,000 influenza cases developed." *Harrisburg Telegraph* (PA), Oct 18, 1918.
"83 deaths in day from influenza." *Evening Star* (Washington, D.C.), Oct 16, 1918.
"El Paso doctors get Rosenow's flu vaccine." *El Paso Herald* (TX), Nov 26, 1918.
"Elmira placed under strict quarantine." *Star-Gazette* (Elmira, NY), Oct 15, 1918.
"Emergency hospital is needed." *Courier* (Fort Collins, CO), Dec 6, 1918.
"Emergency measure hits all persons." *San Francisco Chronicle*, Oct 25, 1918.
"Employees will all be shot." *Lake County Times* (Hammond, IN), Oct 24, 1918.
"Ends the influenza ban." *Kansas City Star* (MO), Nov 14, 1918.
"Epidemic closes public places." *Indianapolis Star*, Oct 7, 1918.
"Epidemic fight goes on." *Kansas City Star* (MO), Oct 20, 1918.
"Epidemic forces drastic action." *Times-Dispatch* (Richmond, VA), Oct 6, 1918.
"Epidemic fought by New England." *Evening Star* (Washington), Sep 26, 1918.
"Epidemic gain causes anxiety among officers." *Idaho Daily Statesman* (Boise), Oct 29, 1918.
"Epidemic in Marion." *Sumter Item* (SC), Jan 20, 1919.
"Epidemic is over." *Alexandria Gazette* (VA), Oct 31, 1918.

"Epidemic problem puzzling experts." *Lincoln Journal Star* (NE), Dec 17, 1918.
"Escondido wears flu masks again." *San Diego Union*, Jan 13, 1919.
"Everybody his own quarantine officer, Dr. Raunick." *Harrisburg Telegraph* (PA), Oct 15, 1918.
"Everybody may have to wear mask in fight on influenza." *Deseret News* (Salt Lake City), Oct 24, 1918.
"Everybody must wear flu masks." *Daily Star-Mirror* (Moscow, ID), Oct 30, 1918.
"Everything is closed tight by the flu." *Bismarck Tribune* (ND), Oct 9, 1918.
"Exclusive pictures of stricken Rheims." *Sun* (NY), Feb 27, 1916.
"The exercise of vigilance." *Mansfield News* (OH), Oct 8, 1918.
"Expert flays flu mask." *Los Angeles Times*, Feb 1, 1919.
"Experts tell how to combat flu." *Chicago Tribune*, Dec 14, 1918.
"An exploded theory." *Tucson Citizen* (AZ), Dec 20, 1918.
"Extend the quarantine." *Bisbee Review* (AZ), Dec 5, 1918.
"Extends flu quarantine." *Watchman & Southron* (Sumter, SC), Oct 26, 1918.
"The face mask." *Des Moines Tribune* (IA), Nov 30, 1918.
"Face mask need urged on women." *Detroit Free Press*, Oct 22, 1918.
"Face masks must be worn by those afflicted." *Ogden Standard* (UT), Oct 26, 1918.
"Face masks worn by draft board." *Detroit Free Press*, Oct 19, 1918.
"Face masks worn in office of local draft board." *Daily News Leader* (Staunton, VA), Oct 12, 1918.
"Facing hazards bravely." *Independent Record* (Helena, MT), Dec 16, 1918.
"Facts on influenza." *Ogden Standard* (UT), Feb 3, 1920.
"Fair closed." *Wichita Beacon* (KS), Oct 10, 1918.
"Fairfax." *Richford Gazette* (VT), "Feb 21, 1919.
"Fairfield doctors at odds." *Bridgeport Telegram* (CT), Oct 21, 1918.
"Fargo is closed tight." *Fargo Forum* (ND), Oct 9, 1918.
"Fear of epidemic from Spanish grip scouted by officials." *New York Tribune*, Aug 17, 1918.
"Few churches plan services." *Indianapolis Star*, Nov 23, 1918.
"Few new cases of influenza are reported." *Grand Forks Herald* (ND), Oct 17, 1918.
"Fewer new cases reported for day." *Scranton Republican* (PA), Oct 24, 1918.
"50,000 cases foreseen by Dr. Hutchinson." *San Francisco Examiner*, Oct 21, 1918.
"Fight flu wear a mask." *Concordia Empire* (KS), Dec 5, 1918.
"Fine Taylor $100." *Paducah Sun-Democrat* (KY), Jan 29, 1919.
"Fined for no mask." *Reno Gazette* (NV), Nov 5, 1918.
"First arrests made for not wearing masks." *Arizona Republican* (Phoenix), Nov 30, 1918.
"5 arrested for not observing flu regulation." *Medford Mail Tribune* (OR), Dec 11, 1918.
"Five victims of Spanish influenza." *Idaho Daily Statesman* (Boise, ID), Oct 27, 1918.
"Flu and masks." *Oregon Journal* (Portland), Jan 17, 1919.
"Flu again on the ascendancy here." *Seattle Star*, Oct 25, 1918.
"Flu appears both here and at Olaa." *Hilo Tribune*, Jan 21, 1919.
"Flu ban at Statesville." *Charlotte Observer* (NC), Feb 14, 1919.
"Flu ban continues in effect." *Parisian* (Paris, TN), Mar 5, 1920.
"Flu ban is lifted." *Knoxville Sentinel* (TN), Feb 3, 1919.
"Flu ban is off except the masks." *Seattle Star*, Nov 11, 1918.
"Flu ban lifted in Juneau by order of mayor." *Alaska Empire* (Juneau), Nov 27, 1918.
"Flu ban off Friday." *Arizona Republican* (Phoenix), Dec 9, 1918.
"Flu ban on again." *Wichita Eagle* (KS), Dec 1, 1918.
"Flu ban on theaters is to be lifted." *St. Louis Star* (MO), Nov 12, 1918.
"Flu ban on; to run four days." *San Diego Union*, Dec 6, 1918.
"Flu ban wholly lifted in county." *Jackson News* (MS), Oct 8, 1918.
"Flu campaign to begin with wide publicity drive." *Hilo Tribune*, Jan 16, 1919.
"Flu cases are on increase in Helena." *Independent Record* (Helena, MT), Oct 27, 1918.
"Flu cases reach low mark; masks doffed at midnight." *San Diego Union*, Dec 24, 1918.
"Flu causes the public schools to be closed." *Maryland Gazette* (Annapolis), Oct 3, 1918.
"Flu closing ban is made more drastic." *St. Louis Star* (MO), Nov 9, 1918.
"Flu coming back." *Jamestown Alert* (ND), Nov 14, 1918.
"Flu cuts store hours." *Baltimore Sun* (MD), Oct 10, 1918.
"Flu defense is up before state health officers." *Virginian Pilot* (Norfolk, VA), Sep 14, 1919.
"Flu drops off." *Indianapolis Star*, Nov 21, 1918.
"Flu epidemic far from over." *Billings Gazette* (MT), Dec 12, 1918.
"Flu epidemic in Fargo." *Fargo Forum* (ND), Oct 7, 1918.
"Flu epidemic is not yet at peak." *Oregon Journal* (Portland), Nov 1, 1918.
"Flu epidemic is spreading here." *Knoxville Sentinel* (TN), Oct 9, 1918.
"Flu epidemic spreads." *Watchman & Southron* (Sumter, SC), Oct 19, 1918.
"Flu flares up in many places throughout PA." *Harrisburg Telegraph* (PA), Nov 20, 1918.
"Flu here and at Bozeman." *Helena Independent* (MT), Oct 17, 1918.

"Flu hysteria not warranted." *Bismarck Tribune* (ND), Dec 12, 1918.

"Flu in Denver becomes more alarming." *Courier* (Fort Collins, CO), Nov 29, 1918.

"Flu is serious." *Topeka State Journal* (KS), Oct 9, 1918.

"Flu is spreading." *Topeka State Journal* (KS), Oct 10, 1918.

"Flu law violations charged in warrants." *Los Angeles Evening Express*, Dec 23, 1918.

"Flu lid come entirely off in city tomorrow." *Chicago Tribune*, Nov 3, 1918.

"Flu lid lifted here." *Helena Independent* (MT), Dec 22, 1918.

"Flu lid on again in Southern Cal cities." *Santa Ana Register* (CA), Nov 27, 1918.

"Flu likely to return says health service." *Arizona Republican* (Phoenix), Sep 17, 1919.

"The flu mask." *Honolulu Star-Bulletin*, Mar 1, 1919.

"The flu mask." *Weekly Pioneer Times* (Deadwood, SD), Feb 13, 1919.

"Flu mask and many other precautions failed." *The Bulletin* (Pomona, CA), Jan 28, 1919.

"Flu mask enforcement." *Arizona Star* (Tucson), Dec 22, 1918.

"Flu mask issue up to board of health." *Salt Lake Tribune*, Nov 30, 1918.

"Flu mask or jail is choice in S.F. today." *San Francisco Examiner*, Jan 20, 1919.

"Flu mask order for Georgia fairs." *Macon Daily Telegraph* (GA), Oct 15, 1918.

"Flu mask order is effective tonight." *Des Moines Tribune* (IA), Dec 2, 1918.

"Flu mask order is modified." *Des Moines Tribune* (IA), Nov 30, 1918.

"Flu mask order is off." *Indianapolis Star*, Nov 24, 1918.

"Flu mask order is rescinded." *Des Moines Tribune* (IA), Dec 3, 1918.

"Flu mask order now effective." *Brazil Times* (IN), Nov 20, 1918.

"Flu mask order stands." *Lima Republican Gazette* (OH), Dec 17, 1918.

"Flu mask order stands." *Indianapolis Star*, Nov 24, 1918.

"Flu mask ordinance is passed." *Sacramento Star* (CA), Oct 29, 1918.

"Flu mask ordinance meets with defeat." *Sacramento Star* (CA), Oct 24, 1918.

"Flu mask scare is false alarm." *Gate City* (Keokuk, IA). Nov 15, 1918.

"Flu mask violators go to police court." *Evening Tribune* (San Diego), Dec 7, 1918.

"Flu mask wearers get bawling out." *San Francisco Examiner*, Nov 22, 1918.

"Flu masking ordinance is turned down." *Oakland Tribune* (CA), Jan 21, 1919.

"Flu masks abolished." *Clinton Messenger* (OK), Dec 19, 1918.

"Flu masks appear in Pendleton today." *East Oregonian* (Pendleton), Jan 7, 1919.

"Flu masks are doomed." *Town Talk* (Alexandria. LA), Oct 29, 1918.

"Flu masks are now ordered to be worn." *Santa Fe New Mexican*, Nov 22, 1918.

"Flu masks are to stay." *Hanford Sentinel* (CA), Dec 17, 1918.

"Flu masks can now be discarded while out in open air." *Alaska Empire* (Juneau), Dec 28, 1918.

"Flu masks come off today." *Fresno Morning Republican* (CA), Feb 3, 1919.

"Flu masks come off tomorrow at hour of twelve." *Stockton Evening Record* (CA), Nov 27, 1918.

"Flu masks do little good, says health board." *Oregon Daily Journal* (Portland), Jan 27, 1919.

"Flu masks for bond captains." *Charlotte Observer* (NC), Oct 15, 1918.

"Flu masks, forced vaccination urged." *Los Angeles Evening Express*, Jan 23, 1919.

"Flu masks go on what-not shelf." *Shreveport Times* (LA), Nov 15, 1918.

"Flu masks in San Francisco be resumed." *San Bernardino County Sun* (CA), Dec 8, 1918.

"Flu masks in use by local firm." *Macon News* (GA), Oct 15, 1918.

"Flu masks must be worn." *Indianapolis Star*, Nov 19, 1918.

"Flu masks must be worn." *Indianapolis Star*, Nov 19, 1918.

"Flu masks must be worn by all." *Brazil Times* (IN), Nov 25, 1918.

"Flu masks must be worn here." *Brazil Times* (IN), Nov 19, 1918.

"Flu masks no longer required on the streets." *Medford Mail Tribune* (OR), Dec 23, 1918.

"Flu masks off in Pendleton." *La Grande Observer* (OR), Jan 13, 1919.

"Flu masks ordered by health board." *Des Moines Register* (IA), Nov 29, 1918.

"Flu masks scorned by councilmen, but session is brief." *Macon News* (GA), Oct 23, 1918.

"Flu masks to aid in city fight." *Los Angeles Record*, Oct 24, 1918.

"Flu masks to be worn." *St. Louis Post-Dispatch* (MO), Jan 9, 1919.

"Flu may last all winter." *Arizona Republican* (Phoenix), Oct 28, 1918.

"Flu ordinance is repugnant." *Los Angeles Times*, Jan 24, 1919.

"Flu ordinance will be enforced." *Goldfield News* (NV), Dec 14, 1918.

"Flu prevention and treatment." *Evening Sun* (Baltimore, MD), Oct 8, 1918.

"Flu puts 9 more to bed." *Leader-Telegram* (Eau Claire, WI), Oct 15, 1918.

"Flu quarantine." *News of Henderson County* (Hendersonville, NC), Dec 24, 1918.

"Flu quarantine clamped down again." *Kennewick Courier-Reporter* (WA), Oct 24, 1918.

"Flu quarantine imposed." *Muscatine Journal* (IA), Nov 28, 1918.

"Flu quarantine in Augusta." *Washington Herald* (Washington, D.C.), Jan 12, 1918.

"Flu quarantine is lifted at Woodruff." *Greenville News* (SC), Feb 7, 1918.

"Flu quarantine is modified." *Public Ledger* (Maysville, KY), Nov 7, 1918.
"Flu quarantine is raised in Pocatello." *Salt Lake Tribune*, Dec 22, 1918.
"Flu quarantine may be lifted in 10 days." *Jackson News* (MS), Oct 21, 1918.
"Flu quarantine on again at Statesville." *News and Observer* (Raleigh, NC), Jan 13, 1919.
"Flu quarantine ordered by state." *Des Moines Register* (IA), Sep 30, 1919.
"Flu quarantine proves failure." *Tennessean* (Nashville, TN), Dec 8, 1918.
"Flu quarantine to be raised here Friday." *Alliance Herald* (NE), Nov 14, 1918.
"Flu quarantine to become stricter." *Journal Gazette* (Mattoon, IL), Oct 16, 1918.
"Flu quarantine useless." *Lincoln Star* (NE), Dec 27, 1918.
"Flu quarantine will be lifted." *West Virginian* (Fairmont), Nov 6, 1918.
"Flu regulations are pulled tight." *Seattle Star*, Oct 26, 1918.
"Flu serum in hands of all doctors here." *Bismarck Tribune* (ND), Nov 7, 1918.
"Flu serum no good, says Ohio newspaper." *Public Ledger* (Maysville, KY), Dec 19, 1918.
"Flu serum useless." *Elk Mountain Pilot* (Irwin, CO), Feb 27, 1919.
"Flu situation." *Journal* (Logan, UT), Dec 24, 1918.
"Flu situation is clearing up." *Albuquerque Morning Journal* (NM), Nov 23, 1918.
"Flu situation is not yet improved." *Coshocton Tribune* (OH), Nov 19, 1918.
"Flu situation reported today." *Journal* (Logan, UT), Nov 18, 1918.
"The flu situation serious." *Keowee Courier* (Pickens, SC), Oct 23, 1918.
"Flu under control." *Daily Arkansas Gazette* (Little Rock), Oct 21, 1918.
"Flu vaccine used successfully here." *Idaho Springs Sifting-News* (CO), Dec 13, 1918.
"Flying squadron of speakers." *Bridgeport Telegram* (CT), Oct 17, 1918.
"For not wearing masks." *Mountainair Independent* (NM), Nov 14, 1918.
"Force vaccination upon Havre people." *Great "Falls Tribune* (MT), Dec 2, 1918.
"Forty-six violators of flu mask order." *Lima Times Democrat* (OH), Dec 16, 1918.
"4 more deaths, 17 new cases." *Lexington Herald* (KY), Nov 2, 1918.
"Four feet or flu mask is dictum here." *East Oregonian* (Pendleton), Jan 6, 1919.
"Four maskless men are nipped." *Escanaba Morning Press* (MI), Dec 8, 1918.
"Four simple rules for combating influenza." *Knoxville Sentinel* (TN), Mar 21, 1919.
"14 theater men arrested at Terre Haute." *Indianapolis Star*, Nov 29, 1918.
"Free vaccine for flu prevention." *Glasgow Courier* (MT), Aug 29, 1919.
"Free vaccine to all people." *Webster City Freeman* (IA), Dec 16, 1918.

"Free whiskey for those who need stimulant." *Harrisburg Telegraph* (PA), Oct 18, 1918.
"Further agitation of flu ban." *Montgomery Advertiser* (AL), Dec 10, 1918.
"Further modification of quarantine proclamation." *Idaho Republican* (Blackfoot, ID), Dec 13, 1918.
"Gas masks on phones to ward off influenza." *Evening Star* (Washington, D.C.), Oct 8, 1918.
"Gas masks on phones to ward off influenza." *Evening Star* (Washington, D.C.), Oct 8, 1918.
"Gas masks used as influenza preventive." *New York Tribune*, Sep 27, 1918.
"Gas will win the war." *Evening Star* (Washington, D.C.), May 10, 1918.
"Gauze face masks." *New Britain Herald* (CT), Oct 11, 1918.
"Gauze mask order in Provo modified." *Sentinel* (Grand Junction, CO), Dec 20, 1918.
"Gauze masks not street essential." *Great Falls Tribune* (MT), Oct 29, 1918.
"Gauze masks to be worn by people as safeguard." *Americus Times-Recorder* (GA), Oct 15, 1918.
"Gauze masks to every policeman." *Boston Globe*, Oct 5, 1918.
"Gauze masks to ward off influenza." *Quad City Times* (Davenport, IA), Oct 18, 1918.
"Gauze muzzle is opposed by doctors." *Salt Lake Tribune*, Dec 3, 1918.
"Germ screen." *Chicago Tribune*, Oct 6, 1918.
"German gas visits Swiss." *Evening Star* (Washington, D.C.), May 13, 1918.
"Get your mask or your money will be needed." *Alaska Empire* (Juneau), Nov 16, 1918.
"The girl in the gas mask." *Richmond Palladium* (IN), Jan 17, 1918.
"Good effect is noted in fight against flu." *Arizona Republican* (Phoenix), Nov 21, 1918.
"Government physicians advised of influenza quarantine." *Honolulu Star Bulletin*, Oct 22, 1918.
"Governor orders inspection of trains." *Reno Gazette* (NV), Oct 23, 1918.
"Grand jury to hold sessions in flu masks." *Atlanta Constitution*, Oct 24, 1918.
"Grasping for a straw." *Bisbee Review* (AZ), Nov 19, 1918.
"Grip crisis in N.Y. over, but fight goes on." *New York Sun*, Oct 13, 1918.
"Grippe situation now well in hand." *Times-Dispatch* (Richmond, VA), Oct 11, 1918.
"Guards placed to protect Ogden." *Ogden Standard* (UT), Dec 7, 1918.
"Guilford wins fight to keep schools shut." *Star Tribune* (Minneapolis), Oct 22, 1918.
"Gypsy Smith from trenches." *Montgomery Advertiser* (AL), Nov 1, 1918.
"Hampton again puts on influenza quarantine." *Courier* (Waterloo, IA), Dec 21, 1918.
"Happy Atlantans throng theaters." *Atlanta Constitution* (GA), Oct 27, 1918.
"Hassler urges people of city to wear masks." *San Francisco Chronicle*, Dec 18, 1918.

"Haynes blocks all efforts to compel wearing of flu masks." *Sacramento Star* (CA), Oct 28, 1918.
"Headway of the epidemic checked." *Boston Globe*, Oct 2, 1918.
"Health authorities every resource to check disease." *Buffalo Enquirer* (NY), Oct 14, 1918.
"Health board acts." *West Virginian* (Fairmont), Oct 7, 1918.
"Health board decides not to shut saloon." *Racine Journal-News* (WI), Oct 21, 1918.
"Health board discusses flu." *Evansville Press* (IN), Nov 22, 1918.
"Health board issues rigid closing order." *Mansfield News* (OH), Oct 7, 1918.
"Health board orders wearing of flu masks." *Muscatine Journal* (IA), Dec 12, 1918.
"Health board recommends anti-flu mask." *Leader-Telegram* (Eau Claire, WI), Oct 29, 1918.
"Health condition in Portland is almost normal." *Oregon Journal* (Portland), Oct 20, 1918.
"Health experts plan great war on influenza." *Chicago Tribune*, Dec 11, 1918.
"Health officer condemns masks." *Sheridan Post* (WY), Nov 3, 1918.
"Health officer favors masks." *Reno Gazette* (NV), Dec 12, 1918.
"Health officer over zealous." *Wyoming State Journal* (Lander, WY), Oct 25, 1918.
"Health officer's bulletin." *Wyoming State Journal* (Laramie), Dec 13, 1918.
"Health officers instruct public." *Oregon Journal* (Portland), Oct 8, 1918.
"Health regulations." *Vernal Express* (UT), Jan 17, 1919.
"Health rule on flu likely for 10 days." *Indianapolis Star*, Oct 9, 1918.
"Health rules." *Indianapolis News*, Nov 25, 1918.
"Heard about town." *Richmond Register* (KY), Jan 7, 1919.
"Helena board keeps lid on flu." *Billings Gazette* (MT), Dec 17, 1918.
"Hello girls wearing masks." *Macon Daily Telegraph* (GA), Oct 20, 1918.
"Help control the epidemic." *Scranton Republican* (PA), Oct 26, 1918.
"Here are terms of new flu ordinance." *East Oregonian* (Pendleton), Jan 4, 1919.
"Holding city well in hand." *Argus Leader* (Sioux Falls, SD), Oct 14, 1918.
"Hooded terrors." *Abbeville Press and Banner* (SC), Oct 18, 1918.
"Hornady declares that masks must be worn for protection." *Birmingham News* (AL), Dec 15, 1918.
"Hospital grew in a night." *Boston Globe*, Sep 29, 1918.
"Hot Springs holds up the flu with masks." *Argus-Leader* (Sioux Falls, SD), Nov 5, 1918.
"How Boston fights spread of epidemic." *Des Moines Register* (IA), Oct 12, 1918.
"How grip spreads and how to dodge it." *Bangor Daily News* (ME), Oct 7, 1918.
"How well do you know friends." *Knoxville Sentinel* (TN), Jan 18, 1919.
"How you would look in a flu mask." *Wyoming State Tribune* (Cheyenne), Nov 26, 1918.
https://chroniclingamerica.loc.gov. Accessed Dec 1, 2022.
https://www.statista.com/statistics/189959/housing-units-with-telephones. Accessed Jan 11, 2023.
"Hutchinson says wearing masks is way to curb flu." *Fort Worth Star Telegram* (TX), Dec 11, 1918.
"Idaho state news items." *Rathdrum Tribune* (ID), Jan 3, 1919.
"Immune to influenza." *Sioux City Journal* (IA), Dec 4, 1918.
"Increase of influenza brings appeal to public." *Fort Wayne Journal Gazette* (IN), Dec 5, 1918.
"Influenza." *Ogden Standard* (UT), Oct 14, 1918.
"Influenza again." *Crittenden Press* (Marion, KY), Feb 6, 1920.
"Influenza ban is lifted here." *Reno Gazette* (NV), Nov 15, 1918.
"Influenza ban is raised by city officers." *Alaska Empire* (Juneau), Dec 30, 1918.
"Influenza ban is raised by proclamation." *Statesman Journal* (Salem, OR), Jan 26, 1919.
"Influenza ban is taken off." *Alma Record* (MI), Nov 28, 1918.
"Influenza ban lifted." *Topeka Capital* (KS), Nov 9, 1918.
"Influenza ban raised at last." *Harrisburg Telegraph* (PA), Nov 9, 1918.
"Influenza being held in check by determined fight." *Buffalo Enquirer* (NY), Oct 15, 1918.
"Influenza cards on many homes." *The State* (Columbia, SC), Jan 26, 1919.
"Influenza cases here total 939." *Bridgeport Telegram* (CT), Oct 12, 1918.
"Influenza cases show sharp drop." *Buffalo Evening News* (NY), Oct 18, 1918.
"Influenza checked." *Orlando Sentinel* (FL), Oct 18, 1918.
"Influenza closes the university." *Daily Star-Mirror* (Moscow, ID), Oct 21, 1918.
"Influenza closes Travis County." *Austin American* (TX), Oct 12, 1918.
"Influenza conditions better at Aberdeen." *Argus Leader* (Sioux Falls, SD), Dec 30, 1918.
"Influenza deaths in Boston fewer." *Boston Globe*, Sep 28, 1918.
"Influenza deaths 78 in 24 hours." *Evening Star* (Washington, D.C.), Oct 15, 1918.
"Influenza encyclopedia. San Antonio." https://influenzaarchive.org. Accessed Dec 20, 2023.
"The influenza epidemic." *Brooklyn Eagle* (NY), Oct 13, 1918.
"The influenza epidemic." *Newport Mercury* (RI), Oct 5, 1918.
"Influenza epidemic worse at Brigham." *Salt Lake Tribune*, Dec 12, 1918.
"Influenza fight must be real, official warning." *San Diego Union*, Oct 19, 1918.
"Influenza finds Camp Lee alert." *Evening Public Ledger* (Philadelphia), Sep 17, 1918.
"Influenza for poor of state." *Morning Tulsa World* (OK), Oct 11, 1919.

"Influenza gain not alarming." *Detroit Free Press*, Dec 7, 1918.

"Influenza gains among civilians." *Star Tribune* (Minneapolis), Oct 9, 1918.

"Influenza gains slowly in city." *Star Tribune* (Minneapolis), Oct 10, 1918.

"Influenza grip on city." *Evening Journal* (Wilmington, DE), Oct 9, 1918.

"Influenza here burning out Copeland says." *New York Tribune*, Oct 22, 1918.

"Influenza here now on decrease." *Tacoma Ledger* (WA), Oct 24, 1918.

"Influenza improving." *Newport Mercury* (RI), Oct 19, 1918.

"Influenza in fifty more homes here." *Rutland Daily Herald* (VT), Oct 7, 1918.

"Influenza in nine camps." *Bisbee Review* (AZ), Sep 21, 1918.

"Influenza is not abating." *San Francisco Examiner*, Oct 21, 1918.

"Influenza is subsiding." *Chattanooga Daily Times* (TN), Oct 17, 1918.

"Influenza is waning." *Star Tribune* (Minneapolis), Oct 17, 1918.

"Influenza is waning here." *Miami Herald* (FL), Oct 9, 1918.

"Influenza jump due to exposures threaten masks." *Journal Times* (Racine, WI), Nov 21, 1918.

"Influenza lid is shut down tight in city of Havre." *Great Falls Tribune* (MT), Nov 20, 1918.

"The influenza mask." *Courier-Journal* (Louisville, KY), Oct 29, 1918.

"Influenza mask hides faces in Fresno crowds?" *Fresno Morning Republican* (CA), Oct 19, 1918.

"Influenza mask is proposed in Chicago." *Champaign News* (IL), Sep 27, 1918.

"Influenza mask measure drawn." *Oregon Journal* (Portland), Jan 14, 1919.

"Influenza mask menace, Salt Lake experts say." *Salt Lake Tribune*, Dec 3, 1918.

"Influenza mask worn by Boston police." *Miami News* (FL), Oct 18, 1918.

"Influenza masks." *Holyoke Daily Transcript* (MA), Oct 2, 1918.

"The influenza masks and treatment." *Muncie Evening Press* (IN), Nov 22, 1918.

"Influenza masks have appeared in Knoxville." *Journal and Tribune* (Knoxville, TN), Oct 16, 1918.

"Influenza masks made for the local doctors." *Greensboro Daily News* (NC), Oct 10, 1918.

"Influenza masks now popular in Kalamazoo." *Battle Creek Enquirer* (MI), Dec 15, 1918.

"Influenza masks worn in Sacramento." *Sacramento Bee* (CA), Oct 23, 1918.

"Influenza toll may be swelled by bad weather." *Virginian Pilot* (Norfolk, VA), Oct 4, 1918.

"Influenza not bad in Reno now; care needed." *Reno Gazette* (NV), Oct 22, 1918.

"Influenza on decline." *Seattle Star*, Nov 4, 1918.

"Influenza on wane, Tuesday reports show." *San Francisco Chronicle*, Jan 22, 1919.

"Influenza patients are quarantined." *Brownsville Herald* (TX), Sep 10, 1918.

"Influenza patients now in quarantine." *Evening Herald* (Klamath Falls, OR), Dec 13, 1918.

"Influenza precepts reviewed by the State Board of Health." *Tampa Times* (FL), Jan 17, 1919.

"Influenza preventives split health meeting." *Bangor Daily News* (ME), Dec 13, 1918.

"Influenza quarantine." *Courier-Journal* (Louisville, KY), Dec 2, 1918.

"The influenza quarantine." *New York Times*, Oct 1, 1918.

"Influenza quarantine air tight here." *Kings Mountain Herald* (NC), Oct 24, 1918.

"Influenza quarantine ended." *Houston Post* (TX), Oct 26, 1918.

"Influenza quarantine here ordered raised." *Evening Herald* (Albuquerque, NM), Nov 28, 1918.

"Influenza quarantine in Butte lifted." *Missoulian* (Missoula, MT), Nov 9, 1918.

"Influenza quarantine is declared against Juneau." *Alaska Empire* (Juneau), Dec 18, 1918.

"Influenza quarantine is in effect." *Herald-Press* (St. Joseph, MI), Dec 11, 1918.

"Influenza quarantine is lifted at Helena." *Great Falls Tribune* (MT), Jan 10, 1919.

"Influenza quarantine modified at Kemmerer." *Sheridan Enterprise* (WY), Dec 30, 1918.

"Influenza quarantine to be lifted Thursday." *Charlotte Observer* (NC), Nov 4, 1918.

"Influenza quarantine to be raised Saturday." *Chandler Tribune* (OK), Nov 7, 1918

"Influenza quarantine to continue." *Woodward News-Bulletin* (OK), Oct 25, 1918.

"Influenza regulations." *Ogden Standard* (UT), Nov 28, 1918.

"Influenza regulations which must be obeyed." *Ogden Standard* (UT), Nov 27, 1918.

"Influenza serum a success." *Carson City Appeal* (NV), Oct 8, 1918.

"Influenza serum is being made in Tulsa." *Tulsa World* (OK), Oct 24, 1918.

"Influenza serum now discovered." *Wheeling Intelligencer* (WV), Oct 2, 1918.

"Influenza serum shot into Gary and steel forces." *Evening World* (NY), Oct 23, 1918.

"Influenza serums." *Bridgeport Times* (CT), Oct 28, 1918.

"Influenza serums." *Shoshone Journal* (ID), Nov 1, 1918.

"Influenza situation becomes more serious." *Las Vegas Age* (NV), Nov 9, 1918.

"Influenza situation has improved notably, cases on decrease." *Greenville News* (SC), Oct 12, 1918.

"Influenza situation looks unpromising." *Bourbon News* (Paris, KY), Oct 22, 1918.

"Influenza spreads, need for doctors and nurses urgent." *Buffalo Courier* (NY), Oct 13, 1918.

"Influenza still spreading in county and city." *Butte Miner* (MT), Oct 18, 1918.

"The influenza still with us." *Shepherdstown Register* (WV), Oct 24, 1918.

"Influenza vaccine free." *Ardmoreite* (Ardmore, OK), Oct 3, 1920.

"Influenza vaccine still experiment." *Sun* (NY), Oct 27, 1918.

"Influenza vaccine to be used." *Bridgeport Telegram* (CT), Oct 16, 1918.

"Influenza vaccine to check epidemic." *Iron County Record* (Cedar City, IA), Nov 29, 1918.

"Influenza worst it has been here." *Tacoma Ledger* (WA), Oct 28, 1918.

"Inoculated against the danger of influenza." *L'Anse Sentinel* (MI), Dec 20, 1918.

"Inspector again advises use of gauze masks." *Ogden Standard* (UT), Nov 19, 1918.

"Inspector asks suspension of flu mask fines." *Macon News* (GA), Nov 6, 1918.

"Interesting health questions." *Richmond Times-Dispatch* (VA), Mar 16, 1919.

"Jackson closes churches." *Jackson News* (MS), Oct 8, 1918.

"Jackson to remain closed for a week." *Jackson News* (MS), Oct 25, 1918,

"Jacksonville is much improved." *Tampa Bay Times* (St. Petersburg, FL), Oct 25, 1918.

"Jail terms given mask slackers by Napa judge." *Sacramento Bee* (CA), Nov 1, 1918.

"Jepson issues order." *Wheeling Intelligencer* (WV), Oct 7, 1918.

"Jim Chinaman fails to wear a mask and is fined." *Ogden Standard* (UT), Dec 9, 1918.

"Juneauites to take off masks at midnight." *Alaska Empire* (Juneau), Nov 30, 1918.

"Jury to pass on masks and lid in fighting flu." *Chicago Tribune*, Dec 13, 1918.

"K.U. doctor says many flu masks defective." *Topeka Capital* (KS), Oct 29, 1918.

"Keep down spread of influenza." *Buffalo Evening News* (NY), Oct 16, 1918.

"Keep will!" *Cincinnati Enquirer* (OH), Oct 4, 1918.

"Kentuckians don masks." *Chattanooga News* (TN), Oct 2, 1918.

"Keystone takes drastic measures of prevention." *Rapid City Journal* (SD), Oct 24, 1918.

King, Fay. "Ward off influenza by wearing mask on street." *San Francisco Examiner*, Oct 21, 1918.

"Kings Co. hospital bars flu masks; called dangerous." *Brooklyn Eagle* (NY), Oct 4, 1918.

"The Ku Klux Klan comes to town." *Brooklyn Eagle* (NY), Oct 20, 1918.

"La Crosse closed up." *Green Bay Press Gazette* (WI), Oct 23, 1918.

"Lander business men refuse to close for influenza quarantine." *Billings Gazette* (MT), Oct 27, 1918.

"Laundry and factory girls to be masked." *Leader-Telegram* (Eau Claire, WI), Oct 13, 1918.

Laurie, Annie. "S.F. feels good without mask." *San Francisco Examiner*, Nov 22, 1918.

"Laws compelling wearing of masks are recommended." *Oregon Journal* (Portland), Jan 13, 1919.

"Let us be consistent." *Tucson Citizen* (AZ), Nov 19, 1918.

"Lid goes on again in Keota." *Times* (Davenport, IA), Dec 21, 1918.

"Lid to be shut tighter." *West Virginian* (Fairmont), Oct 28, 1918.

"The lid will be lifted Friday." *Miami Herald* (FL), Oct 31, 1918.

"Lift ban under protest." *Kansas City Star* (MO), Oct 14, 1918.

"Lift flu ban soon is plan." *News Journal* (Mansfield, OH), Nov 6, 1918.

"Lima to wear muzzles." *Lima Republican Gazette* (OH), Dec 12, 1918.

"Limit on trade hours downtown." *St. Louis Star* (MO), Oct 23, 1918.

"Limit shoppers." *Salina Evening Journal* (KS), Dec 6, 1918.

"Lincoln flu death rate low." *Lincoln Star* (NE), Feb 18, 1919.

"Linthicum advises influenza masks." *Evansville Press* (IN), Nov 22, 1918.

"Little disease prevalent in city." *Billings Gazette* (MT), Dec 14, 1918.

"Local and otherwise." *Concord Tribune* (NC), Oct 16, 1918.

"Local news." *Sentinel* (Grand Junction, CO), Jan 22, 1919.

"A long visit." *Arizona Republican* (Phoenix), Dec 4, 1918.

"Look like gas masks." *Chattanooga News* (TN), Oct 10, 1918.

"Los Angeles lifted the flu quarantine." *Modesto Morning Herald* (CA), Dec 3, 1918.

"Los Angeles will not wear flu masks." *Pomona Progress* (CA), Oct 25, 1918.

"Loveland physician dies of influenza." *Sentinel* (Grand Junction, CO), Oct 30, 1918.

"Lumberton lifts flu quarantine." *Wilmington Morning Star* (NC), Oct 16, 1918.

"Macon discards masks Wednesday." *Macon News* (GA), Nov 6, 1918.

"Madison adopts flu quarantine." *La Crosse Tribune* (WI), Dec 3, 1918.

"Make flu serum." *Topeka State Journal* (KS), Dec 17, 1918.

"Make it universal." *Lima Times Democrat* (OH), Dec 13, 1918.

"Makes denial of flu story." *Seattle Star*, Nov 12, 1918.

"Malady continues on the wan in Salt Lake." *Deseret News* (Salt Lake City), Nov 26, 1918.

"Mandatory order issued by city board of health." *Miami Herald* (FL), Oct 10, 1918.

"Manning advises use of influenza masks." *Evening World-Herald* (Omaha, NE), Oct 17, 1918.

"Many are wearing influenza masks." *Vicksburg Evening Post* (MS), Oct 1, 1918.

"Many cases of influenza in Lewiston and Auburn." *Lewiston Daily Sun* (ME), Sep 28, 1918.

"Many flareups of influenza in state." *Pittsburgh Post-Gazette*, Nov 21, 1918.

"Many flu masks are being worn." *Daily Times* (Davenport, IA), Dec 2, 1918.

"Many schools in state re-opened." *Montgomery Advertiser* (AL), Nov 5, 1918.

"Marion may wear masks." *Mansfield News* (OH), Dec 16, 1918.

"Market house merchants shy at gauze masks." *Chattanooga Daily Times* (TN), Oct 18, 1918.

"Mask against influenza." *Daily Free Press* (Kinston, NC), Nov 4, 1918.

"Mask law is refused by council." *Los Angeles Record*, Jan 22, 1919.

"Mask order is issued." *Huntington Herald* (IN), Dec 10, 1918.

"Mask order was obeyed in city by 95 per cent." *Arizona Republican* (Phoenix), Nov 28, 1918.

"Mask order will remain in effect." *Indianapolis News*, Nov 23, 1918.

"Mask precautions advised for city." *Birmingham News* (AL), Dec 6, 1918.

"Mask violators fined by Smith." *Fresno Morning Republican* (CA), Nov 1, 1918.

"Masked nabobs dine and smoke at club." *Lima Republican Gazette* (OH), Dec 14, 1918.

"Maskless folk are taught lesson by health sleuths." *San Francisco Chronicle*, Nov 2, 1918.

"Masks." *Hawaii Tribune-Herald* (Hilo), Mar 5, 1919.

"Masks against flu." *Alexandria Gazette* (VA), Oct 18, 1918.

"Masks are here for influenza." *Alaska Empire* (Juneau), Nov 1, 1918.

"Masks are worn." *Oshkosh Northwestern* (WI), Oct 2, 1918.

"Masks as sensible as gum shoes." *Leader-Telegram* (Eau Claire, WI), Oct 30, 1918.

"Masks become more popular." *Daily Times* (Davenport, IA), Dec 3, 1918.

"Masks de rigeur in public places." *Tucson Citizen* (AZ), Nov 19, 1918.

"Masks for doctors and nurses in epidemics." *Norwich Bulletin* (CT), Oct 10, 1918.

"Masks in church Sunday program." *Lima Republican Gazette* (OH), Dec 13, 1918.

"Masks may be ordered for Reno." *Reno Gazette* (NV), Dec 3, 1918.

"Masks off at Newcastle." *Indianapolis News*, Nov 22, 1918.

"Masks off Wednesday." *Escanaba Morning Press* (MI), Dec 10, 1918.

"Masks on people brave influenza." *Bisbee Review* (AZ), Oct 30, 1918.

"Masks on street." *Evening Missourian* (Columbia), Oct 17, 1918.

"Masks ordered worn to guard against the flu." *Medford Mail Tribune* (OR), Dec 9, 1918.

"Masks proposed for car riders." *Tacoma Ledger* (WA), Oct 11, 1918.

"Masks should be seen on streets." *Ogden Standard* (UT), Oct 17, 1918.

"Masks, sprays, drugs and vaccines useless." *Santa Fe New Mexican*, Sep 20, 1919.

"Masks still required in stores, shows." *Tucson Citizen* (AZ), Dec 3, 1918.

"Masks voted out by council." *Custer County Republican* (Broken Bow, NE), Nov 14, 1918.

"Masks will be worn as influenza safeguards." *Oregon Journal* (Portland), Jan 12, 1919.

"Mass meeting is urged." *Montgomery Advertiser* (AL), Dec 7, 1918.

"A matter of life and death." *Evening Journal* (Wilmington, DE), Jul 31, 1919.

"May be necessary to re-establish flu quarantine." *Lincoln Star* (NE), Nov 27, 1918.

"May close all public places." *Evening Journal* (Wilmington, DE), Oct 1, 1918.

"May close all public places to check flu." *Buffalo Enquirer* (NY), Oct 7, 1918.

"May close city tight as means to end epidemic." *Arizona Republican* (Phoenix), Nov 18, 1918.

"May reopen schools soon." *Los Angeles Times*, Oct 24, 1918.

"May wear masks." *St. Joseph Gazette* (MO), Dec 1, 1918.

"Mayo Brothers have flu serum." *Evening Times-Republican* (Marshalltown, IA), Oct 17, 1918.

"Mayo influenza vaccine is offered." *Evening World* (NY), Oct 19, 1918.

"Mayor issues a drastic order." *Miami Herald* (FL), Oct 22, 1918.

"Mayor will lift the ban." *Kansas City Star* (MO), Nov 8, 1918.

"Meade men must wear gas masks during routine." *Washington Times* (Washington, D.C.), Jun 14, 1918.

"Medical men protest lifting epidemic ban." *Times-Dispatch* (Richmond, VA), Nov 1, 1918.

"Medicos vote to back health man." *Birmingham News* (AL), Dec 10, 1918.

"Members of board must wear gauze masks." *Times-Dispatch* (Richmond, VA), Oct 11, 1918.

"Missoula quarantine partly lifted today." *Butte Miner* (MT), Nov 20, 1918.

"Modesto again wearing masks." *Hanford Sentinel* (CA), Jan 16, 1919.

"Modesto is to discard influenza mask." *Fresno Morning Republican* (CA), Nov 20, 1918.

"Modesto orders wearing of influenza masks." *Sacramento Bee*, Dec 14, 1918.

"Modify store closing orders at Monroe." *Shreveport Times* (LA), Oct 22, 1918.

"More about vaccination." *Albuquerque Morning Journal* (NM), Jan 2, 1919.

"More flu masks worn." *Tribune* (Seymour, IN), Nov 23, 1918.

"More influenza cases in state." *Daily Arkansas Gazette* (Little Rock), Jan 20, 1919.

"More steps to down the flu." *Columbus Ledger* (GA), Oct 20, 1918.

"Must change face mask." *Evening Herald* (Rock Hill, SC), Oct 17, 1918.

"Must close." *Kentucky Advocate* (Danville, KY), Oct 7, 1918.

"Must make bids thru a flu mask." *Wichita Beacon* (KS), Oct 22, 1918.

"Must quarantine influenza cases." *West Virginian* (Fairmont), Oct 9, 1918.

"Must report influenza." *Los Angeles Times*, Oct 6, 1918.

"Must tell why you are on the streets today." *Arizona Republican* (Phoenix), Nov 20, 1918.

"Must wear flu masks." *Fort Wayne Sentinel* (IN), Dec 3, 1918.

"Must wear flu masks." *Natchez Democrat* (MS), Oct 19, 1918.

"Must wear masks." *Reno Gazette* (NV), Oct 28, 1918.

"Must wear masks in lobbies." *Sacramento Bee* (CA), Nov 19, 1918.

"Must wear masks in town even if riding in autos." *Petaluma Argus Courier* (CA), Nov 5, 1918.

"Nashville ban lifted." *Knoxville Sentinel* (TN), Oct 30, 1918.

"Nation and state gets ready." *Santa Fe New Mexican*, Sep 18, 1919.

"Needs in fight on epidemic supplied." *Pittsburgh Post-Gazette*, Oct 8, 1918.

"New cases of flu drop down to 36." *Tacoma Ledger* (WA), Nov 3, 1918.

"New cases of influenza at low record." *San Francisco Examiner*, Jan 26, 1919.

"New flu vaccine produced at University of Missouri." *Omaha Bee*, Dec 14, 1918.

"New hours for retail stores." *Indianapolis Star*, Oct 14, 1918.

"New influenza serum." *Brattleboro Reformer* (VT), Oct 23, 1918.

"New order closes stores and plants." *Beatrice Sun* (NE), Nov 30, 1918.

"New ordinance being drafted." *East Oregonian* (Pendleton), Jan 3, 1919.

"New York health boss says chiffon veil is mask against flu." *Des Moines Register* (IA), Oct 16, 1918.

"Newcastle to don masks." *Star Press* (Muncie, IN), Nov 21, 1918.

"Newsboys plead for gauze masks." *Scranton Republican* (PA), Oct 28, 1918.

"Nine new families reported for influenza." *East Oregonian* (Pendleton), Jan 29, 1920.

"19 die of influenza in nearby camps." *Sun* (NY), Sep 22, 1918.

"90 new cases of influenza here." *Tacoma Ledger* (WA), Oct 30, 1918.

"No cause for alarm." *Jackson Daily News* (MS), Dec 13, 1918.

"No church tomorrow." *Baltimore Sun* (MD), Oct 12, 1918.

"No convention no platform." *Richford Gazette* (VT), Oct 18, 1918.

"No decrease in influenza here figures show." *Arizona Republican* (Phoenix), Oct 30, 1918.

"No federal court account of flu." *Macon Daily Telegraph* (GA), Oct 18, 1918.

"No flu masks need be worn on streets of city." *Arizona Republican* (Phoenix), Dec 3, 1918.

"No influenza in U.S." *Alexandria Gazette* (VA), Jul 16, 1918.

"No mask; pinched." *Indianapolis Star*, Nov 21, 1918.

"No need to close things in Lincoln." *Lincoln Journal Star* (NE), Oct 8, 1918.

"No occasion for alarm." *Star Herald* (Kosciusko, MS), Oct 18, 1918.

"No thirsty rush as lid lifted." *Evening Public Ledger* (Philadelphia), Oct 30, 1918.

No title. *Bisbee Review* (AZ), Nov 1, 1918.

No title. *Bisbee Review* (AZ), Nov 6, 1918.

No title. *Clinton Messenger* (OK), Dec 12, 1918.

No title. *Junction City Union* (KS), Dec 4, 1918.

No title. *Mountainair Independent* (NM), Nov 7, 1918.

No title. *Reno Gazette* (NV), Oct 23, 1918.

No title. *Shreveport Journal* (LA), Nov 5, 1918.

"Norfolk officials decide on strict flu quarantine." *Lincoln Star* (NE), Dec 14, 1918.

"Normal hours of business be observed." *Miami Herald* (FL), Oct 27, 1918.

"Not to close city says mayor." *Tulsa Daily World* (OK), Dec 14, 1918.

"Not to restore quarantine." *Albuquerque Morning Journal* (NM), Dec 13, 1918.

"Not yet over the flu peak in Helena." *Independent Record* (Helena, MT), Oct 25, 1918.

"Notice." *Idaho Republican* (Blackfoot, ID), Nov 1, 1918.

"Nov 11 date of opening." *Oklahoma News* (Oklahoma City), Nov 2, 1918.

"Now the influenza mask." *Kansas City Times* (MO), Oct 22, 1918.

"Nurses are masked against influenza." *Minneapolis Journal*, Oct 3, 1918.

"Nurses are wanted to help fight flu." *Macon Daily Telegraph* (GA), Oct 15, 1918.

"Nurses needed to handle flu." *Tampa Times* (FL), Oct 19, 1918.

"Nurses wear flu masks." *Winona News* (MN), Oct 24, 1918.

"Oakland mayor pays influenza mask fine." *Stockton Evening Record* (CA), Jan 17, 1919.

"Off again on again worse again." *Douglas Island News* (Douglas, AK), Dec 20, 1918.

"Officials again refuse to lift influenza ban." *St. Louis Star* (MO), Nov 1, 1918.

"Officials say flu epidemic is over; masks not needed." *Oregon Journal* (Portland), Feb 10, 1919.

"Ohio happenings." *Marysville Journal Tribune* (OH), Dec 19, 1918.

"One as dangerous as other." *Mansfield News* (OH), Oct 9, 1918.

"186 arrests on first mask day." *San Francisco Chronicle*, Jan 21, 1919.

"192 new cases of influenza." *St. Louis Star* (MO), Oct 9, 1918.

"175 mask slackers arrested in city." *San Francisco Chronicle*, Nov 2, 1918.

"110 arrested for not wearing flu masks." *San Francisco Examiner*, Oct 28, 1918.

"100,000 influenza masks are needed." *Atlanta Constitution*, Oct 4, 1918.

"100,000 shots of anti-flu serum set for each day." *Rock Island Argus* (IL), Oct 21, 1918.

"1,000 flu cases in Madison." *Wisconsin State Journal* (Madison), Oct 10, 1918.

"1,726 new cases." *Buffalo Courier* (NY), Oct 13, 1918.

"1,332 new case spur flu fight." *Sun* (NY), Jan 24, 1920.

"Only two new cases of influenza in Burley." *Herald-Bulletin* (Burley, ID), Jan 31, 1919.

"Open clinic to check influenza spread." *Evening Journal* (Wilmington, DE), Oct 1, 1918.

"Opening with masks rejected by movies." *Star Tribune* (Minneapolis), Nov 2, 1918.

"Opposes wearing of flu masks by public." *South Bend Tribune* (IN), Nov 20, 1918.

"Opposing wearing influenza masks." *Spokesman-Review* (WA), Nov 7, 1918.

"Order barbers and clerks to wear flu masks." *Billings Gazette* (MT), Oct 22, 1918.

"Order extended on places that must be closed." *Independent Record* (Helena, MT), Oct 24, 1918.

"Order of health dept." *Labor Bulletin* (CO), Oct 12, 1918.

"Order to close schools stands." *Indianapolis News*, Nov 20, 1918.

"Ordinance requires all in San Diego to wear masks." *Evening Tribune* (San Diego), Dec 10, 1918.

"Outdoor meetings barred in effort to stop influenza." *Evening Star* (Washington, D.C.), Oct 9, 1918.

"Over 175 cases of influenza." *Charlotte News* (NC), Oct 3, 1918.

"Parents urged to keep their children home." *Republic* (Columbus, IN), Nov 20, 1918.

"People take action, make regulations." *Arizona Republican* (Phoenix), Nov 19, 1918.

"People urged to wear masks everywhere." *San Francisco Examiner*, Oct 20, 1918.

"Philadelphia is bone dry." *Sun* (NY), Oct 5, 1918.

"Philipp may issue sweeping order." *Racine Journal-News* (WI), Oct 10, 1918.

"Phone operators now wear masks on job." *Shreveport Times* (LA), Oct 24, 1918.

"Physicians give anti-flu vaccine." *West Virginian* (Fairmont), Oct 23, 1918.

"Physicians use influenza masks." *Winona Daily News* (MN), Sep 28, 1918.

"Physicians wear masks to avoid the infection." *Bridgeport Times* (CT), Sep 27, 1918.

"Picture shows ordered closed." *Ardmoreite* (Ardmore, OK), Oct 10, 1918.

"Plague holds entire county in its grip." *Coshocton Tribune* (OH), Nov 17, 1918.

"Plague spreading over a large area." *Sun* (NY), Oct 5, 1918

"Plan a program for flu fight." *Tampa Times* (FL), Dec 12, 1918.

"Pneumonia wards filled." *Lincoln Journal Star* (NE), Oct 19, 1918.

"Poison gas in warfare." *Ogden Standard* (UT), Jan 26, 1918.

"Police prosecutor gets names." *Akron Beacon Journal* (OH), Oct 22, 1918.

"Police restrict liquor business." *Evening Journal* (Wilmington, DE), Oct 31, 1918.

"Politics in Pennsylvania." *Harrisburg Telegraph* (PA), Nov 5, 1918.

"Possibly flu ban lifted next week." *Bucyrus Evening Telegraph* (OH), Dec 18, 1918.

"Post office clerks wearing flu masks." *Coshocton Tribune* (OH), Nov 18, 1918.

"Postmaster Chance among mask-wearers." *Evening Star* (Washington, D.C.), Oct 15, 1918.

"Predicts return of flu." *Burlington Free Press* (VT), Sep 17, 1919.

"Predicts return of flu epidemic." *Bangor Daily News* (ME), Sep 17, 1919.

"A proclamation by the mayor." *Muncie Evening Press* (IN), Oct 24, 1918.

"Progress in mask drive." *Kansas City Star* (MO), Oct 23, 1918.

"Proposed quarantine of entire city." *Evening Tribune* (San Diego), Oct 31, 1918.

"Provo will partially lift flu mask ban." *Provo Post* (UT), Dec 17, 1918.

"Public and parochial schools are ordered closed." *Daily Times* (Davenport, IA), Dec 2, 1918.

"Public gathering places closed." *Atlanta Constitution* (GA), Oct 8, 1918.

"Public gatherings forbidden." *Honolulu Advertiser*, Jan 24, 1918.

"Public gatherings in city." *Rapid City Journal* (SD), Oct 8, 1918,

"Public places closed." *Albuquerque Morning Journal* (NM), Oct 6, 1918.

"Public places not to be closed yet." *Detroit Free Press*, Oct 16, 1918.

"Publicity is found to be aid in fight against influenza." *Honolulu Advertiser*, Jan 18, 1919.

"Quarantine and use of masks ridiculed as flu preventives." *Tampa Tribune* (FL), Dec 13, 1918.

"Quarantine again at Niagara Falls." *Buffalo Enquirer* (NY), Nov 18, 1918.

"Quarantine against flu." *Herald-Press* (St. Joseph, MI), Dec 10, 1918.

"Quarantine at Gregory lifted." *Rapid City Journal* (SD), Nov 7, 1918.

"Quarantine ends here late Friday." *Decatur Herald* (IL), Nov 7, 1918.

"Quarantine for influenza not favored by city." *Harrisburg Telegraph* (PA), Dec 10, 1918.

"Quarantine goes to dances here." *Bisbee Review* (AZ), Jan 9, 1919.

"Quarantine in Harrisburg to be off Tuesday." *Harrisburg Telegraph* (PA), Oct 30, 1918.

"Quarantine is off." *Richford Gazette* (VT), Nov 1, 1918.

"Quarantine lid goes on at 9 o'clock." *Des Moines Tribune* (IA), Oct 10, 1918.

"Quarantine lifted." *Middletown Transcript* (DE), Oct 26, 1918.

"Quarantine on epidemic." *Green Bay Press Gazette* (WI), Dec 2, 1918.

"Quarantine on influenza is observed here." *Harrisburg Telegraph* (PA), Oct 4, 1918.

"Quarantine on Spanish flu to be more rigid." *Albuquerque Morning Journal* (NM), Oct 24, 1918.

"Quarantine order is essential as disease spreads." *Buffalo Enquirer* (NY), Oct 12, 1918.

"Quarantine over state is ordered." *Greenville News* (SC), Oct 8, 1918.
"Quarantine placed in the city." *Rapid City Journal* (SD), Oct 25, 1918.
"Quarantine raised." *Buffalo Times* (NY), Nov 1, 1918.
"Quarantine rules are slackened here." *Streator Times* (IL), Dec 13, 1918.
"Quarantine rules to be lifted here Monday." *Arkansas Democrat* (Little Rock), Oct 30, 1918.
"Quarantine to be raised Monday." *Buffalo Times* (NY), Nov 1, 1918.
"Quarantine to be strict." *Stevens Point Journal* (WI), Dec 4, 1918.
"Quarantine to prevent spread of influenza." *Reno Gazette* (NV), Oct 11, 1918.
"Quarantine unnecessary if influenza masks are used." *Arizona Star* (Tucson), Nov 24, 1918.
"Quarantine will not stop flu, doctor declares." *Lima Republican Gazette* (OH), Dec 11, 1918.
"Raising the embargo on wearing masks." *Tonopah Bonanza* (NV), Jan 7, 1919.
"Recurrence of influenza is not at danger point." *Harrisburg Telegraph* (PA), Jan 24, 1919.
"Red Cross asks city officials to warn public." *Idaho Daily Statesman* (Boise), Jan 4, 1919.
"Refused to don flu mask." *Hanford Sentinel* (CA), Nov 24, 1918.
"Regulation for control of influenza." *Helena Independent* (MT), Oct 8, 1918.
"Regulations for flu modified." *Douglas Island News* (Douglas, AK), Dec 6, 1918.
"Remove lid on meetings." *Argus Leader* (Sioux Falls, SD), Nov 27, 1918.
"Reopen in January." *Rathdrum Tribune* (ID), Dec 13, 1918.
"Reports on flu in state received." *Atlanta Constitution* (GA), Oct 20, 1918.
"Request to all ladies." *Sumter Daily Item* (SC), Oct 5, 1918.
"Resolution in favor of influenza quarantine." *Winston-Salem Journal* (NC), Oct 29, 1918.
"Restrictions on the flu quarantine tightened." *Chillicothe Gazette* (OH), Oct 24, 1918.
"Resumes normal activity." *Des Moines Register* (IA), Oct 29, 1918.
"Revise flu quarantine." *Albion News* (NE), Nov 28, 1918.
"Reynolds calls face mask best epidemic check." *Chicago Tribune*, Oct 18, 1918.
"Rigid grip test as schools open." *Evening Public Ledger* (Philadelphia), Oct 26, 1918.
"Rotarians are enforcing rules." *Tampa Tribune* (FL), Oct 22, 1918.
"Royer's order isolates city of Lancaster." *Harrisburg Telegraph* (PA), Nov 2, 1918.
"S.F. dons gas mask to stop flu ravages." *San Francisco Examiner*, Oct 23, 1918.
"S.F. may doff flu masks Friday morning." *San Francisco Examiner*, Jan 28, 1919.
"Sacramento puts ban on flu mask." *Santa Barbara Daily News* (CA), Dec 17, 1918.
"Safety first is slogan of Juneau people." *Alaska Empire* (Juneau), Nov 5, 1918.
"Safety first!" *Tampa Times* (FL), Nov 5, 1918.
"Safety measures being taken." *Douglas Island News* (Douglas, AK), Nov 15, 1918.
"Saloonman is arrested by city." *Harrisburg Telegraph* (PA), Oct 8, 1918.
"Saloons restricted; Laurel races to end." *Baltimore Sun* (MD), Oct 12, 1918.
"Salt Lake takes off quarantine." *Ogden Standard* (UT), Dec 7, 1918.
"San Diego removes flu restrictions." *Long Beach Press* (CA), Nov 15, 1918.
"San Francisco and the masks." *Butte Miner* (MT), Dec 1, 1918.
"San Francisco again puts on health masks." *San Francisco Chronicle*, Jan 18, 1919.
"San Francisco waits go give decision." *Modesto Morning Herald* (CA), Dec 12, 1918.
"San Francisco's first dry year." *Bakersfield Morning Echo* (CA), Oct 9, 1920.
"Sandersville to re-open schools." *Macon News* (GA), Dec 29, 1918.
"Sanitary campaign on to stop influenza." *Chattanooga News* (TN), Oct 9, 1918.
"Saturday night ban is removed." *Harrisburg Telegraph* (PA), Nov 8, 1918.
"The saving grace of common sense." *Muncie Evening News* (IN), Dec 16, 1918.
"Say flu masks handicap." *Des Moines Register* (IA), Nov 30, 1918.
"Says barbers and dentists should wear flu masks." *Gazette* (Cedar Rapids, IA), Dec 25, 1918.
"Says physicians regard flu masks as absurd." *St. Louis Star* (MO), Dec 13, 1918.
"School attendance is 10 per cent less." *Fort Worth Star Telegram* (TX), Oct 30, 1918.
"Schools are closed." *Arizona Republican* (Phoenix), Jan 6, 1919.
"Schools close as influenza plague gains." *Detroit Free Press*, Oct 22, 1918.
"Schools, churches and entertainment." *Burlington Free Press* (VT), Oct 5, 1918.
"Schools, churches and theaters to be freed." *Racine Journal-News* (WI), Nov 1, 1918.
"Schools, churches, theaters and dance halls." *Racine Journal-News* (WI), Oct 5, 1918.
"Schools, churches, theaters closed." *La Crosse Tribune* (WI), Oct 10, 1918.
"Schools closed by the influenza." *Morning News* (Wilmington DE), Nov 23, 1918.
"Schools closed." *Kemmerer Camera* (WY), Mar 26, 1919.
"Schools do not open on Monday." *Maryland Gazette* (Annapolis), Oct 26, 1918
"Schools open Monday." *Diamond Drill* (Crystal Falls, MI), Nov 16, 1918.
"Schools should not be closed." *Birmingham News* (AL), Dec 7, 1918.
"Schools to be shut because of influenza." *St. Louis Star* (MO), Oct 7, 1918.
"Scores of arrests follow flu mask ordinance." *Arizona Star* (Tucson), Dec 17, 1918.
"Scots in France Wearing Gas Masks." *Meridian Times* (ID), Jun 2, 1916.

"Scouts do good work." *Deseret News* (Salt Lake UT), Oct 21, 1918.
"Second arrest influenza law." *Arizona Republican* (Phoenix), Oct 27, 1918.
"See end of influenza scourge." *Los Angeles Times*, Feb 9, 1919.
"Send the children to school." *Richford Gazette* (VT), Nov 22, 1918.
"760 new flu cases sets high record." *St. Louis Star* (MO), Nov 28, 1918.
"$7000 fines paid in flu mask cases." *Oakland Tribune* (CA), Nov 4, 1918.
"Short state notes." *Bennet Sun* (NE), Nov 7, 1918.
"Shows to run, churches open." *Detroit Free Press*, Oct 13, 1918.
"Simmons urges state influenza mask law." *Sacramento Bee* (CA), Jan 25, 1919.
"Six deaths today's toll." *Bismarck Tribune* (ND), Oct 24, 1918.
"65 die of influenza here." *Washington Herald* (DC), Oct 13, 1918.
"Slight improvement in the influenza epidemic." *Wheeling Intelligencer* (WV) Oct 23, 1918.
"Slight increase in new flu cases." *Macon Daily Telegraph* (GA), Oct 30, 1918.
"Society girls busy making flu masks." *Deseret News* (Salt Lake), Oct 18, 1918.
"Soda fountains will be closed." *Virginian Pilot* (Norfolk), Oct 8, 1918.
"Soldier boys in Spokane must don masks now." *Spokane Chronicle* (WA), Oct 26, 1918.
"Some doctors question the efficacy of closing." *Battle Creek Enquirer* (MI), Dec 13, 1918.
"Spanish flu has Boston in tragic grip." *Seattle Star*, Sep 26, 1918.
"Spanish flu much like grip." *Evening Times-Republican* (Marshalltown IA), Sep 30, 1918.
"Spanish flu rigid quarantine." *Sentinel* (Grand Junction CO), Nov 5, 1918.
"Spanish influenza." *Mountainair Independent* (NM), Nov 7, 1918.
"Spanish influenza." *Ogden Standard* (UT), Nov 23, 1918.
"Spanish influenza – three-day fever, the flu." *Muskogee Times-Democrat* (OK), Oct 17, 1918.
"Spanish influenza and how to combat it." *Daily Telegram* (Long Beach CA), Oct 12, 1918.
"Spanish influenza cases have jumped." *Tampa Tribune* (FL), Oct 21, 1918.
"Spanish influenza here officials fear." *New York Tribune*, Sep 12, 1918.
"Spanish influenza here." *New York Sun*, Sep 12, 1918.
"Spanish influenza not epidemic here." *Atlanta Constitution*, Oct 10, 1918.
"Spanish influenza quarantine." *Lenoir Topic* (NC), Oct 18, 1918.
"Spanish influenza strikes two more residents of city." *Honolulu Advertiser*, Oct 30, 1918.
"Spanish influenza vaccine is provided." *Capital Journal* (Salem OR), Oct 17, 1918.
"Spanish influenza widespread but not severe." *Sun* (NY), Aug 4, 1918.

"Spartanburg folk wearing face masks." *The State* (Columbia SC), Oct 16, 1918.
"Speed up flu law." *Topeka State Journal* (KS), Sep 15, 1919.
"Spray is ordered as guard against spread of disease." *San Diego Union*, Oct 17, 1918.
"Spread of flu in Helena is unabated." *Independent Record* (Helena MT), Oct 29, 1918.
"Springfield lifts the influenza ban." *Mansfield News* (OH), Nov 1, 1918.
"St. Paul closed by influenza spread." *Minneapolis Journal*, Nov 4, 1918.
"Start fight to stamp out the influenza here." *Arizona Republican* (Phoenix), Nov 20, 1918.
"State board put quarantine on city and county." *Greenville News* (SC), Oct 8, 1918.
"State board urges masks." *Sacramento Bee* (CA), Oct 21, 1918.
"State board's influenza advice." *Greenville Sun* (TN), Oct 8, 1918.
"State flu ban to be lifted." *Independent Record* (Helena MT), Dec 16, 1918.
"State flu ban will be lifted." *Indianapolis Star* (IN), Nov 1, 1918.
"State grip decree closes up Detroit." *Detroit Free Press*, Oct 19, 1918.
"State health board doubts efficacy of influenza masks." *Sacramento Bee* (CA), Nov 14, 1918.
"State health officials order wearing of masks." *Spokane Chronicle* (WA), Nov 7, 1918.
"State will not be quarantine for flu." *Arkansas Democrat* (Little Rock AR), Jan 20, 1919.
"Statewide quarantine ordered by Dr. Duke." *Guthrie Leader* (OK), Oct 10, 1918.
"Stay at home." *Bismarck Tribune* (ND), Oct 14, 1918.
"Steps taken to check disease." *Roanoke Leader* (AL), Oct 23, 1918.
"Sterilize mask every two hours." *Detroit Free Press*, Oct 27, 1918.
"Stop gatherings." *Kansas City Star* (MO), Oct 7, 1918.
"Store people called on to make their own masks." *Ogden Standard* (UT), Nov 29, 1918.
"Storm council, demand repeal flu mask edict." *Medford Mail Tribune* (OR), Dec 18, 1918.
"Strict influenza quarantine." *Bedford Mail* (IN), Nov 21, 1918.
"Strict quarantine ordered for flu." *Clearwater Record* (NE), Jan 3, 1919.
"Stringent rules against epidemic." *Casper Press* (WY), Dec 7, 1918.
"Successful influenza vaccine is not found." *Tulsa World* (OK), Oct 11, 1918.
"A sure cure for the flu." *Middletown Transcript* (DE), Oct 26, 1918.
"Swat flu mask; also Hutchinson." *Los Angeles Times*, Nov 8, 1918.
"Sweeping quarantine against influenza." *Banner* (Cambridge MD), Oct 4, 1918.
"Take steps to halt influenza." *Shreveport Times* (LA), Oct 8, 1918.
"Tampa acts to head off epidemic here." *Tampa Times* (FL), Oct 8, 1918.

"Tampa Electric Co., take precautions." *Tampa Times* (FL), Oct 19, 1918.

"Tampa schools open Monday." *Orlando Evening Star* (FL), Nov 7, 1918.

"Teachers call for more pay." *Evening Public Ledger* (Philadelphia), Jan 3, 1919.

"Teachers may be paid during the epidemic." *Montgomery Advertiser* (AL), Oct 26, 1918.

"Teachers to help combat influenza among children." *Buffalo Courier* (NY), Oct 17, 1918.

"Teachers will dray pay for flu period." *Sentinel* (Grand Junction CO), Nov 21, 1918.

"Teachers will get full pay." *Chickasha Express* (OK), Oct 24, 1918.

"Telephone flu mask is latest stroke." *Omaha Evening Bee* (NE), Oct 19, 1918.

"Ten commandments for the prevention of flu." *News and Observer* (Raleigh NC), Oct 21, 1918.

"Tent hospitals as last resort." *Harrisburg Telegraph* (PA), Oct 7, 1918.

"Test case of flu mask order." *Spokesman-Review* (Spokane WA), Nov 9, 1918.

"Thanksgiving offer." *Arizona Republican* (Phoenix), Nov 28, 1918.

"Theater men to resist mask rule." *Logansport Pharos-Tribune* (IA), Dec 7, 1918.

"Theaters and movies closed." *Chicago Tribune*, Oct 15, 1918.

"Theaters downstate warned not to open." *Decatur Herald* (IL), Nov 1, 1918.

"Theaters join fight on flu infection." *Indianapolis Star*, Sep 29, 1918.

"Theaters to come under mask order." *Macon Daily Telegraph* (GA), Oct 17, 1918.

"They're wearing gas masks in El Paso." *El Paso Times* (TX), Oct 6, 1918.

"Third Saturday night closing is ordered at 6:30." *Harrisburg Telegraph* (PA), Oct 26, 1918.

"This is last day of wearing the mask in Salt Lake City." *Deseret News* (Salt Lake), Dec 17, 1918.

"This mask bunk." *Goodwin's Weekly* (Salt Lake), Dec 7, 1918.

"Those exposed to flu should wear masks." *Buffalo Enquirer* (NY), Oct 12, 1918.

"Thousands hit by flu mask order Monday." *Seattle Star*, Oct 28, 1918.

"Thousands of gauze masks doing service." *Chattanooga News* (TN), Oct 11, 1918.

"Thousands take anti-flu serum as a precaution." *Oregon Journal* (Portland), Oct 27, 1918.

"Three shot in struggle with mask slacker." *San Francisco Chronicle,* Oct 29, 1918.

"Three thousand masks needed immediately." *Chattanooga News* (TN), Oct 11, 1918.

"3,000 wear masks at football game." *Birmingham News* (KY), Nov 3, 1918.

"Time to act now if Hilo hopes to escape the flu." *Hilo Tribune,* Jan 15, 1919.

"Timely warning given by health officer Locke." *Public Ledger* (Maysville KY), Oct 23, 1918.

"To check disease." *Alexandria Gazette* (VA), Oct 5, 1918.

"To confer on state closing." *Lansing State Journal* (MI), Oct 18, 1918.

"To lift lid Saturday Night." *Times Advocate* (Escondido CA), Nov 9, 1918.

"To lift the lid." *Topeka State Journal* (KS), Oct 30, 1918.

"To re-open Thursday." *Evening Missourian* (Columbia), Oct 28, 1918.

"To return single no-flu mask fine." *Arizona Republican* (Phoenix), Dec 4, 1918.

"To the citizenship of Clinton." *Custer County Chronicle* (Clinton OK), Dec 5, 1918.

"Toledo lifts quarantine." *Cincinnati Enquirer* (OH), Nov 2, 1918.

"Topeka to wear masks." *Topeka Daily Capital* (KS), Oct 19, 1918.

"Town board of health rules and regulations." *Northern Herald* (Cody WY), Oct 23, 1918.

"Town quarantined." *Custer Chronicle* (Custer City SD), Oct 26, 1918.

"Trains to be met by committee." *Morning Union* (Grass Valley CA), Oct 25, 1918.

"Twenty thousand influenza masks wanted." *Baltimore Sun* (MD), Oct 2, 1918.

"Twenty-five special officers." *Stockton Evening Record* (CA), Nov 15, 1918.

"29,002 cases Spanish flu army's report." *Washington Herald* (DC), Sep 26, 1918.

"200 deaths in city." *Evening Journal* (Wilmington DE), Oct 4, 1918.

"249 new cases show increase." *Indianapolis Star*, Nov 23, 1918.

"Two new cases of influenza in this city today." *Topeka State Journal* (KS), Sep 17, 1919.

"Two thousand cases develop at Billings." *Great Falls Tribune* (MT), Oct 24, 1918.

"Uncle Sam has gas mask which would get Hun." *Ogden Standard* (UT), Dec 14, 1918.

"Uncle Sam's advice on flu." *Asbury Park Press* (NJ), Oct 12, 1918.

"Uncle Sam's advice on flu." *Daily Herald* (Biloxi MS), Oct 15, 1918.

"Uncle Sam's advice on flu." *Newport Mercury* (RI), Oct 12, 1918.

"Uncle Sam's advice on flu." *Rutland Daily Herald* (VT), Oct 14, 1918.

"Uncle Sam's Advice." *Rathdrum Tribune* (ID), Oct 18, 1918.

"University women make masks." *Evening Missourian* (Columbia), Oct 30, 1918.

"Until November three." *Richford Gazette* (VT), Oct 25, 1918.

"Up to each city." *Gate City* (Keokuk IA), Oct 24, 1918.

"Urges use of masks to curb influenza." *Times-Dispatch* (Richmond VA), Oct 9, 1918.

"U.S. Health warns against flu vaccines." *Eureka Sentinel* (NV), Dec 7, 1918.

"Use mask and avoid all crowds, they say." *Evening Missourian* (Columbia), Dec 23, 1918.

"Use more masks." *Topeka State Journal* (KS), Oct 30, 1918.

"Use thermometer at M. S." *Sioux City Journal* (IA), Dec 10, 1918.

"Using flu masks." *Daily Democrat Forum* (Maryville MO), Oct 31, 1918.

"Utah County lifts ban Dec 27." *Provo Post* (UT), Dec 20, 1918.

"Vaccinate class one." *Gate City* (Keokuk IA), Oct 23, 1918.

"Vaccination against pneumonia." *Topeka State Journal* (KS), Nov 12, 1918.

"Vaccination first rule against flu." *Seattle Star*, Dec 13, 1918.

"Vaccination station here." *Gate City* (Keokuk IA), Dec 4, 1918.

"Vaccine for flu." *Topeka Stat Journal* (KS), Dec 10, 1918.

"Vaccine for school is not recommended." *Ogden Standard* (UT), Dec 17, 1918.

"Vaccine given R&V workers." *Rock Island Argus* (IL), Oct 26, 1918.

"Vaccine used to curb spread of influenza." *Rogue River Courier* (Grants Pass OR), Oct 24, 1918.

"Value of vaccination against influenza." *Arizona Republican* (Phoenix), Nov 17, 1918.

"Views on cure for influenza differ widely." *Pittsburgh Post-Gazette*, Dec 13, 1918.

"Violated flu mask ordinance." *Hanford Sentinel* (CA), Nov 28, 1918.

"Violates flu rule, pays fine." *Montgomery Advertiser* (AL), Oct 29, 1918.

"Vote early." *Sentinel* (Grand Junction CO), Nov 4, 1918.

"Want ordinance to penalize violators." *Evening Tribune* (San Diego), Oct 24, 1918.

"Warning." *Ogden Standard* (UT), Nov 30, 1918.

"Warns against needless travel." *Daily Arkansas Gazette* (Little Rock), Nov 27, 1918.

"Warns of Spanish flu." *Baltimore Sun* (MD), Sep 14, 1918.

"Weapons against influenza." *Greenville Daily News* (SC), Dec 7, 1918.

"Wear a gauze mask and smile; help the fight against influenza." *Seattle Star*, Oct 30, 1918.

"Wear a mask against the flu." *Evening Capital* (Annapolis MD), Sep 30, 1918.

"Wear a muslin mask to balk influenza." *New Britain Herald* (CT), Sep 30, 1918.

"Wear cheese cloth mask." *Winona News* (MN), Oct 17, 1918.

"Wear flu masks board suggests." *Kenosha Evening News* (WI), Dec 7, 1918.

"Wear masks at Bedford." *Indianapolis News*, Nov 1, 1918.

"Wear masks – keep off the flu." *Columbus Enquirer-Sun* (GA), Oct 20, 1918.

"Wear masks to escape plague." *Shoshone Journal* (ID), Jun 14, 1918.

"Wear ward masks." *Muskogee Times-Democrat* (OK), Oct 9, 1918.

"Wear your mask." *Alaska Empire* (Juneau), Nov 14, 1918.

"Wearing anti-flu masks." *Salina Evening Journal* (KS), Oct 31, 1918;

"Wearing flu masks made compulsory." *Quad City Times* (Davenport IA), Dec 4, 1918.

"Wearing flu masks mandatory in Provo." *Salt Lake Telegram*, Oct 19, 1918.

Index

Abbeville (SC) 85
Abele, John G. 216
Abercrombie, T. F. 87
Aberdeen (SD) 146–147
Adams, G.B. 28
advice, medical 8
advice, official 45, 178; contradictory 143
Akron (NY) 53
Akron (OH) 117
Alabama 96–99
Alaska 198–200
Albemarle (NC) 83
Albuquerque (NM) 176
alcohol: rules 71–72; sales, by prescription 61–62
Alexandria (VA) 78
Alger, Mrs. Russell 115
Alma (MI) 32, 113
Amarillo (TX) 111
Amble, C.J. 176
American Journal of Public Health 85–86
American Public Health Association (Chicago) 44, 70, 95, 97, 103, 105, 121, 127, 134–135, 159, 195; conclusion 134–135
Annapolis (MD) 72
Anti-Mask League of San Francisco 236–237
antiseptics 73, 94, 166
Appleton, Henry 233
Ardmore (OK) 109
Arizona 186–195
Arkansas 108
Arkansas Board of Health 108
arrests 62, 115, 122, 123, 129, 172, 177, 184, 186, 191, 192, 204, 211
arrests: massive 228, 233, 236; theater owners 124; totals (CA) 237
Ascher, J.A. 197
Asheville (NC) 83
Ashland (OH) 116
Atlanta (GA) 87–88
Auer, Edward 22

Augusta (GA) 87
Austin (TX) 111
automobiles, inside of 227
Ayer (MA) 45
Ayer Board of Health 45

Babcock, E.V. 65
Babcock, H.C. 93
Baltimore (MD) 72
Bangor Board of Health 43–44
banks 162, 168, 170, 206–207
barbers 51, 58, 60, 69, 79, 95, 103, 104, 111, 133, 141, 149, 165, 184, 225; refuse 81
Barbour, Max 168, 170
Bauman, James E. 117
Beard, C.Y. 173
Beatrice (NE) 160
Beatty, T.B. 181
Beaumont (TX) 111
Belfast (ME) 44
Bell Telephone Company 107
Bingham, P.H. 107
Bird, R.E. 164
Birmingham (AL) 96–98
Bisbee (AZ) 187–188, 189–190
Bismarck (ND) 144–145
Bissell, William G. 56
Black, Mrs. Eugene R. 91
Blackfoot (ID) 171
blacks, rules 93
Blake, John D. 72
blame the victim 175, 201, 202, 206, 219
Blue, Rupert 10–11, 28, 73–74
Blue, Rupert, and masks 11
Blum, George 234
Boise (ID) 171
Bolton, Ralph 154
Bon Marché store 29, 202
Boone, D.W. 118
Boston (MA) 48–49
Bowes, Timothy W. 26
Boy Scouts: as police 93; as propagandists 181
Boyd, Charles 227
Boykin, W.D. 84
Bozeman (MT) 167

Bracken, H.M. 140
Brady, William 12
Bremerton navy yard 25
Bridgeport (CT) 40
Briggs, Jessie 162
Brigham City (UT) 180
Bright, J. Fulmer 79
Brooklyn (NY) 58–59
Brown, Ben 102
Brown, Orville H. 27, 186
Brown, W.P. 32
Brown, Walter H. 40–41
Brownlow, Louis 75
Brumbaugh, Martin 64
Buck, George S. 52
Buerkele, John G. 220
Buffalo (NY) 52–53, 53–56
Buffalo Forge 56
Buffalo Health Department 53–56
Buffalo Police Department 56
Bullen, Roy 178
Bunch, Rollin H. 127
Bureau for the Guidance of the Public 8
Burton, E.G. 120–121
Burton, S.L. 12
business: hours 107; lobbying 226; protests 124, 174–175; usages 75–76, 157–158, 165
Butler, W.P. 147
Butte (MT) 167, 169
Byington Frank 196

California 216–237
California Board of Health 217, 224
Camden (NJ) 67
Camp Devens (MA) 9, 45
Camp Dix (NJ) 24
Camp Gordon (GA) 91
Camp Greene (NC) 81
Camp Lee (VA) 8
Camp Meade (MD) 17
camps, army 8–9
cantonments 9, 45
Carlson, A.J. 115
Carnes, A.W. 111

277

Index

Carter, C.F. 99
Carter, Thomas J. 164
Casey, E.L. 208
celebrities, for propaganda 101
chairs, removed 133
Chance, Merritt 76
Chandler, G.C. 107
Chaplin, Charlie 46
Charleston (TN) 101
Charleston (WV) 81
Charlotte (NC) 81, 83
Chartres-Martin, E.P. 220
Chattahoochee Valley Fair 88
Chattanooga (TN) 100, 102–103
Chattanooga Railway and Light Company 103
Chetwynd, J.W. 117
Chicago 132–134
Chicago Health Department 21
children: arrest threats 100–101; banned 119; confined to home 84; forced masking 90; loitering 146; movements banned 114; restrictions 94, 100, 162, 216
chiropractors 173
Cincinnati (OH) 120
citizens, duties 88
Citizens' League of Los Angeles 226
Clark, A.W. 165
Clark, H.L. 164–165
Clay, G.H. 158
Cleveland (OH) 118
Clifton (NJ) 51
Clinton. Fred S. 110
closures: Blue Protocols 10; financial costs 125; rationales 45–46; total 155, 221
clothing, treatment 148
clothing and formaldehyde 205
Cochraine, W.R. 100
Cody (WY) 172
Coffey, L.H. 82
Cogswell, W.F. 167
colds, head 92, 172
Coleville (PA) 62
College Park (GA) 89
Collier, F.H. 159
Colorado 173–176
Columbia (MO) 157
Columbia (SC) 85
Columbus (GA) 88
Columbus (IN) 125
Commercial National Bank 75
commercial tie-ins 17–19
company employees, as police 69
Comstock, Willard 81
Concord (NC) 83
Concordia (KS) 165
congregating 116, 144
Connecticut 40–42

Connecticut Department of Health 40
Converse, G.M. 79
Copeland, Royal 7, 8, 9, 20–21, 38, 51–53, 60–61, 115, 178
Copeland, W.E. 194
Cornwell, John J. 80
Corput, G.M. 106
Coshocton (OH) 119
coughing and sneezing 49
Cowgill, James 157
Cox, James M. 117
Criss, H.L. 80
Critchlow, J.F. 182
Crosby, Daniel 228
Custer County (ID) 172
Custer County (OK) 110
customers, limited floor space 164, 210, 211

D.H. Holmes Company 28
Dallas (TX) 111
Dallas County Medical Society 96
Dalton, Charles F. 23
dances 44, 123, 132, 168, 180, 213
dancing, floor space limits 213
Dargavel, Hugh 104
Davenport (IA) 148–149
Davie, John L. 228
Davies, Gordon 117
Davis, W.D. 111
Decatur (IL) 133
deGravelles, C.C. 28
DeLamater, H. 157
Delaware 71–72
Delaware Board of Health 71
Delaware Hospital 20
dentists 51, 73, 111
Denver 173–175
Denver, as example 166
Denver Board of Health 173–174
Derivaux, C.A. 101
Des Moines (IA) 147–149
Detroit (MI) 113–115
diagnostics 12
disease, reportable 44
disinfectants 133, 212
District of Columbia 73–77
District of Columbia Commissioners 74
Douglas (AZ) 195, 198
Dowell, Spright 96
Dowling, J.D. 97
Dowling, Oscar 106
Drake, St. Clair 22, 132
Duhigg, T.F. 154
Duke, John W. 109

E.S. Wakelin Grocery Co. 192–193
East Liverpool (OH) 117

Eau Claire (WI) 138
editorial cartoon 76
editorial: comments 58, 60, 74, 82, 105, 120; comments, anti 100, 159, 186, 190, 238; comments, for 41–42, 122, 183, 202–204
El Paso (TX) 111, 112
Elko (NV) 196
Ellegood, Robert E. 71
Ellwood City (PA) 69
Elmira (NY) 53
Ely (NV) 196
employee hours, staggered 60, 113
Erickson, Abel 227
Escanaba (MI) 114–115
Escondido (CA) 218, 228
examples, setting of 181
Exchange National Bank 206–207

Fairfield (CT) 41
Fairfield, J.H. 168
Fairmont (WV) 24
Fairmont Board of Health 80
Fargo (ND) 144–145
Fayetteville (AR) 108
fear, induced 42–43, 74, 83, 119–120, 126, 176, 184, 200–201, 229–230
federal government role 11–12
Fee, James A. 209
Fess, Simeon D. 11–12
financial losses, from rules 64, 155
fines 62, 104, 117, 122, 123, 194–195, 221, 223, 228
Finley, G.W. 124
Fitzgerald, J. 58
Flannaghan, Roy K. 78
Flint (MI) 114
Florida 92–95
flu, diagnostics 43
flu mask vs gas masks 74
football game 105, 165
Fort Collins (CO) 174
Fort Wayne (IN) 126
Fort Worth (TX) 111
four-foot rule 210–211
Frantz, A.E. 71
Frazer, T. Atchison 38–39
fresh air 11
Fresno (CA) 222–223
Freyermuth, E.G. 125
Frost, D.F. 126
fruit pits 16
fumigation 53, 119, 177
funerals 61, 93, 179

Gainesville (GA) 87
Gallagher, Andrew J. 237
Gannon, A.J. 156

Index

Garner, Samuel 72–73
Garrison, C.W. 108
Gary, Elbert H. 23–24
Gates, C.E. 211
Geiger, J.C. 108
Georgia 87–92
Georgia Board of Health 87, 89
Germany 7–8
germicides 56, 138
germs, travel length 49
Gilbert, J.D. 25
Giles, James 92
Gilleland, J.L. 200
Girvin, Henry J. 56
Goodman, Guy T. 116
Goodwin's Weekly 186
Gram, Franklin C. 52
Grass Valley (CA) 222
Great Falls (MT) 168
Great Lakes Naval Training Station 9
Green Bay (WI) 137
Greene, Finlay H. 53
Greensboro (NC) 83
Greenville (SC) 84
Grimshaw, Charles B. 22
grip 7–8
Grosjean, Mrs. C.E. 236
Grote, Carl A. 97
Guilford, H.M. 140
gunplay, noncompliance 227, 233

Haile, Mrs. W.T. 219
Hall. J.W. 31
Halloween, controlled 64
handkerchiefs, in lieu of 47, 56, 124–125
Hanford (CA) 227
Hanson, Ole 201–202
Harding, Warren 11–12
Harper A.A. 136
Harris, L.I. 8
Harrisburg (PA) 62–64
Harrisburg (PA) Health Board 66
Hassler, William C. 169, 229–234, 236–237
Havre (MT) 168–169
Hawaii 237–239
Hayes, Edward 224
Hayne, James A. 84, 85
Haynes, John R. 226
health officer, special 174
health pass 81–82, 116–117, 169, 179, 186–187, 196
hectoring: 130, 232; public speaking 40
Heiser, Victor G. 116
Helena (MT) 167–168, 170
Hennepin County Medical Society 140
Hill, W.H. 127

Hilo (HI) 238
Hobby, W.P. 110
Hold, Harry H. 79
Holyoke Board of Health 46
Honolulu (HI) 238–239
Hornady, J.R. 98
Hoskins, J.K. 88
hospital, open-air 47
Houston, Frank 189
Hubbard, Charles H. 110
Hubbard, Daniel D. 7
Hubbard, Leslie E. 174
Huebsch Laundry 138
Huffaker, H.D. 102
Huntington, W.K. 172
Hurty, J.N. 124
Hutcheson, Sherman 227
Hutchinson, Woods 112, 121, 225
hyperbole 98

Idaho 171–172
Illinois 132–135
Illinois Department of Health 132
impositions, sudden 102
Inches, James W. 113, 114
Indiana 123–132
Indiana Board of Health 123
Indianapolis (IN) 123, 128
Indianapolis Board of Health 130
industrial usages 56, 69, 138
instructions: from media 52; masks 121, 138
Iowa 147–154

Jackson (MS) 99
Jacksonville (FL) 94
Jenkins, Park B. 145
Jepson, S.L. 80
Johnson, Henry C. 34
Johnston, R.M. 110–111
Jones, Hampson 72
Jordan, George A. 159
Juneau (AK) 198

Kalamazoo (MI) 114, 115
Kansas 163–166
Kansas City (MO) 156, 157
Kansas City Railway Company 157–158
Kealy, P.J. 156
Keegan, J.F. 40
Kellogg, W.H. 181, 217
Kelly, E.R. 29
Kemmerer (WY) 173
Kennedy, J.P. 87
Kennewick (WA) 200
Kentucky 104–105
Kentucky Board of Health 104
Keokuk (IA) 32, 150
Keystone (SD) 145–146

Kiel, Henry 154–155
King, Fay 229
King, William 111
Kings County Hospital 58
Kings Mountain (NC) 82
Kinston (NC) 83
Kirtley, C.L. 172
kissing 62
Klamath Falls (OR) 209
Kleinman, Dan 189
Knight, C.P. 102
Knoxville (TN) 100, 101
Kolf, E.F. 134
Kolynos company 17–19

La Crosse (WI) 137
Lamb, Ellis 110
Lancaster (PA) 65
Lansing (MI) 114
Larkin Company 56
Last, Henry 186
Las Vegas (NV) 196
laundry workers 176
Laurie, Annie 235
Laux, F.S. 123
Lawrence (KS) 165
Leary, Timothy 26
Leathers, W.S. 99
legal proceedings 64, 90–91, 104, 117, 164, 172, 177–178, 185–186, 191, 208, 221
Lenoir (NC) 81
Lewiston (ME) 44
Lewistown (MT) 168
Lexington (MO) 165
Lilly, G.W. 122
Lima (OH) 119
Lima Board of Health 122–123
Lincoln (NE) 160
liquor outlets 46
Little Rock (AR) 108
local vs state 69–70, 113, 117–118, 131–132, 140–141, 148, 173, 200
Locke, J.S. 104
Logan (UT) 178, 180
loitering 99, 172
Los Angeles (CA) 218, 225–226
Louisiana 106–107
Louisville (KY) 105
loyalty 88
Lumberton (NC) 81
Lunger, J.S. 119

Machada, Chris Mrs. 219
Macon (GA) 89
Madison (WI) 136
Maine 43–45
malnutrition 7
mandate vs. persuasion 57, 97
mandates, difficult 75
Mansfield (OH) 116

Manufacturers' Association of East Chicago 25
Marchant, George 149
Marion (OH) 117, 118
Marion (SC) 84
Martin, Willsie 172
Maryland 72–73
Maryville (MO) 156–157
masks: Bridgeport (CT) 40–42, care of 138; changing of 133; criticisms 44–45, 80; disposal 128; flu vs. gas 17; gas 12–16; industrial 13–16; instructions 85; as lucky charms 145; make one 41, 56, 85, 217; pre-flu 12–14; reversing 79; technical aspects 116; treatment of 40, 42
Massachusetts 45–50
Matheson, Carleton 223
Mayo, William James 21
Mayo Brothers Clinic 21
McBride, J.S. 21, 200
McCalla, L.P. 172
McCarthy, J.L. 196
McCrann, W.J. 161
McElroy, Sylvan 92
McGurran, C.J. 144
McKay, Donald 92
Medbury, C.S. 152
Medford (OR) 211
media: coverage 10; lies 83; reports, false 69; hype 109; propaganda 97; publicity 90
medical exams, forced, children 67
medical visits, forced 172
medicated masks 89, 103, 119–120
Melts, J. 89
Mesa (AZ) 189
Meyer, Karl F. 37
Miami (FL) 93–94
Miami Board of Health 93
Michigan 113–116
Michigan Health Board 113
Middleton (DE) 71
Millard, Ezra 162
Miller, Henry D. 233
Mills, W.F. 175
Minneapolis (MN) 140–141
Minneapolis Board of Education 141
Minneapolis Street Railway Company 140
Minnesota 140–143
Minty, F.W. 145
Mississippi 99–100
Missoula (MT) 167
Missouri 154–160
Modesto (CA) 227
Moline (IA) 149–150
Monroe (LA) 107

Montana 167–171
Montgomery, R.C. 172
Montgomery County Health Bureau 96
Montgomery Ward and Company 157
Montrose (CO) 174
Moore, Edwin C. 192
Moore, W.E. 145
Morgan, Herman G. 128–130
Morningside College 150
Moscow (ID) 172
Mountainair (NM) 176
Mulvihill, Joseph 235
Muncie (IN) 127
Murdy, R.L. 147
Murray (UT) 183
Murray (KY) 104
Muscatine (IA) 148
Muskogee (OK) 109
Mustard, Harry S. 75

Napa (CA) 227
Nashville (TN) 100–101
Nebraska 160–163
Nebraska Board of Health 161
neighbors, visit 92
Nesbitt, Charles 117
Nevada 195–197
New Hampshire 45–45
New Haven (CT) 41
New Jersey 51
New Jersey Board of Health 51
New Mexico 176–178
New Mexico Health Department 178
New Mexico Normal University 32
New Orleans (LA) 106
New York 51–61
Newcastle (IN) 125
Niagara Falls (NY) 53
Nichols, A.B. 189
Norfolk (VA) 79
North Carolina 81–84
North Dakota 143–145
North Dakota Bureau of Health 144
nose spray 219
nursing mothers 141

Oakland (CA) 228
O'Brien, Daniel 234
office workforce 182
officers, special 218
officials: hectoring 126; local, remove 117–118
Ogden (UT) 32, 178–179, 183
Ogden vs Salt Lake City 179
Ohio 116–123
Ohio Board of Health 117
oil spray 56
Oklahoma 109–110

Oklahoma City Health Department 110
Olin, R.M. 113
Omaha (NE) 161–162
opposition 151–153, 154–155, 169–170
orders rescinded 131–132, 147, 151–152, 153–154, 155, 161, 175, 208, 225, 234
Oregon 209–216
Oregon Board of Health 209
origins of influenza and masking 7–11
Orlando (FL) 92
Orlando Board of Health 92
overcrowding 11

Pace, Stephen 88
Paris (KY) 104
Parke, William H. 20
Parrish, George 212
Parsons, J.G. 145
Pasadena (CA) 218, 228
Pastors' Union of Lima 122
patients, names and addresses published 209
Pendleton Oregon 209–211
Pennsylvania 61–70
Pennsylvania Department of Health 61
persuasion 134, 138, 229
persuasion vs mandate 212–213
Petaluma (CA) 227
Peters, Andrew 26
Peters, William 21
Philadelphia 64
Philadelphia Electric Company 26
Phoenix (AZ) 188–189
physicians: against 41, 103, 107, 114, 116, 125, 147, 168, 178, 182; charges 219; for 159–160, 197; refuse 81
Pickford, Mary 101
Pickle, E.E. 211
Pinson, Louis 210
Pittsburgh (PA) 24, 69–70
placarding 86, 124, 127, 146, 176; businesses 173
pneumonia 21, 29
Pocatello (ID) 172
police: Boston 48–49; Buffalo 56; dead bodies 111; extras 144; hotel raids 224; patrols 200; raids 191, 204; special 210; special mask force 126
politicians: local, disputes 65–66; non-compliance 90
Pomeroy, J.L. 217
Port Huron (MI) 114
Porter, Kirk B. 237
Portland (ME) 44
Portland (OR) 212–214

Portsmouth (NH) 45
post office, customer limits 146
Powers, L.M. 225
preventions 187, 204
Proctor and Gamble 158
protests 211–212
Provo (UT) 180
psychological aspects 127
public libraries 136
public pressure against 42
public relations campaign 76
Pueblo (CO) 174
purchases, done quickly 116

quarantine: travel 81–82; residential 124, 127, 132, 146, 160, 176, 176; residential, arrests 219; residential, honor 133
Quong, Louie 186

Racine (WI) 136
Racine County Medical Association 136
Rader, C.M. 208
Raleigh (NC) 83
Rapid City (SD) 145
Raunick, J.M. 61, 63
Rautros, A. 25
Ray (AZ) 186
Red Cross 17, 46, 73, 74, 84, 115; labor unpaid 73
reimposition, of lockdowns 69–70, 84, 87, 101, 104, 115, 125, 148, 156, 175, 198, 199, 218, 236
Rendall, John L. 152
Reno (NV) 195–196
Reno Board of Health 195
reportable disease 217
restaurants, rules for 61, 122
Reston, Louis 129
retail, sales events 108
Reynolds, A.R. 134
Rhode Island 43–43
Rhode Island Board of Health 43
Rice, N.J. 237
Richards, C.W. 109
Richmond (VA) 78–79
Riddell, C.M. 206
Riverton (WY) 172–173
Roanoke (AL) 96–97
Robertson, John Dill 132
Robie, I.H. 143
Robin, W.H. 106
Robinson, W.E. 146
Robles. H.C. 79
Rodgers, Joe 227
Rolph, James 235
Root and VanDervoort company 27
Rose, Mary 90

Rosenow, Edward C. 21–26
Rotary Club members, as police 94
Royer, B. F. 61
rules for the elite 234–235
Russian flu 1890 7–8

Sacramento (CA) 217, 223–224
Salem (OR) 216
sales events 178
Salina (KS) 165–166
saloons 133; breaking rules 61
Salt Lake City (UT) 179–181
San Antonio (TX) 111
San Diego (CA) 219–222
San Francisco (CA) 228–237; as example 169, 200, 214–216, 217; influence of 98
Sanderson, W.E. 37
sanitary cards 107
Saturday night hours 62
Schmitz, Eugene 236
school teachers, full pay 174
schools: close or open 45, 61
Schultz, Walter H. 94
scientific comments 226–227
scientists, lying 129
Scott, Walter 53
Scranton (PA) 69
seating: schools, staggered 195; staggered 104, 119, 143, 210
Seattle (WA) 200
Selma (AL) 96
Seneca Iron and Steel Company 56
Serras, James 184
serums 20
Sexton, L.L. 238
Seymour (IN) 125–126
Shepherdstown (WV) 81
Sherman W.O. 134
Sherman. Dewitt C. 56
Shisler, J.W. 93
Shorten, George 32
Shreveport (LA) 107
Sieb, John 136
Simmons, G.C. 223–224
Sioux Falls Health Board 145
skating rinks 132
Skinner and Eddy shipyards 25
Sleeper, Albert 113
sleeping, outdoors 178
Sloane, L.O. 198
Smart, George 111
Smith, Clarence 86
Smith, Harry 206
smoking, and masks 70
soldiers 81; as examples 101
Sommer, E.A. 212
Sorkness, Paul 144
South Bend (IN) 125
South Carolina 84–86
South Dakota 145–147

South Dakota Board of Health 145
Southern Fair (GA) 91
space per person 119
space, minimum rule 126
Spain 7–8
Spartanburg (SC) 85
speakers, flying squad 41
speakers, public 128
Spiller, Charles 126
spitting 51
Spokane (WA) 200–201
Springfield (OH) 118
St. Louis (MO) 154, 159
Starkloff, Max D. 154
Starr, E.B. 118
state fair 89
state, blaming victims 137–138
statistics 163, 224
Staunton (VA) 79
Stephens, William 223
sterilize 128
Steubenville (OH) 117
Stockton (CA) 225
Stockton, Charles G. 52
stores: capacity limits 136, 137; closed 82, 148, 160–161, 172–173; customer limits, by space 174; food 82; hours 73; policed 156; windows open 101
Strauss, F.B. 29, 34, 143
Streator (IL) 133
street sprinkling 91–92, 114
streetcars: capacity 87, 106, 117, 148, 156; conductors 176; fumigation 62; limits on 136; police on 176; windows 63, 78, 123, 205; windows removed 113
streetlights, turned off 106
Stubbs, Jesse 90
Sumner, Guilford H. 148
Sumter (SC) 84
surgeons, and masks 129
Swanson, W.H. 182

Tacoma 204, 206
Tampa (FL) 92
Tampa Electric Company 94
Tate, Frank 155
Taylor, S.J. 84
teachers, comments 67
telephone operators 107
telephones 162; masking of 74
Tennessee 100–103
Tennessee Board of Health 100
Terre Haute (IN) 124
Texas 110–112
theater managers 154, 175
Theater Owners' Association of Los Angeles 225
theaters, reactions 87
Thielcke, George E. 4

Thomas, W.E. 91
throat gargles 158
Tiedeman, D.W. 87
Tobin, Charles A. 119
Toledo (OH) 118
Tonawanda (NY) 53
Tonopah (NV) 196
Toole Glen 89–90
Topeka (KS) 164–165
trains 196
travel, bans 116–117
travel restrictions 65, 100, 146, 148, 174, 179, 186, 189, 191–192, 196
trips, needless 108
True, Frank H. 226
Tucson (AZ) 190–191
Tufts College (MA) 20
Tulsa (OK) 25, 110
Tuttle, Thomas D. 37, 201, 209
typhoid vaccine 20

U. S. Army Medical School 29
United States Congress 72
United States Post Office 76, 107
United States Public Health Service 11–12, 32–33, 80
United States Public Health Service, and masks 51
United States Steel Corporation 23–24
University of Minnesota 141
University of Missouri 157
Utah 178–186
Utah Board of Health 178, 180–181

vaccinations 20–39; children 30, 34; community 32; compulsory 169; compulsory at university 32; false and exaggerated claims 32–33; false data 31; first 20–21; local doctors 24
vaccine vs. serum 27
vaccines: conflict of interest 28, 30–31; corporation use and force 23–30; criticisms 29; in stores 22; media lies 21–28; numbers of 34; production of 37–38; value of 27–28
Van Metze, Maurice 150
Vare, Edwin H. 64
veils, as masks 60–61, 222, 229
Vermont 42–43
Vermont Board of Health 42–43
Vernal (UT) 180
Victor (MT) 168
Vidalia (MS) 99–100
Virginia 78–80
Virginia Board of Health 78
Virginia Council of Defense 78
Virginia State Fair 78
virus, size 127, 147
viruses, travel in groups 129
visiting friends 104, 111
Voyles, H. 124

Walla Walla (WA) 208
Ward, H.D. 85
Washington (state) 200–209
Washington (D.C.) 74–78
Washington State Board of Health 207
Watkins, Warner 27
Watson, John W. 93
Weber, Andy 69
weddings 93
Welch, William S. 72
Wentworth Military Academy 165
West Virginia 80–81
Western Union 103
whiskey supplied 63
White, D.A. 231
White, H.F. 84–85
Wichita (KS) 164, 166
Wickersham, James 198
Widchinsky, Norman 152
Wilkes, B.A. 110
Wilkinson, Melville L. 155
Williams (AZ) 187
Williams, C.L. 91
Williams, Ennion G. 78
Wilmington Board of Health 71
Wilson, G.W. 204
Wilson, Robert D. 205
windows open 101
Winona (MN) 141
Winston-Salem (NC) 82
Winter Park (FL) 94
Wisconsin 136–139
Wiser, James 233
Wood W.L. 78
Woodman, Frederic T. 225
Woodruff (SC) 84
Woodward, William C. 44, 45, 49
Woolsey, C.H. 204
World War I 7–8
World War I, celebrations 175
Wyoming 172–173
Wyoming Board of Health 173

zinc sulfate 56

www.ingramcontent.com/pod-product-compliance
Ingram Content Group UK Ltd.
Pitfield, Milton Keynes, MK11 3LW, UK
UKHW011454070425
457209UK00025B/245